Introduction to Sports Biomech

Introduction to Sports Biomechanics: Analysing Human Movement Patterns is a genuinely accessible and comprehensive guide to all of the biomechanics topics covered in an undergraduate sport and exercise science degree.

Now in a fully revised and updated third edition, the book explores both the qualitative and quantitative analysis of human movement, covering the following key topics:

- Movement patterns – the essence and purpose of sports biomechanics
- Qualitative analysis of sports movements
- Sports movement patterns and the geometry of motion
- Quantitative motion analysis in sports biomechanics
- What causes sports movements? Forces and moments of force
- The anatomy of human movement

Every chapter contains cross references to key terms and definitions, learning objectives and summaries, study tasks to confirm and extend understanding, and suggestions for further reading.

In addition to the printed textbook, readers of this new edition will also have access to an Interactive eTextbook version, a new kind of ebook that can be used on both mobile and desktop devices, offering students an unparalleled level of interactivity. Featuring video, data files, pop-up definitions, hyperlinks, self-test quizzes and interactive labelling and sorting tasks, this new electronic edition brings the subject of sports biomechanics to life like no other textbook. With downloadable resources also provided for instructors, including PowerPoint slides and answer guidelines, this remains an essential course text for students of sport and exercise, human movement sciences, ergonomics, biomechanics, physical education, and sports performance and coaching.

Roger Bartlett was Professor of Sports Biomechanics in the School of Physical Education, Sport and Exercise Sciences, University of Otago, New Zealand until he retired in August 2013; he formerly held professorships at Manchester Metropolitan University, Staffordshire University and Sheffield Hallam University, all in the UK. He is an Invited Fellow of the International Society of Biomechanics in Sports and an Honorary Fellow of the British Association of Sport and Exercise Sciences, of which he was Chairman 1991–1994. He is a former editor-in-chief of the *Journal of Sports Sciences* and *Sports Biomechanics*. He is co-author of *Sports Biomechanics: Reducing Injury Risk and Improving Sport Performance* and co-editor of several other sport science books.

Introduction to Sports Biomechanics

Analysing Human Movement Patterns

Third edition

Roger Bartlett

Routledge
Taylor & Francis Group

LONDON AND NEW YORK

First edition published 1997
Second edition published 2007
This edition published 2014
by Routledge
2 Park Square, Milton Park, Abingdon, Oxon OX14 4RN

and by Routledge
711 Third Avenue, New York, NY 10017

Routledge is an imprint of the Taylor & Francis Group, an informa business

British Library Cataloguing-in-Publication Data
A catalogue record for this book is available from the British Library

Library of Congress Cataloging-in-Publication Data

Bartlett, Roger
Introduction to sports biomechanics : analysing human movement patterns / by Roger Bartlett.
    pages cm
  1. Sports—Physiological aspects. 2. Human mechanics. 3. Biomechanics. I. Title.
  RC1235.B36   2014
  612.7'6—dc23   2013023821

ISBN: 978-0-415-63243-0 (pbk)

Typeset in Adobe Garamond
by Apex CoVantage, LLC

Printed and bound by CPI Group (UK) Ltd, Croydon, CR0 4YY

To my Bringers of Hope – Jo S. and my 'star' students in my time at the University of Otago, particularly Jo T., Peter L., Stephanie L., Anna S., and Deirdre A.

Contents

Figures

Tables

Boxes

Preface

The cover name for the third edition of this book is the same as that for the second edition. After a major change from the first edition to the second, and after teaching, researching and consulting in sports biomechanics for over 35 years, my definition of sports biomechanics is now, simply, 'the study and analysis of human movement patterns in sport'. The focus, structure and contents of this book reflect an important change in sports biomechanics over the last fifteen years. In the early part of the third millennium, more students who graduate with a degree focused on sports biomechanics go on to work as movement analysts or performance analysts with sports organisations or client groups in exercise and health than enrol for a research degree. The requirements on them are usually to undertake mostly qualitative, rather than quantitative, analysis of movement. Indeed, I often use the term 'movement analyst' instead of 'sports biomechanist' to reflect this shift from quantitative to qualitative analysis, and to broaden the term somewhat, as will be apparent later.

So, qualitative analysis is again the main focus of the first three chapters of this edition; however, everything in these chapters is also relevant for quantitative movement analysis – you cannot be a good quantitative movement analyst without first being a good qualitative analyst. The last three chapters again focus on quantitative analysis; as in the second edition, measurement methods are incorporated within those chapters and are covered only in the detail needed for undergraduate students. I have added an introduction to on-line motion analysis systems in Chapter 4 as these are now much more commonly found in sports biomechanics laboratories than when the second edition was published.

So what do sports biomechanists – or movement analysts – do? We study and analyse human movement patterns in sport; we do it to help people perform their chosen sporting activity better or to reduce the risk of injury. We also do it because it is so fascinating, otherwise so many of us would not still be doing it. And it is intellectually challenging and personally gratifying – if you can contribute to reducing an athlete's injury risk or to improving his or her performance, it gives you a warm feeling of satisfaction. It sounds exciting and indeed it is; sports biomechanics – like sport itself – is rarely boring. So, let us start the journey.

This edition is intended to be even more reader friendly than the second edition. Each chapter starts with an outline of learning outcomes, and knowledge assumed, which is cross-referenced mostly to other parts of the book. At the end of each chapter, a summary is provided of what was covered along with ten study tasks, including an in-depth interactive case study. Hints are given about how to go about each task, including referring to video clips, data tables and other material available on the book's website for instructors and, for the first time with this edition, in the Interactive eTextbook for students; links are provided to sets of multiple-choice questions for each chapter. The instructors' website and the Interactive eTextbook are both hugely important pedagogical resources. These resources also include PowerPoint slides for lecturers to use as a basis for their lectures and exemplar solutions to all of the study tasks. Further reading material is also recommended at the end of each chapter; a glossary of important terms is included at the end of the book (not, as for the second edition, at the end of each chapter).

The production of any textbook relies on the co-operation of many people. I would never have started this book without a period of six-months' study leave, which was supported by the Dean of the School of Physical Education, Sport and Exercise Sciences, Prof Doug Booth, and the Dean of the Division of Sciences, Prof Keith Turner; many thanks to you both. I would like to acknowledge the help of Simon Whitmore and Adam Micklethwaite at the publishers, Routledge. The help of all those in the School who were involved in the assembling of video and photographic material is gratefully acknowledged. Chris Sullivan, the School's technical manager, took most of the photographs in this edition of the book, and facilitated the involvement of other technical staff, for which many thanks; Julie Mink's patient involvement in all aspects of the video material was particularly invaluable as was Nigel Barrett's help with the force plate recordings and various aspects of Simi Motion (and as a video 'participant'). All colleagues, friends, students and others who acted as participants in the video or photo sessions, or who helped with data collection, are thankfully acknowledged: Dr Melanie Bussey (most of whose glossaries for the second edition are also incorporated here) and her son Jackson; Stephanie Lovelock (who also kindly read and provided useful feedback on Chapters 5 and 6); Sasha Wong; Rens Meerhoff; Rhys Thorp; Penny Roy; Melanie Button (and her mother Angela Button for accompanying her); David Hadcroft; Neil Anderson; Sam Mepham; Mario Ray; Ryan Duffy; Alice Foote; Gary Morrow of Macandrew Bay Lawn Bowling Club (and Westpac Stadium, Dunedin, for allowing us to use one of their rinks without charge); and, from the second edition, Neil Davis and Jo Trezise. I gratefully acknowledge Associate Professor Stefan Lindinger's (University of Salzburg) provision of material for several figures in Chapter 5 and for the pressure measurement material in the Interactive eTextbook. I also acknowledge my PHSE302 students at the University of Otago, whose qualitative analyses using Siliconcoach I have put in the Interactive eTextbook: Jamie Douglas, Mi Jung Jeon, Stephanie Lovelock, Rebekah Ronke and Sara Stannard. I should not need to add that any errors in any aspect of the book are entirely my responsibility. Last, but by no means least, I extend my heartfelt gratitude to Jo Stuthridge, without whose invaluable psychological support this book would never have seen the light of day.

Roger Bartlett, New Zealand

Introduction

The first three chapters of this book focus mainly on qualitative analysis of sports movements. Chapter 1 starts by outlining my approach to sports biomechanics and establishing that our focus in this chapter is the qualitative analysis of human movement patterns in sport. This includes consideration of the planes and axes of movement and the principal movements in all three cardinal planes. We will then touch on the constraints-led approach to studying human movements, and go on to look at examples of walking, running, jumping, throwing, striking and kicking, including the sub-division of these fundamental movements in to phases. In these movements, we will compare movement patterns between ages, sexes and tasks. The chapter concludes with a comparison of qualitative and quantitative analysis, looking at their background, uses, and strengths and weaknesses.

Chapter 2 considers how qualitative biomechanical analysis of movement is part of a multidisciplinary approach to movement analysis. We will look at several structured approaches to qualitative analysis of movement, all of which have, at their core, the identification of critical features of the movement studied. We will identify four stages in a structured approach to movement analysis, consider the main aspects of each stage and note that the value of each stage depends on how well the previous stages have been implemented. We will see that the most crucial step in the whole approach is how to identify the critical features of a movement, and we will look at several ways of doing this, none of which is foolproof. We will work through a detailed example of the best approach, using deterministic models, consider the 'movement principles' approach, and how to deal with subjectively judged sports.

Chapter 3 covers the principles of kinematics – the geometry of movement – which are important for the study of movement in sport. Our focus will be very strongly on movement patterns and their qualitative interpretation. Several other forms of movement pattern will be introduced, explained and explored, including time series graphs, angle–angle diagrams, phase planes, continuous relative phase and cross-correlation functions. We will consider the types of motion and the model appropriate to each. The importance of being able to interpret graphical patterns of linear or angular displacement and to infer from these the geometry of the velocity and acceleration patterns will be stressed. We will look at several ways of assessing joint coordination using angle–angle diagrams and, through phase planes, relative phase, and cross-correlation functions. We will briefly touch on the strengths and weaknesses of these various approaches.

Chapters 4 to 6 focus mainly on quantitative analysis of sports movements. Chapter 4 covers the use of videography in the study of sports movements, including the equipment and methods used. The necessary features of video equipment for recording movements in sport will be considered, along with the advantages and limitations of two- and three-dimensional recording of sports movements. We will outline the possible sources of error in recorded movement data and describe experimental procedures that minimise recorded errors in two- and three-dimensional movements. We will introduce the use of on-line motion analysis systems for recording sports movements. The need for smoothing or filtering of kinematic data will be covered, and the ways of performing this will be touched on. We will also outline the requirement for accurate body segment inertia parameter data and how these can be obtained, and some aspects of error analysis. We will present a cautionary tale of unreliable data as a warning about the analysis of data containing unacceptable measurement errors. Projectile motion will be considered and equations presented to calculate the maximum vertical displacement, flight time, range and optimum projection angle of a simple projectile for specified values of the three projection parameters. Deviations of the optimal angle for the sports performer from the optimal projection angle will be explained. We will also look at the calculation of linear velocities and accelerations caused by rotation and conclude with a brief consideration of three-dimensional rotation.

Chapter 5 deals with linear 'kinetics', which are important for an understanding of human movement in sport and exercise. This includes the definition of force, the identification of the various external forces acting in sport and how they combine, and the laws of linear kinetics and related concepts, such as linear momentum. We will address how friction and traction influence movements in sport and exercise, including reducing and increasing friction and traction. Fluid dynamic forces will also be considered and we will outline the importance of lift and drag forces on both the performer and on objects for which the fluid dynamics can impact on a player's movements. We will emphasise both qualitative and quantitative aspects of force-time graphs. The segmentation method for calculating the position of the whole-body centre of mass of the sports performer will be explained. The vitally important topic of rotational kinetics will be covered, including the laws of rotational kinetics and related concepts such as angular momentum and the ways in which rotation is generated and controlled in sports motions. The use of force plates in sports biomechanics will be covered, including the equipment and methods used, and the processing of force plate data. The procedures for calibrating a force plate will be outlined, along with those used to record forces in practice. The different ways in which force plate data can be processed to obtain other movement variables will be covered. The value of contact pressure measurements in the study of sports movements will also be considered. Some examples will be provided of the ways in which pressure data can be presented to aid analysis of sports movements.

Chapter 6 focuses on the anatomical principles that relate to movement in sport and exercise. The functions of the skeleton, the types of bone, bone fracture and typical surface features of bone will be covered. We will then look briefly at the tissue structures involved in the joints of the body, joint stability and mobility, and the identification of the features and classes of synovial joints. The features and structure of skeletal muscles will be considered along with the ways in which muscles are structurally and functionally classified, the types and mechanics of muscular contraction, how tension is produced in muscle and how the total force exerted by a muscle can be resolved into components depending on the angle of pull. The use of electromyography in the study of muscle activity in sports biomechanics will be considered, including the equipment and methods used, and the processing of EMG data. Consideration will be given to why the electromyogram (EMG) is important in sports biomechanics and why the recorded EMG differs from the physiological EMG. We will cover the relevant recommendations of SENIAM and the equipment used in recording the EMG, along with the main characteristics of an EMG amplifier. The processing of the raw EMG signal will be considered in terms of its time domain descriptors and the EMG power spectrum and the measures used to define it. We will conclude by examining how isokinetic dynamometry can be used to record the net muscle moment (or torque) at a joint.

GUIDE TO THE INTERACTIVE eTEXTBOOK AND INSTRUCTOR eRESOURCE

With Routledge Interactive, you can access your Interactive eTextbook at home, on campus or on the move, whether online or offline. Your eTextbook offers note sharing and highlighting functionality, as well as exclusive interactive content to enhance your learning experience. The notes you make on your Interactive eTextbook will synchronize with all other versions, creating a personalized version that you can access wherever and whenever you need it.

Throughout the text you will see icons in the margin where further multimedia resources are available via your Interactive eTextbook. These include:

A wealth of downloadable video content, demonstrating biomechanical movements and activities across a range of sporting disciplines

Specially-tailored interactive exercises to test your knowledge and understanding of key topics

As well as this tailor-made content, you can also benefit from the following features of the eTextbook platform:

- **Search** to find what you need to know.
- Check the meaning of key terms with the integrated pop-up **glossary**.
- Follow **hyperlinks** to navigate more easily.
- Add **Notes** to the text, and share them with the rest of the class.

FOR INSTRUCTORS

Instructor resources are located on the "Instructors" tab of RoutledgeInteractive.com:
http://cw.routledge.com/textbooks/routledgeinteractive/instructors.asp
On this site you will find:

- Downloadable zip files containing all of the **video clips** from the Interactive eTextbook
- **PowerPoint slides** to help with your lectures
- **Answers** to the Study Task questions from the Interactive eTextbook

1 Movement patterns – the essence of sports biomechanics

Knowledge assumed
Familiarity with human movement in sport
Ability to undertake simple analysis of videos of sports movements

INTRODUCTION

What were my reasons for choosing the same title for this book and the same name for this chapter as those for the second edition published in 2007? Well, in 2007 my definition of sports biomechanics had become, and remains today, after teaching, researching and consulting in the discipline for over 35 years, quite simply, 'the study and analysis of human movement patterns in sport'.

Nothing about 'the scientific methods of mechanics' or 'the effects of various forces' or 'Newton's laws' or 'vectors' or . . . ? No, nothing like that – just 'the study and analysis of human movement patterns in sport'! It sounds rather exciting, doesn't it? Indeed it is – a wealth of fascination. So, let us begin our journey.

Having offered my definition of sports biomechanics, it becomes obvious what sports biomechanists do – we study and analyse human movement patterns in sport. But why do we do it? Well, the usual reasons are:

- To help people perform their chosen sporting activity better. We should note here that this does not just apply to the elite athlete but to any sportsperson who wants to improve his or her performance.
- To help reduce the risk of injury.

From a pedagogical perspective, we might add:

- To educate new generations of sports biomechanists, performance analysts, coaches and teachers.

And, from a personal viewpoint:

- Because it is so fascinating. Yes, it is fascinating, otherwise so many of us would not still be doing it. It is also intellectually challenging and personally gratifying – if you can contribute to reducing an athlete's injury risk or to improving his or her performance, it gives you a warm glow.

Most sports biomechanics textbooks, including the first edition of this one, have strongly reflected the mathematical, engineering or physics backgrounds of their authors and their predominant research culture. Hence the mechanical focus that is evident, particularly in earlier texts, as well as a strong emphasis on quantitative analysis in sports biomechanics. However, during the last years of the second millennium and since, the 'real world' of sport outside of academia has generated – from coaches, athletes and other practitioners – an increasing demand for good qualitative movement analysts. Indeed, I will often use the term 'movement analyst' instead of 'sports biomechanist' to reflect this shift from quantitative to qualitative analysis, and I will broaden the term somewhat, as will be apparent later. So, qualitative analysis is our main focus in this chapter – and the next two. However, everything in these chapters is also relevant for quantitative movement analysts – you cannot be a good quantitative movement analyst without first being a good qualitative analyst.

BOX 1.1 LEARNING OUTCOMES

After reading this chapter you should be able to:

- think enthusiastically about analysing movement patterns in sport
- understand the fundamentals of defining joint movements anatomically
- define the cardinal planes and axes of movement, and name and describe all of the principal movements in those planes in sport and exercise
- appreciate the differences – and the similarities – between qualitative and quantitative analysis of sports movements
- describe, from video observation or pictorial sequences, some fundamental sports movements, such as walking, running, jumping, throwing, striking and kicking
- appreciate why breaking those movements into phases can help simplify their description and later analysis
- be familiar with finding and using supplementary information – particularly videos
- feel enthusiastic about progressing to Chapters 2 and 3.

DEFINING HUMAN MOVEMENTS

In this section, we look at how we can define human movements. To specify unambiguously the movements of the human body in sport, exercise and other activities, we need to use an appropriate scientific terminology. Terms such as 'bending knees' and 'raising arms' are acceptable, at least in principle, in everyday language, including when communicating with sport practitioners. However, 'raising arms' is ambiguous and we should strive for precision. 'Bending knees' is often thought to be scientifically unacceptable – a view with which I profoundly disagree as I consider that simplicity is always preferable, particularly in communications with non-scientists. We need to start by establishing the planes in which these movements occur and the axes about which they take place, along with the body postures from which we define these movements. These planes, axes and postures are summarised in Box 1.2. We will then look at the main movements in the three cardinal planes, in the following section. We will return to other anatomical aspects of human movement in Chapter 6.

Sports biomechanists, particularly for two-dimensional movement analysis, normally use the convention that the fully extended position of most joints is 180°; when most joints flex, this angle decreases. Other biomechanists sometimes use an alternative convention in which a fully extended joint is 0°, so that flexion increases the joint angle; a similar definition is normally used by three-dimensional motion analysis systems. We will use the former convention throughout this book, in which most, but not all, of the movements we will analyse will be in the sagittal plane – flexion reduces the joint angle, extension increases it.

BOX 1.2 PLANES OF MOVEMENT, AXES OF MOVEMENT AND POSTURES FROM WHICH MOVEMENTS ARE DEFINED

Various terms are used to describe the three mutually perpendicular, intersecting planes in which many, though not all, joint movements occur. The common point of intersection of these three planes is most conveniently defined as either the centre of the joint being studied or the centre of mass of the whole human body. In the latter case, the planes are known as cardinal planes – the sagittal, frontal and transverse planes – as depicted in Figure 1.1 and described below.

Movements at the joints of the human musculoskeletal system are mainly rotational and take place about a line perpendicular to the plane in which they occur. This line is known as an axis of rotation. Three axes – the anteroposterior, mediolateral and longitudinal axes – can be defined by the intersection of pairs of the planes of movement, as in Figure 1.1. The main movements about these three axes for a particular joint are flexion and extension about the sagittal axis, abduction and adduction about the frontal axis, and internal and external (medial and lateral) rotation about the longitudinal axis. The descriptions of these planes and axes below apply to the reference postures (Figure 1.2), standing upright.

- The sagittal plane is a vertical plane passing from the rear (posterior) to the front (anterior) dividing the body into left and right halves, as in Figure 1.1(a). It is also known as the anteroposterior plane. Most sport and exercise movements that are almost two-dimensional, such as running and long jumping, take place in this plane.
- The frontal plane is also vertical and passes from left to right, dividing the body into posterior and anterior halves, as in Figure 1.1(b). It is also known as the coronal or the mediolateral plane.
- The transverse plane divides the body into top (superior) and bottom (inferior) halves, as in Figure 1.1(c). It is also known as the horizontal plane, but this can be a confusing name when a sports performer is not standing upright, for example in a layout somersault, as the cardinal planes move with the performer.
- The mediolateral (or frontal) axis (Figure 1.1(a)) passes horizontally from left to right and is formed by the intersection of the frontal and transverse planes.
- The anteroposterior (or sagittal) axis (Figure 1.1(b)) passes horizontally from posterior to anterior and is formed by the intersection of the sagittal and transverse planes.
- The longitudinal axis (Figure 1.1(c)) passes vertically from inferior to superior and is formed by the intersection of the sagittal and frontal planes. It is also known as the vertical axis, but this can be a confusing name when a sports performer is not standing upright, for example in a layout somersault, as the cardinal axes move with the performer.

Figure 1.1 Cardinal planes and axes of movement. Left: (a) sagittal plane and mediolateral axis; Middle: (b) frontal plane and anteroposterior axis; Right: (c) transverse plane and longitudinal axis.

A precise description and analysis of human movement requires the definition of a reference position or posture, from which these movements are specified. The two positions we use, demonstrated by the athlete in Figure 1.2, are the fundamental (Figure 1.2(a)) and anatomical (Figure 1.2(b)) reference positions. With the exception of the forearms and hands, the fundamental and anatomical reference positions are the same. The fundamental position of Figure 1.2(a) is similar to a 'stand to attention'. The forearm is in its neutral position, neither pronated ('turned in') nor supinated ('turned out'). In the anatomical position of Figure 1.2(b), the forearm has been rotated from the neutral position of Figure 1.2(a) so that the palm of the hand faces forwards. Movements of the hand and fingers are defined from the anatomical reference position, movements of the forearm (radioulnar joints) are defined from the fundamental reference position and movements at other joints can be defined from either reference position.

Figure 1.2 Reference postures (positions). Left: (a) fundamental reference position; Right (b) anatomical reference position.

MOVEMENTS IN THE CARDINAL PLANES

Movements in the sagittal plane about the mediolateral axis

- Flexion, shown in Figure 1.3, is initiated by movement away from the middle of the body. It is generally a 'bending' movement, in which the angle between two body segments decreases. Usually, the movement is forwards, except for the knee, ankle and toes; when the knee flexes, the calf moves backwards. The term hyperflexion is sometimes used to describe flexion of the upper arm beyond the vertical; it is cumbersome and is completely unnecessary if the range of movement is quantified.
- Extension, also shown in Figure 1.3, is the return movement from flexion. It is generally a 'straightening' movement. The movement of the whole arm about the shoulder joint from the anatomical reference position is called flexion and its return to that position is

Figure 1.3 Movement of forearm about the elbow joint in the sagittal plane – flexion and extension.

called extension. The continuation of extension beyond the anatomical reference position, for the shoulder and some other joints, is called hyperextension; only a little hyperextension is possible at the hip joint. The return movement from a hyperextended position is usually called flexion in sports biomechanics, although in strict anatomical terms it is described, somewhat cumbersomely, as reduction of hyperextension.

- Dorsiflexion and plantar flexion are normally used to define sagittal plane movements at the ankle joint. In dorsiflexion, the foot moves upwards towards the anterior surface of the calf; in plantar flexion, the foot moves downwards towards the posterior surface of the calf.

Movements in the frontal plane about the anteroposterior axis

- Abduction, shown in Figure 1.4, is a sideways movement away from the middle of the body or, for the fingers, away from the middle finger. These movements are not possible, or very restricted, for some joints, such as the elbow and knee. Abduction of

Figure 1.4 Abduction and adduction of the arm about the shoulder joint and the thigh about the hip joint.

the upper arm, particularly past the horizontal, also involves upward rotation of the scapula (see below). Abduction of the thigh often involves lateral pelvic tilt to the opposite side (see below).

- Radial flexion – also known as radial deviation – denotes the movement of the middle finger away from the middle of the body and can also be used for the other fingers.
- The term hyperabduction is sometimes used to describe abduction of the upper arm beyond the vertical.
- Adduction, also shown in Figure 1.4, is the return movement from abduction towards the middle of the body or, for the fingers, towards the middle finger.
- Ulnar flexion, also known as ulnar deviation, denotes the movement of the middle finger towards the middle of the body and can also be used for the other fingers.
- Continuation of adduction, normally only for the upper arm at the shoulder joint and the thigh at the hip joint, beyond the reference position is usually called

hyperadduction. This is only possible when combined with some flexion of the upper arm, thigh or trunk.

- The return movement from a hyperadduction position is often called abduction in sports biomechanics, although in strict anatomical terms it is described, again rather cumbersomely, as reduction of hyperadduction.

- Lateral flexion to the right or to the left, shown in Figure 1.5(a), is the sideways bending of the trunk, neck or head to the right or left and, normally, the return movement from the opposite side.

- Eversion and inversion refer to the raising of the lateral and medial border of the foot (the sides of the foot furthest from and nearest to the middle of the body) with respect to the other border. Eversion cannot occur without the foot tending to be displaced into a toe-out, or abducted, position; likewise, inversion tends to be accompanied by adduction. The terms pronation and supination of the foot, shown in Figures 1.5(b) and (c), are widely used in describing and evaluating running gait, and may already be familiar to you for this reason. Pronation of the foot involves a combination of eversion and abduction (Figure 1.5(b)), along with dorsiflexion of the ankle. Supination involves inversion and adduction (Figure 1.5(c)) along with plantar flexion of the ankle. These terms should not be confused with pronation and supination of the forearm (see below). When the foot is bearing

Figure 1.5 Some other movements in the frontal plane about the anteroposterior axis. Left: (a) lateral flexion of the trunk; Right top: (b) pronation of the foot; Right bottom: (c) supination of the foot.

weight, as in running, its abduction and adduction movements are restricted by friction between the shoe and the ground. Medial and lateral rotation of the lower leg is then more pronounced than in the non-weight-bearing positions of Figures 1.5(b) and (c).

Movements in the transverse plane about the longitudinal axis

- External and internal rotation, shown in Figure 1.6, are the outwards and inwards movements of the arm (or leg) about their longitudinal axes – these movements are also known, respectively, as lateral (or outward) and medial (or inward) rotation. External and internal rotation of the forearm are referred to, respectively, as supination and pronation.
- Rotation to the left and rotation to the right are the rather obvious terms for transverse plane movements of the head, neck and trunk.
- Horizontal flexion and extension (or horizontal abduction and adduction), shown in Figure 1.7, define the rotation of the arm about the shoulder joint or the leg about the hip joint from a position of 90° abduction. In sports biomechanics, movements from any position in the transverse plane towards the anterior are usually called horizontal flexion (or abduction) and those towards the posterior horizontal extension (or adduction). (In strict anatomical terms, these movements are named from the 90° abducted position; the return movements towards that position are called reduction of horizontal flexion and extension respectively.)

Figure 1.6 Internally (medially) and externally (laterally) rotated positions of the arm about the shoulder joint.

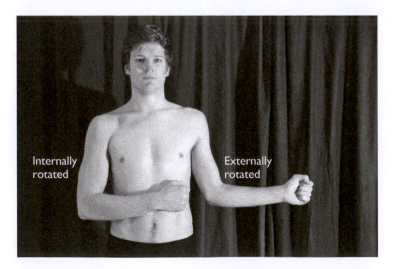

Figure 1.7 Horizontal flexion (left arm moving towards anterior of trunk) and horizontal extension (right arm moving towards posterior of trunk) of the abducted arm about the shoulder joint.

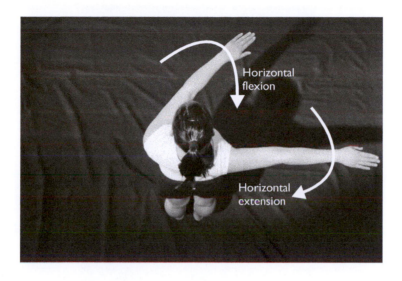

Movements of the thumb

The movements of the thumb, shown in Figures 1.8(a) to (c), may appear to be confusingly named.

- Abduction and adduction (Figure 1.8(a)) are used to define movements away from and towards the palm of the hand in the sagittal plane from the anatomical reference position (Figure 1.2(b)); hyperadduction is the continuation of adduction beyond the starting position.
- Extension and flexion (Figure 1.8(b)) refer to frontal plane movements away from and towards the index finger; hyperflexion (Figure 1.8(c)) is the movement beyond the starting position.
- Opposition is the movement of the thumb to touch the tip of any of the four fingers of the same hand. It involves abduction and hyperflexion of the thumb, along with flexion of the involved finger at some combination of the metacarpophalangeal (knuckle) joint and the interphalangeal joints (the joints between adjacent phalanges of any finger).

Circumduction of the arm and leg

The movement of the arm or leg to describe a cone is called circumduction and is a combination of flexion and extension with abduction and adduction. Several attempts have been made to define movements in diagonal planes, for example the golf swing, but none has been adopted universally.

Figure 1.8 Movements of the thumb. Top: (a) abduction-adduction; Middle: (b) flexion-extension; Bottom: (c) hyperflexion.

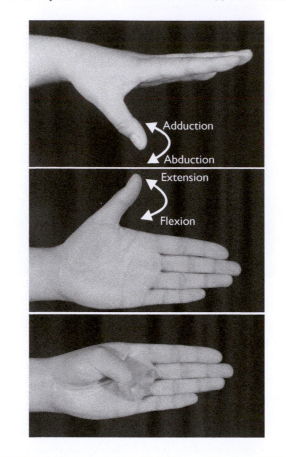

Movements of the shoulder girdle

Some movements of the shoulder girdle are shown in Figure 1.9, along with the upper arm movements with which they are usually associated.

- Elevation and depression are upward and downward linear movements of the scapula, as in a simple shrug of the shoulders; these movements of the scapula are approximately in the frontal plane, although they are generally accompanied by some upward and downward rotation of the scapula, respectively.
- Upward (Figure 1.9(a)) and downward rotation of the scapula are defined by the turning of the distal end of the scapula – that further from the middle of the body – with respect to the proximal end – that nearer the middle of the body.

Figure 1.9 Shoulder girdle movements. Top left: (a) upward rotation; Top right: (b) protraction; Bottom left: (c) retraction (note the asymmetry between the left and right shoulders for this person); Bottom right: (d) posterior tilt.

- Protraction (Figure 1.9(b)) and retraction (Figure 1.9(c)) describe the movements of the scapula away from and towards the vertebral column. These are not simply movements in the frontal plane but also have anterior and posterior components owing to the curvature of the thorax.
- Posterior and anterior tilt are the upwards and downwards movement, respectively, of the inferior angle – the lower tip – of the scapula away from (Figure 1.9(d)) or towards the thorax.

Movements of the pelvis

Changes in the position of the pelvis are brought about by the motions at the lumbo-sacral joint, between the lowest lumbar vertebra and the sacrum, and the hip joints. Movements at these joints, shown in Figure 1.10, permit the pelvis to tilt forwards, backwards and sideways (laterally) and to rotate horizontally.

- Forward (or anterior) tilt, from the position in Figure 1.10(a) to that in Figure 1.10(b), involves increased inclination in the sagittal plane about the mediolateral axis.

Figure 1.10 Pelvic girdle movements. Top left: (a) neutral position; Top right: (b) forward tilt; Bottom left: (c) backward tilt; Bottom right: (d) lateral tilt.

This results from lumbosacral hyperextension and, in the standing position, hip flexion. The lower part of the pelvic girdle where the pubic bones join – the symphysis pubis – turns downwards and the posterior surface of the sacrum turns upwards.

- Backward (or posterior) tilt, from the position in Figure 1.10(a) to that in Figure 1.10(c), involves decreased inclination in the sagittal plane about the mediolateral axis. This results from lumbosacral flexion and, in the standing position, hip extension. The symphysis pubis moves forwards and upwards, and the posterior surface of the sacrum turns somewhat downwards.
- Lateral tilt is the movement of the pelvis in the frontal plane about the sagittal axis such that one iliac crest is lowered and the other is raised. This can be demonstrated by standing on one foot with the other slightly raised directly upwards off the ground, keeping the leg straight (Figure 1.10(d)). The tilt is named from the side of the pelvis that moves downwards; in lateral tilt of the pelvis to the left, the left iliac crest is lowered and the right is raised. This is a combination of right lateral flexion of the lumbosacral joint, abduction of the left hip and adduction of the right.
- Rotation or lateral twist is the rotation of the pelvis in the plane about the transverse longitudinal axis. The movement is named after the direction towards which the front of the pelvis turns.

SOME FUNDAMENTAL MOVEMENTS

The Interactive eTextbook contains many video clips of various people performing some of the movements that are fundamental to sport and exercise. These people include young children, young and older adults, males and females, who are shown walking, running, jumping, throwing, striking objects and kicking in various conditions. These conditions include: locomotion on a level and inclined treadmill and overground; standing vertical and long jumping; underarm, sidearm and overarm throwing and striking; and different types of kicking. Some of these movements are performed with markers to identify centres of rotation of joints. An in-depth study of these videos is recommended to all readers who wish to become competent movement analysts; such study is required to complete the study tasks later in the chapter, and you are all encouraged to attempt these. The video sequences shown in the figures below have been extracted from the clips using the qualitative analysis packages Siliconcoach (www.siliconcoach.com) and Kinovea; the latter of these is free and can be downloaded from www.kinovea.org. If you do not already have access to a qualitative biomechanical analysis package, then I suggest that you download Kinovea, familiarise yourself with it and use it for the relevant study tasks in this chapter.

When analysing any human movement, ask yourself, 'What are the "constraints" on this movement?' The constraints can be related to the sports task, the environment or the organism. This 'constraints-led' approach serves as a very strong basis on which to develop an understanding of why we observe particular movement patterns. In the video examples and the sequences in the figures below, an environmental constraint might be the equipment used – balls, rackets and so on; environmental constraints are external ones that are usually related to space or time. Task constraints are specific to the sports task or activity. Running overground and running on a treadmill are task constraints (although they have also been seen as environmental constraints). Jumping vertically to achieve maximum height is clearly a task constraint. Organismic constraints are, basically, biomechanical constraints internal to the individual; they relate to a given individual's body characteristics, which affect his or her movement responses to the task and environmental constraints. Organismic constraints are affected by, among many other things, genetic make-up, age, biological sex, fitness, injury record and stage of rehabilitation, and pathological conditions. Not surprisingly, the movement patterns observed when one individual performs a specific sports task will rarely be identical to those of another person; indeed, the movement patterns from repetitions of that task by the same individual will also vary – this becomes more obvious when we quantitatively analyse those movements, but can be seen qualitatively in many patterns of movement, as in Chapter 3. These variable responses, often known as movement variability, can and do affect the way that movement analysts look at sports movements. The qualitative descriptions in the following sections will not, therefore, apply to every adult, but will apply to many so-called 'normals'. The developmental movement patterns of maturing children up to a certain age, as seen in Figures 1.14 and 1.18, show differences from the movement patterns for an adult.

A first step in the analysis of a complex motor skill is often the establishment of the phases into which the movement can be divided for analysis. For example, the division of a throwing movement into separate, but linked, phases is useful because of the sheer complexity of many throwing techniques. The phases of the movement should be selected so that they have biomechanically distinct roles in the overall movement, which are different from those of the preceding and succeeding phases. Each phase then has clearly defined biomechanical functions and easily identified phase boundaries, often called key events. Although phase analysis (see also Appendix 1.1) can help the understanding of movement patterns, an essential feature of all sports movements is their wholeness; this should always be borne in mind when undertaking any phase analysis of a movement pattern.

In the fundamental movements that I cover below, I have: identified the phases of the movement; described the most important joint rotations for that fundamental movement, particularly those in the sagittal plane; related those joint rotations to the movement phases; and noted any important biomechanical features of the overall movement. (You should adopt a similar approach to your video analysis.) To identify these features of a movement, a movement analyst needs to have good observational skills – it is very important for you to develop these skills. Practise them on the video clips in the Interactive eTextbook, so that you can undertake, successfully, the study tasks at the end of this chapter.

Walking

Walking is a fundamental skill, not only for everyday life but also for sports, particularly team games, in which changes from walking to running and vice versa are common. Walking is a cyclic activity in which one stride follows another in a continuous pattern. We define a walking stride as being from touchdown of one foot to the next touchdown of the same foot, or from toe-off to toe-off: in a video recording, toe-off is sometimes easier to identify than touchdown. Toe-off is normally defined as the first frame after the foot breaks contact with the ground and touchdown as the first frame after the foot touches the ground. In walking, there is a single-support phase, when one foot is on the ground, and a double-support phase, when both are. The single-support phase starts with toe-off of one foot and the double-support phase starts with touchdown of the same foot. The duration of single support is typically much longer than that of the double-support phase, the average ratio is almost 4:1 for the whole walking stride from the first left foot touchdown in Figure 1.11; this ratio depends very much on walking speed. Alternatively, we can consider each leg separately. Each leg then has stance and swing phases, with similar functions to those in running (see below). In normal walking at a person's preferred speed, the stance phase for one leg occupies about 60 per cent of the whole stride and the swing phase around 40 per cent (see, for example, Figures 1.11 and 1.12). In normal walking, the average durations of stance and swing will be very similar for the left and right sides. In pathological gait, there may be a pronounced difference between the two sides, leading to arrhythmic gait patterns. The young female walking at her preferred speed overground (Figure 1.11) and on a level treadmill (Figure 1.12) has identical stride and swing and stance phase durations for the two forms of walking; this is not necessarily typical, given the different task constraints between overground and treadmill walking.

It should be noted for the still frame sequences in this chapter that the frame rate for the interlaced digital video cameras used for the sequences in this book is 25 Hz, so that the time interval between frames is 0.04 s. For illustration purposes, I chose the video frame that was closest to each key event, so the timings match that particular frame. When you view the video sequences in the Interactive eTextbook, for example to complete the study tasks for this chapter, you may feel confident enough to estimate the occurrence of a key event to one half of a frame (0.02 s) but there will, of course, not be an actual video frame to correspond to your estimation. For example, in Figure 1.13 you might reasonably suggest that a good estimate of left foot toe-off would be midway between the two frames in the third line, at 0.66 s.

The Interactive eTextbook contains many video clips from side and rear views of people walking. These video clips enable you to look at differences between males and females, between young and older adults and young children, between overground and treadmill locomotion and between different speeds and treadmill inclines. Figures 1.11 to 1.14 contain still images from a selection of these video clips. Observing these figures, you should note, in general, the following typical patterns of flexion and extension of

Figure 1.11 Young adult female walking overground at her preferred speed in trainers. Top left: (a) left foot touchdown (0 s); Top right: (b) right foot toe-off (0.12 s); Second line left: (c) left foot mid-stance (0.24 s); Second line right: (d) right foot touchdown (0.52 s); Third line left: (e) left foot toe-off (0.60 s); Third line right: (f) right foot mid-stance (0.72 s); Bottom left: (g) left foot touchdown (1.0 s); Bottom right: (h) right foot toe-off (1.12 s). Duration of one stride from left foot touchdown to next left foot touchdown, or right foot toe-off to next right foot toe-off is 1.0 s. Duration of right and left foot stance phases each 0.60 s, 60 per cent of stride time; duration of right and left foot swing phases each 0.40 s, 40 per cent of stride time. Average duration of the three double-support phases (touchdown of one foot to toe-off of the next) is 0.11 s; average duration of the two single-support phases (toe-off of one foot to touchdown of the same foot) is 0.4 s; ratio of single support to double support almost 4:1.

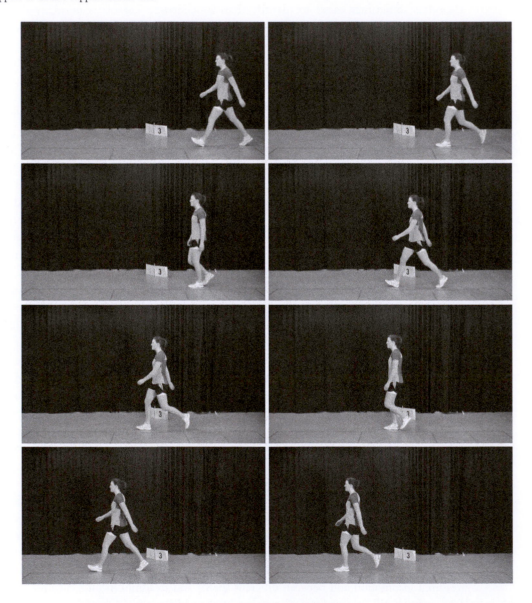

Figure 1.12 The same young adult female as in Figure 1.11 walking on a level treadmill at her preferred speed (here 6 km/h) in trainers. Top left: (a) left foot touchdown (0 s); Top right: (b) right foot toe-off (0.12 s); Second line left: (c) left foot mid-stance (0.24 s); Second line right: (d) right foot touchdown (0.52 s); Third line left: (e) left foot toe-off (0.60s); Third line right: (f) right foot mid-stance (0.72 s); Bottom left: (g) left foot touchdown (1.0 s); Bottom right: (h) right foot toe-off (1.12 s). Duration of one stride from left foot touchdown to next left foot touchdown, or right foot toe-off to next right foot toe-off is 1.0 s, identical to that in Figure 1.11. Duration of right and left foot stance phases each 0.60 s, 60 per cent of stride time; duration of right and left foot swing phases each 0.40 s, 40 per cent of stride time, again identical to those in Figure 1.11. Average duration of the three double-support phases (touchdown of one foot to toe-off of the next) is 0.11 s; average duration of the two single-support phases (toe-off of one foot to touchdown of the same foot) is 0.4 s; ratio of single support to double support almost 4:1, yet again identical to Figure 1.11.

Figure 1.13 Young adult male walking on a 20 per cent grade treadmill at his preferred speed in walking shoes. Top left: (a) left foot touchdown (0 s); Top right: (b) right foot toe-off (0.16 s); Second line left: (c) left foot mid-stance (0.28 s); Second line right: (d) right foot touchdown (0.52 s); Third line left: (e) just before left foot toe-off (0.64 s); Third line right: (f) just after left foot toe-off (0.68 s); Bottom left: (g) right foot mid-stance (0.80 s); Bottom right: (h) left foot touchdown (1.0 s). Interestingly, the duration of one stride from left foot touchdown to next left foot touchdown is 1.0 s, identical to that in Figures 1.11 and 1.12, although the walking speed is slower. Duration of left foot stance phase 0.68 s, 68 per cent of stride time; duration of left foot swing phase 0.32 s, 32 per cent of stride time.

the hip and knee and dorsiflexion and plantar flexion of the ankle for adults (for example, Figure 1.11 and Figure 1.12). You should also study the video clips from which these sequences were taken in the Interactive eTextbook to become familiar with identifying these movements on video. For a typical young, fit adult walking at his or her preferred speed, the hip flexes during the swing phase (e.g. right leg, Figure 1.11(b)) and then begins to extend just before touchdown (e.g. right leg, Figure 1.11(d)); hip extension continues until the heel rises soon before toe-off (e.g. right leg, Figure 1.11(g), is between heel rise and toe-off). The hip then starts to flex for the next swing phase (e.g. right leg, Figure 1.11(g)), roughly when the other foot touches down. The knee is normally slightly flexed at touchdown (e.g. left leg, Figure 1.11(a)) and this flexion continues after touchdown (e.g. left leg, Figure 1.11(b)), although not necessarily in slow walking. Some, but not much, extension follows (e.g. left leg, Figure 1.11(c)) before the knee starts to flex sharply immediately after the heel rises (e.g. left leg, Figure 1.11(d)); this flexion continues through toe-off (e.g. left leg, Figure 1.11(e)) until about half way through the swing (e.g. left leg, Figure 1.11(f)), when the knee extends again, before flexing slightly just before touchdown. The ankle is roughly in a neutral position at touchdown (e.g. left leg, Figure 1.11(a)), as in the reference positions of Figure 1.2. The ankle then plantar flexes until the whole foot is on the ground, when dorsiflexion starts (e.g. left leg, Figure 1.11(b)); this continues until the other leg touches down (e.g. Figure 1.11(d)). Plantar flexion then follows almost to toe-off (e.g. left leg, Figure 1.11(e)), just before which the ankle dorsiflexes quickly to allow the foot to clear the ground as it swings forwards (e.g. left leg, Figure 1.11(f)).

As you should note from Figures 1.11 to 1.14 and from the video clips in the Interactive eTextbook (see specific references in this section and in the study tasks later in this chapter), the sequence of movements described above varies somewhat from person to person, with the surface inclination and the walking speed, and between overground and treadmill walking. The movement pattern for walking on a treadmill at a 20 per cent grade (Figure 1.13) differs from level walking; for example, the trunk is flexed throughout and the knee is more flexed at touchdown. The movement pattern for a five-year-old girl walking at her preferred speed overground (Figure 1.14) is very similar to that of a young female adult (Figure 1.11), except, obviously, that the stride time and the stride length are both shorter.

The movement pattern for a female compared to a male of similar age and body build accommodates the wider female pelvis and increased 'Q angle' (the angle of the rectus femoris muscle relative to the patellar tendon). For frontal plane video comparisons of a male and a female walking, which are needed to highlight such differences, see the video clips available in the Interactive eTextbook.

So, what else would we seek to observe as movement analysts looking at walking patterns (this is often called gait analysis)? We would not only observe differences from the 'normal' pattern described above, but also right–left side differences, variations across strides and how external factors, such as changed task or environmental constraints, affect the gait pattern. We might also seek to discern how the joints within one leg are coordinated and how contralateral limb movements are coordinated (see also

Figure 1.14 Five-year-old girl walking overground at her preferred speed in trainers. Top left: (a) left foot touchdown (0 s); Top right: (b) right foot toe-off (0.12 s); Second line left: (c) left foot mid-stance (0.24 s); Second line right: (d) right foot touchdown (0.44 s); Third line left: (e) left foot toe-off (0.56 s); Third line right: (f) right foot mid-stance (0.64 s); Bottom left: (g) left foot touchdown (0.88 s); Bottom right: (h) right foot toe-off (1.0 s). Duration of one stride from left foot touchdown to next left foot touchdown, or right foot toe-off to next right foot toe-off is 0.88 s. Duration of right and left foot stance phases 0.56 s, 64 per cent of stride time; duration of right foot swing phase 0.32 s, 36 per cent of stride time.

Study Task 10). Studying video sequences, such as those in Figures 1.11 to 1.14, is not necessarily the best, or the easiest, way to observe such movement and coordination patterns, as we shall see in Chapter 3, but it is nevertheless a vitally important skill for movement analysts.

Running

Running, like walking, is a fundamental skill for many sports. It is, like walking, a cyclic activity: one running stride follows another in a continuous pattern. As for walking, we define a running stride as being from touchdown of one foot to the next touchdown of the same foot, or from toe-off to toe-off. Unlike walking (see above), running can, basically, be divided into a stance (or support) phase, when one foot is on the ground, and a swing (or recovery) phase, in which both feet are off the ground (see also Appendix 1.1 for a more detailed phase analysis of running). The runner can only apply force to the ground for propulsion during the stance phase, which defines that phase's main biomechanical function and provides the key events that indicate the start of the phase, touchdown (or foot strike), and its end, toe-off. The swing phase starts at toe-off and ends at touchdown; at this stage, we will consider its function to be to prepare the leg for the next touchdown. In slow running, or jogging, the swing phase will be very short and then increase with running speed.

As for walking, the Interactive eTextbook also contains many side- and rear-view video clips of people running (see specific references in this section and in the study tasks later in this chapter). These illustrate differences between males and females, between younger and older adults and young children, between overground and treadmill locomotion, and between different speeds. Figures 1.15 to 1.18 contain still images from a selection of these video clips. Observing these figures, you should note, in general, the following typical patterns of flexion and extension of the hip and knee and dorsiflexion and plantar flexion of the ankle for adults (for example, Figures 1.15 and 1.16); you should also study the video sequences in the Interactive eTextbook to become familiar with identifying these movements from video. The hip continues to extend early in the swing phase (e.g. right leg, Figure 1.15(b)), roughly until maximum knee flexion, after which it flexes (e.g. right leg, Figures 1.15(c) and (d)) then begins to extend just before touchdown (e.g. right leg, Figure 1.15(e)); extension continues (e.g. right leg, Figure 1.15(f)) until toe-off (e.g. right leg, Figure 1.15(g)). The knee is normally slightly flexed at touchdown (e.g. left leg, Figure 1.15(b)) and this flexion continues (e.g. left leg, Figure 1.15(c)), depending on running speed, to absorb shock, until the hip is roughly over the ankle. Knee extension then proceeds until toe-off (e.g. left leg, Figure 1.15(d)), soon after which the knee flexes as the hip continues to extend (e.g. left leg, Figure 1.15(e)). The knee starts to extend (e.g. left leg, from about Figure 1.15(f)) while the hip is flexing and continues to extend (e.g. left leg, Figure 1.15(g)) almost until touchdown, just before which the knee might flex slightly. The ankle movements vary depending on whether the runner lands on the forefoot or rear foot.

Figure 1.15 Young adult female running overground at her preferred speed in trainers. Top left: (a) right foot toe-off (0 s); Top right: (b) left foot touchdown (0.16 s); Second line left: (c) left foot mid-stance (0.24 s); Second line right: (d) left foot toe-off (0.36 s); Third line left: (e) right foot touchdown (0.52 s); Third line right: (f) right foot mid-stance (0.60 s); Bottom: (f) right foot toe-off (0.76 s). Duration of one stride from right foot toe-off to next right foot toe-off is 0.76 s. Duration of right foot stance phase 0.24 s, 32 per cent of stride time; duration of right foot swing phase 0.52 s, 68 per cent of stride time. Note that the relative and percentage times of phases are more subject to error than for walking because of their shorter durations.

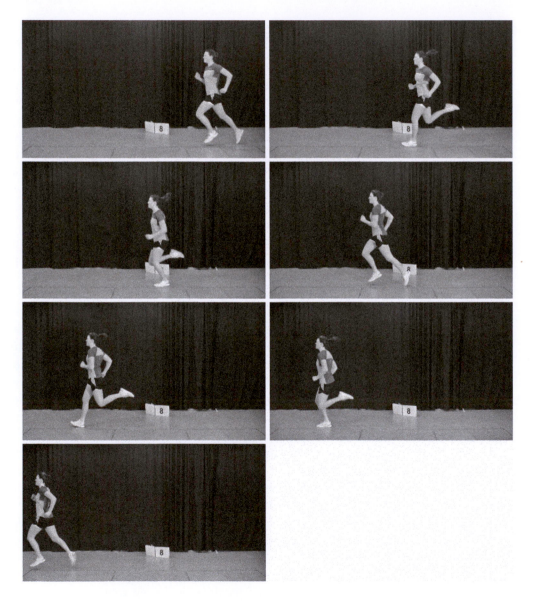

Figure 1.16 Young adult female running on a level treadmill at 13.2 km/h in trainers. Top left: (a) left foot touchdown (0 s); Top right: (b) left foot mid-stance (0.12 s); Second line left: (c) left foot toe-off (0.24 s); Second line right: (d) right foot touchdown (0.36 s); Third line left: (e) right foot mid-stance (0.48 s); Third line right: (f) right foot toe-off (0.60 s); Bottom left: (g) left foot touchdown (0.72 s); Bottom right: (h) left foot mid-stance (0.84 s). Duration of one stride from left foot touchdown to next left foot touchdown is 0.72 s. Duration of left foot stance phase 0.24 s, 33 per cent of stride time; duration of left foot swing phase 0.48 s, 67 per cent of stride time. The percentage phase durations are very similar to those in Figure 1.16. Note that the relative and percentage times of phases are more subject to error than for walking because of their shorter durations.

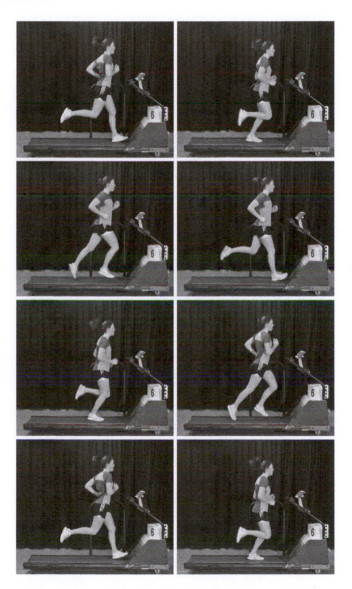

Figure 1.17 Young adult male running on a level treadmill at 12.6 km/h in trainers (he is wearing dark, tight-fitting clothing and white reflective markers to help with quantitative analysis). Top left: (a) left foot touchdown (0 s); Top right: (b) left foot mid-stance (0.12 s); Second line left: (c) left foot toe-off (0.24 s); Second line right: (d) right foot touchdown (0.36 s); Third line left: (e) right foot mid-stance (0.48 s); Third line right: (f) right foot toe-off (0.60 s); Bottom left: (g) left foot touchdown (0.72 s); Bottom right: (h) left foot mid-stance (0.84 s). Duration of one stride from left foot touchdown to next left foot touchdown is 0.72 s. Duration of left foot stance phase 0.24 s, 33 per cent of stride time; duration of left foot swing phase 0.48 s, 67 per cent of stride time. The phase and stride durations are identical to those of Figure 1.16 despite different runners and slightly different speeds. Note that the relative and percentage times of phases are more subject to error than for walking because of their shorter durations.

Figure 1.18 Five-year-old girl running overground in trainers. Top left: (a) right foot toe-off (0 s); Top right: (b) left foot touchdown (0.12 s); Second line left: (c) left foot mid-stance (0.16 s); Second line right: (d) left foot toe-off (0.32 s); Third line left: (e) right foot touchdown (0.44 s); Third line right: (f) right foot mid-stance (0.48 s); Bottom left: (g) right foot toe-off (0.64 s); Bottom right: (h) left foot touchdown (0.72 s). Duration of one stride from right foot toe-off to next right foot toe-off is 0.64 s. Duration of left and right foot stance phases 0.20 s, 31 per cent of stride time; duration of right foot swing phase 0.44 s, 69 per cent of stride time. Note that the relative and percentage times of phases are more subject to error than for walking because of their shorter durations.

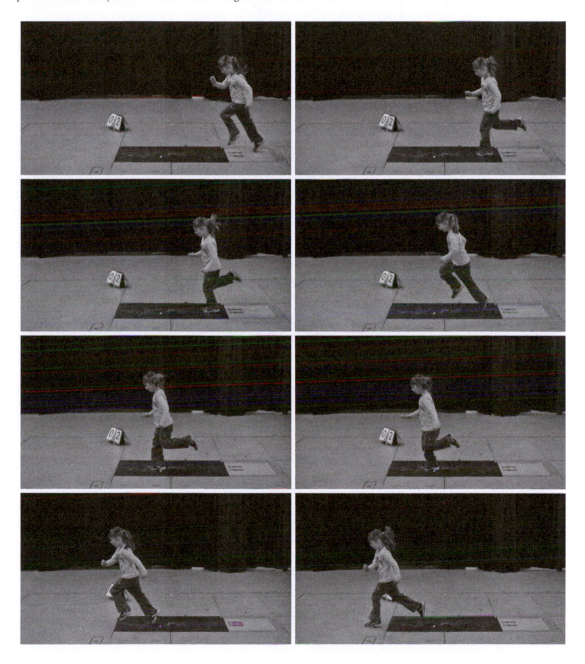

The ankle is roughly in a neutral position at touchdown, as in the reference positions of Figure 1.2. For a rear foot runner, in particular, the ankle then plantar flexes slightly until the whole foot is on the ground (e.g. left leg, Figure 1.15(b), which is shortly after touchdown and the left ankle is seen to be slightly more plantar flexed than before touchdown, e.g. Figure 1.15(a)); dorsiflexion then occurs until mid-stance (e.g. left leg, Figure 1.15(c)). The ankle plantar flexes from mid-stance until toe-off (e.g. left leg, Figure 1.15(d)), as the whole support leg lengthens. At some time during the swing phase, the ankle starts to dorsiflex to a neutral position (this is more noticeable for the left leg of the runner from Figure 1.15 running on a treadmill in Figure 1.16, particularly from Figures 1.16(d) to (e)) and plantar flexes slightly just before touchdown.

As you should note from Figures 1.15 to 1.18, this sequence of movements varies somewhat from person to person (e.g. Figure 1.17), with running speed, and between overground and treadmill running. The movement pattern for a child running (Figure 1.18) is easily seen to be different from that of an adult; for example, the child has greater hip flexion of the swing leg at toe-off of the opposite leg (Figure 1.18(d) and (g)), more forward lean of the trunk (e.g. Figure 1.18(d)) and a 'bouncier' movement (the last of these is more evident from the video clip in the Interactive eTextbook).

So, what else would we seek to observe as movement analysts looking at running patterns? Differences from this normal pattern, certainly, but also right–left side differences, variations across strides, how joint movements are coordinated within a limb as well as between legs and with the arm movements. We might also want to look at how external factors, such as changed task or environmental constraints, affect the running pattern. As we also noted for walking, the study of video sequences, as in Figures 1.15 to 1.18, is not necessarily the best, or easiest, way of analysing movement coordination.

Jumping

Simple standing jumps (as well as throws) can be subdivided biomechanically into three phases: preparation; action; recovery. Each of these phases has specific biomechanical functions. In countermovement jumps from a standing position, such as those in Figures 1.19 to 1.24, the preparation is a lowering phase, which puts the body into an advantageous position for the action (raising) phase and stores elastic energy in the eccentrically contracting (lengthening) muscles, particularly the quadriceps femoris. The action phase, unlike that for throwing, involves a more synchronised than sequential coordination of joint rotations, with all leg joints extending or plantar flexing more or less together. The recovery phase involves both the time in the air and a controlled landing, the latter through eccentric contraction of the leg muscles. Jumps that involve a run-up, such as the long or

Figure 1.19 Standing countermovement vertical jump with hands on hips. Top left: (a) starting position; Top right: (b) body at lowest point; Bottom left: (c) take-off; Bottom right: (d) peak of jump.

high jump, or that have a more complex structure, such as the triple jump, benefit from being divided into more than three phases (see, for example, the running long jump in Chapter 2). In jumps with arm movements, the coordination of the arm actions with those of the legs is very important to performance.

Figure 1.20 Standing countermovement vertical jump with normal arm action. Top left: (a) starting position; Top middle: (b) initial forwards-upwards arm movement; Middle right: (c) arms at highest point behind body; Bottom left: (d) body at lowest point; Bottom middle: (e) take-off; Bottom right: (f) peak of jump. Note that the jumper jumps slightly higher (observe the top of her head) than in the jump in Figure 1.19.

The standing vertical jump

The standing vertical jump looks simple. The extensor muscles of the hips and knees and the plantar flexors of the ankle contract eccentrically to allow the knees and hips to flex and the ankles to dorsiflex simultaneously in the preparation phase, during which the trunk also flexes. The action phase involves the more-or-less simultaneous

Figure 1.21 Standing countermovement vertical jump with 'model' arm action. Top left: (a) starting position; Top right: (b) lowest point; Bottom left: (c) take-off; Bottom right: (d) peak of jump. Note that the jumper jumps almost as high (observe the top of her head) as in the jump with her preferred arm action in Figure 1.20.

extension of the hips and knees and plantar flexion of the ankles through shortening (concentric) contraction of the muscles that extend or plantar flex these joints, driving the body vertically upwards while the trunk extends. This sequence is evident in all of the Figures 1.19 to 1.22. The main difference between the countermovement jump with no arm action in Figure 1.19 and that with a free arm action in Figure 1.20 is that the arm actions in the latter jump, if properly coordinated with those of the legs, will enhance performance of the jump.

Figure 1.22 Standing countermovement vertical jump with abnormal arm action. Top left: (a) starting position; Top right: (b) lowest point; Bottom left: (c) take-off; Bottom right: (d) peak of jump. Note that the jumper jumps about the same height (observe the top of her head, not her hair) as in the jump in Figure 1.19.

You should also compare Figure 1.20, in which the jumper used her normal arm action, with the simpler arm action in Figure 1.21, based on a simple biomechanical 'model', and the reverse, or poorly coordinated, arm action in Figure 1.22. The jumper performs almost as well with the unfamiliar model action as with her normal action, part of which is nearly identical to the model. (The heights of these jumps are more easily identified from the height measure on the front views of these jumps in the Interactive eTextbook.) In contrast,

Figure 1.23 Standing countermovement long jump with hands on hips. Top left: (a) starting position; Top right: (b) body at lowest point; Bottom left: (a) take-off; Bottom right: (d) landing.

the arm action of Figure 1.22, which is roughly the reverse of the model action, causes a decline in jump performance. In the model and normal jumps, the arm and leg movements are well coordinated, unlike in the reverse jump, in which the arm and leg movements are poorly coordinated.

In further analysis of a standing vertical jump, we might first seek to observe coordination of the movements within and between the legs, to see if they flex and extend in true synchrony. We might then look at the coordination between the movements of the legs with those of the arms. The standing vertical jump is often used as a field test of leg power, so the movement needs to be fast and powerful, as well as coordinated, to result in a successful – and high – jump.

Figure 1.24 Standing countermovement long jump with normal arm action. Top left: (a) starting position; Top right: (b) initial forwards-upwards arm movement; Middle left: (c) arms at highest point behind body; Middle right: (d) body at lowest point; Bottom left: (e) take-off; Bottom right: (f) landing. Note that the jumper jumps 40 cm further (four white strips on the ground) than in the jump in Figure 1.23.

The standing long, or broad, jump

The sequence of movements and the principles of the standing long – or broad – jump are very similar to those of the standing vertical jump. However, as the task is now to jump as far as possible horizontally, the jumper needs to partition effort between the vertical and horizontal aspects of the jump, mainly through trunk flexion (forward lean); this somewhat complicates the task. As in the standing vertical jump, the coordinated swing of the arms improves performance, as can be seen by comparing the jump without (Figure 1.23) and with (Figure 1.24) an arm swing. Coordination of all limb actions is again critically important. We would also look for a take-off angle of 35–45° as an indicator of how well the jumper had partitioned effort between the horizontal and vertical components of the jump. We could do this by trying to observe the difference between the height of the jumper's centre of mass – indicated roughly by the height of the hips – at take-off and at landing. The higher the take-off height above the landing height, the smaller the take-off angle should be. If the take-off and landing heights are equal, the optimum take-off angle would be 45° (see also the section on projectile motion in Chapter 4), compared with 90° for a standing vertical jump.

Throwing

This section focuses on the principles of those sports or events in which the participant throws, passes, bowls or shoots an object from the hand or, in the case of lacrosse, from an implement. Some, or all, of these principles relate to: throws from a circle – hammer and discus throws, shot put; crossover skills – javelin throw and cricket bowling; pitching in baseball and softball; shooting and passing movements in basketball, netball, handball, water polo and lacrosse; throwing-to skills in baseball, cricket, soccer, rugby, American and other variants of football; underarm bowling; and dart throwing. Some of these are used as examples in this section. Throws are often described as 'ballistic' movements – ones initiated by muscle activity in one muscle group, continued in a 'coasting' period with no muscle activation, and terminated by deceleration by the opposite muscle group or by passive tissue structures, such as ligaments. As with other ballistic sports movements, many throws can be subdivided biomechanically into three phases: preparation; action; recovery (see also Appendix 1.1). Each of these phases has specific biomechanical functions. The later phases depend upon the previous phase or phases. In a basic throw, the preparation phase puts the body into an advantageous position for the action phase and increases the acceleration path of the object to be thrown. In skilled throwers, the action phase often demonstrates a sequential action of muscles as segments are recruited into the movement pattern at the correct time. The recovery phase involves the controlled deceleration of the movement by eccentric contraction of the appropriate muscles. Throws that have a more complex structure, such as the discus throw, or that involve a run-up, such as javelin throwing or cricket bowling, benefit from being divided into more than three phases (see also Appendix 1.1 for a phase breakdown of the javelin throw).

Throwing movements are often classified as underarm, overarm or sidearm. The last two of these can be viewed as diagonal movement patterns, in which trunk lateral flexion, the trunk bending sideways, is mainly responsible for determining whether the throw is overarm or sidearm. In the overarm pattern, the trunk laterally flexes away from the throwing arm, in a sidearm pattern the trunk laterally flexes towards that arm. Many throwing movements are one-handed; exceptions include the hammer throw, the chest and overhead passes in basketball and netball, and the spiral pass in rugby.

The goal of a throwing movement will generally be distance, accuracy or some combination of the two, acting as a task constraint. The goal is important in determining which of the movement principles discussed in detail in Chapter 2 are more, and which are less, applicable. Some movement analysts distinguish between throw-like movements for distance, in which segmental rotations occur sequentially, and push-like movements for accuracy, in which segmental rotations occur simultaneously or synchronously. Speed-dominated throws for distance, such as the javelin throw, are usually characterised by a proximal-to-distal sequence of joint rotations, in which the movement is initiated by the larger, more powerful muscles of the legs and trunk and continued and ended by the smaller and faster muscles of the arms. The coordination of joint rotations is sequential. Push-like movements, which are usually accuracy dominated – such as the basketball free throw and dart throwing – have a more synchronous coordination of joint rotations. Because of the large mass of the shot, the shot put shows a mixture of these two coordination patterns, with sequential movements of the legs, trunk and shoulder girdle, and a more synchronous coordination of the rotations of the joints of the putting arm. Few throws in sport have no accuracy requirements. Even those, such as javelin, discus and hammer throwing and shot putting, in which the distance of the throw is predominant, have to land in a specified area and have rules that constrain the throwing technique. In throws for distance, the release speed – and, therefore, the force applied to the thrown object – is most crucial, a theme to which we will return in Chapter 4. Very few, if any, throws in sport have no requirement for speed – even the darts throw.

In some throws, the objective is not to achieve maximal distance; instead, it may be accuracy or minimal time in the air. The latter is particularly important in throws from the outfield in baseball and to the wicketkeeper in cricket. In such throws, the release speed, height and angle need to be such that the flight time is minimised within the accuracy and distance constraints of the throw. In accuracy-dominated skills, such as dart throwing and shooting in basketball, the release of the object needs to achieve accuracy within the distance constraints of the skill. The interaction of speed and accuracy in these skills is often expressed as the speed–accuracy trade-off. This can be seen, for example, in a basketball shot, in which the shooter has to release the ball with both speed and accuracy to pass through the basket.

Underarm throws

Curling and softball pitching are underarm throws, as are lawn bowling (Figures 1.25 and 1.26), tenpin bowling and skittles. Underarm throws with one arm are characterised by the shoulder action, which is predominantly flexion, often from a hyperextended position at the end of the preparation phase (backswing); the upper arm can reach a position above the horizontal because of trunk flexion. It should be noted that the end of the preparation phase is defined as the rearmost position of the ball. In the draw shot in lawn bowling (Figure 1.25), in which the bowler tries to place his ball accurately, close to the target ball (the jack), the bowler here has the upper arm partly flexed at the end of the backswing (Figure 1.25(b)). For the faster drive shot (Figure 1.26), in which the bowler is trying to disrupt the opposing team's balls, the upper arm is slightly hyperextended at the end of the preparation phase (Figure 1.26(b)), giving a longer acceleration path for the ball. In the preparation phase, the weight transfers to the rear foot and the front foot steps forwards. Weight transfers onto the front foot during the action phase, as the pelvis and trunk rotate slightly to the left, for a right-handed bowler. The shoulder flexes during the action phase and, at release, the throwing arm is parallel to, or slightly in front of, a vertical line through the right shoulder (there is little elbow rotation in the action phase). Note here the sequential coordination pattern as the right then the left leg are moving forwards while the arm and ball are

Figure 1.25 Underarm 'throw' – experienced male bowling a draw. Top left: (a) starting position; Top right: (b) end of backswing; Bottom left: (c) delivery (ball release); Bottom right: (d) follow through.

Figure 1.26 Underarm 'throw' – experienced male bowling a drive. Top left: (a) starting position; Top right: (b) end of backswing; Bottom left: (c) delivery (ball release); Bottom right: (d) follow through.

still moving backwards towards the end of the preparation phase. In throws in which the ball is released above the ground, as in softball pitching, rather than at, or very near, the ground, as in bowling, the action sequence will differ from that for lawn bowling. For example, far more movements occur outside of the sagittal plane, including pronounced rotation of the pelvis and trunk. Video clips of lawn bowling and other underarm throws, such as the cricket underarm throw and the rugby spiral pass, which is a two-handed throw, are also available in the Interactive eTextbook. You should study carefully the sequences in Figures 1.25 and 1.26 and the video clips in the Interactive eTextbook to observe differences between individuals and tasks in various underarm throwing, or bowling, patterns (see also Study Task 9).

Sidearm throws

Sidearm throws (e.g. Figure 1.27) are sometimes considered to differ from underarm and overarm throws mainly by restricted action at the shoulder joint. The dominant movements are rotation of the pelvis and trunk (Figure 1.27(c) to (d)) with the arm abducted to a position near the horizontal, from which it vigorously inwardly rotates (along with elbow extension) just before ball release (Figure 1.27(c) to (e)). Unlike the other two throwing patterns, in which the movements are mainly in the sagittal,

Figure 1.27 Sidearm throw in cricket. Top left: (a) start of movement; Top right: (b) end of backswing (preparation phase); Middle left: (c) start of main pelvis and trunk rotation; Middle right: (d) upper arm externally rotated; Bottom left: (e) release; Bottom right: (f) follow through.

or a diagonal, plane, transverse plane movements dominate in sidearm throws. The discus throw, some throws in baseball and cricket (Figure 1.27), and some shots in handball are sidearm throws. The hammer throw is probably best characterised as a sidearm throw rather than an underarm throw.

Overarm throws

Overarm throws are normally characterised by external rotation of the upper arm in the preparation phase and by its internal rotation in the action phase. These movements are among the fastest joint rotations in the human body. Many of the other joint movements are similar to those of the underarm throw. The sequence of movements in the preparation phase of a baseball pitch, for example, include, for a right-handed pitcher, pelvic and trunk rotation to the right, horizontal extension and external rotation at the shoulder, elbow flexion and wrist hyperextension. These movements are followed, sequentially, by their anatomical opposite at each of the joints mentioned plus pronation (internal rotation) of the forearm about the radioulnar joints.

Baseball pitching, javelin throwing, throwing from the outfield in cricket and passing in American football are classic examples of one-arm overarm throws. The mass (inertia) and dimensions of the thrown object – plus the size of the target area and the rules of

Figure 1.28 Overarm 'throw' – bowling in cricket. Top left: (a) approach; Top right: (b) start of bound; Middle left: (c) back foot landing; Middle right: (d) front foot landing; Bottom left: (e) release; Bottom right: (f) follow through.

Figure 1.29 Overarm throw – soccer throw-in. Left: (a) start of movement; Middle: (b) end of backswing of ball; Right: (c) release.

the particular sport – are constraints on the movement pattern of any throw. Bowling in cricket (Figure 1.28) differs from other overarm throwing patterns, as the rules restrict elbow straightening (extension) during the latter part of the delivery stride. The predominant action at the shoulder is, therefore, circumduction – a combination of shoulder flexion, extension, abduction and adduction. The soccer throw-in (Figure 1.29) uses a two-handed overarm throwing pattern. The shot put combines overarm throwing with a pushing movement, because of the event's rules and the mass of the shot. Basketball shooting (e.g. Figure 1.30) and netball shooting use various modifications to the overarm throwing pattern, depending on the rules of the game and the circumstances and position of the shot – including release speed and accuracy requirements. Passing in basketball, in which accuracy is also crucial, varies from the overarm pattern of the overhead and baseball passes to the highly modified pushing action of the chest pass; the overhead and chest passes are also important in netball. In dart throwing, the dominant requirement for accuracy restricts movements in the action phase mostly to elbow extension, some shoulder abduction (and perhaps flexion), as well as wrist adduction (ulnar deviation). You should study carefully the video clips of overarm throws in the Interactive eTextbook to observe, for example, differences between males and females in their overarm throwing patterns and differences in movement patterns between activities with different task constraints (see specific references in this section and in the study tasks later in this chapter).

Figure 1.30 Free throw in basketball. Top left: (a) start of preparation phase; Top right: (b) end of preparation phase; Bottom left: (c) release; Bottom right: (d) recovery.

Striking and kicking

There are many similarities between striking and kicking, and throwing. The basic three-phase approach can often be used for striking skills, although in striking skills with a bat, racket, club or stick the preparation phase is often called the backswing (see also Appendix 1.1). As in throwing, the preparation phase evokes the stretch–shortening cycle in the stretched muscles, making for a more effective and powerful action phase. The three-phase structure fits well those skills, such as a golf swing, in which the striking action is performed from a stationary position. There are often, however, as in the javelin throw, earlier phases, in which the player gets into position to play, for example, a stroke in tennis or badminton, or takes the run-up to a place kick. An additional complication in many striking and some kicking skills is that the ball, or other struck object, is generally moving before being kicked or struck. This involves sensory-perceptual and motor responses that are not present in many throws (consideration of these is beyond the scope of this book).

Most striking and kicking actions are performed for distance, so that the coordination of joint rotations is sequential, rather than synchronous. Because most striking skills involve an object held in the hand (exceptions to this include volleyball, boxing and fives, and, uniquely, heading in soccer), the longitudinal axis rotations of the arm, including supination and pronation of the radioulnar joints of the forearm, are more important than in throwing. These long axis rotations often depart from the strict proximal-to-distal sequence. In the tennis serve (Figure 1.31) and badminton smash, for example, upper arm flexion-abduction is followed by elbow extension, then wrist adduction, upper arm internal rotation, wrist flexion and forearm pronation. In a punt (Figure 1.32) – in rugby, American and Australian Rules football – the non-kicking foot is stabilised on the ground; the pelvis, which is here the proximal segment, tilts forwards and rotates away from the kick (Figure 1.32(b)), while the hip hyperextends and abducts, the knee flexes and the ankle plantar flexes during the preparation phase (which ends around Figure 1.32(c)). In the kicking, or action, phase, the pelvis tilts backwards, the hip flexes while the knee is still flexed, then the knee extends; the ankle usually remains partly plantar flexed at impact (as in Figure 1.32(d)). The foot speed should be maximal at impact. The pelvis continues to tilt backwards in the recovery phase while the hip continues to flex (Figure 1.32(e)). These phases are usually preceded by a relatively short run-up, which generates an initial speed for the whole body (from Figure 1.32(a)). Some striking skills, such as a tennis volley (Figure 1.33), and instep kicking for accuracy, as in a soccer pass, have a more synchronous than sequential coordination of joint rotations or involve only some joints in the segment chain. This can be seen from comparing the tennis serve in Figure 1.31 with the tennis volley in Figure 1.33.

Striking skills, like throwing skills, can be classified as overarm, sidearm and underarm. Examples of overarm striking skills are the tennis serve (Figure 1.31), the volleyball spike and the badminton smash. Sidearm striking movements include the drive in badminton and the tennis forehand (Figure 1.33) and backhand volley. Underarm striking

Figure 1.31 Tennis serve. Top left: (a) start of movement; Top middle: (b) ball release; Top right: (c) ball at peak height; Bottom left: (d) end of backswing; Bottom middle: (e) impact; Bottom right: (f) follow through.

 movements include the badminton lob, the dig in volleyball, and the forward defensive shot in cricket. The golf swing is probably most usefully characterised as a diagonal striking movement. Overarm, sidearm and underarm striking movements often have a similar structure to similarly classified throws, usually with the added complication of an object held in the hand. Example videos of several striking and kicking skills are contained in the Interactive eTextbook and are worth your attention (see specific references in this section and in the study tasks later in this chapter).

Figure 1.32 Rugby punt. Top left: (a) start of run; Top right: (b) foot plant, start of backswing; Middle left: (c) end of backswing; Middle right: (d) impact; Bottom left: (e) follow through to maximum hip flexion; Bottom right: (f) recovery.

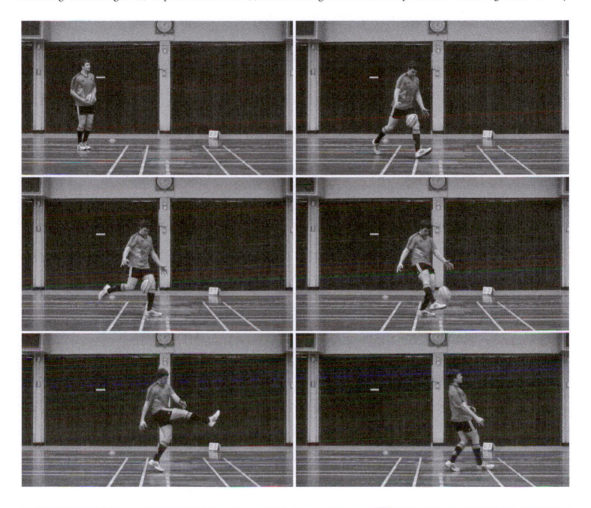

Figure 1.33 Tennis forehand volley. Top left: (a) start of movement; Top right: (b) end of backswing; Bottom left: (c) impact; Bottom right: (d) follow through.

MOVEMENT PATTERNS

Most of you (readers of this book) will be undergraduate students in the earlier stages of your career. You will be familiar with human movement patterns from sport – when viewed live, as a performer, coach or spectator – whether these are movement patterns of individuals or of teams as a whole. An example for an individual sport can be presented as a sequence of still video frames, as in Figures 1.11 to 1.33; most packages for qualitative video analysis make it easy to observe, and to compare, such movement patterns.

Video recordings and still video sequences are probably the most complex representations of sports movements that you will come across. It is only your familiarity with sports videos that enables you to understand such patterns – watch a video of a game or sporting activity for which you do not know the rules (task constraints), and the complexity of movement patterns observed on video becomes obvious. This is true not only for the movements of the segments and joints of the body of one sports performer, which sports biomechanists generally focus on, but also for the movement patterns of players within a team (shown, for example, by tracking the players using the global positioning system, GPS). The latter will not be considered further in this book – sports biomechanists are rarely involved in analysing such movement patterns.

To appreciate why I say that video recordings are complex: did you find it easy to follow all the flexion and extension descriptions for walking and running in the previous section? Could you easily perceive within-leg and between-leg coordination patterns in walking, or arm and leg coordination patterns in running, using the sequences above or videos from the Interactive eTextbook? If your answers to these questions are a resounding 'YES', then you are already a talented qualitative movement analyst! Many of us struggle at times to extract what we want from video or selected video frame sequences; for one thing they contain so much information that is irrelevant to the patterns which the movement analyst wishes to observe. So, what alternative representations of a movement are available, not only to the quantitative analyst but also to the qualitative analyst? We will answer this important question in Chapter 3.

QUALITATIVE AND QUANTITATIVE MOVEMENT ANALYSIS

Sports biomechanists use two main approaches to analysing human movement patterns in sport – qualitative and quantitative analysis. This chapter has focused on qualitative analysis. A third approach fits somewhere between the two and is often known as semi-quantitative analysis. These approaches will be developed and explained more fully in later chapters; meanwhile, Box 1.3 gives a bullet-pointed outline of each, focusing on the two main approaches, including why they are used and by whom, as well as some advantages and drawbacks of each. It is important to note that the idea that qualitative analysis is descriptive while quantitative analysis is analytical is mistaken. Both, when done well, involve description and analysis.

BOX 1.3 COMPARISON OF QUALITATIVE AND QUANTITATIVE MOVEMENT ANALYSIS

Qualitative analysis

What do we use for this?

- Video recording or observation.
- Other movement patterns, such as graphs (see Chapter 3), focusing on their patterns, not their quantification.
- Software packages for qualitative biomechanical analysis (see Chapter 2).

Who uses this?

- Teachers, coaches, athletes, physiotherapists, gait analysts and judges of 'artistic' sports, such as ice dance and gymnastics.
- 'Performance analysts' working with athletes and others.

- Movement coordination researchers (this one might surprise you but it shouldn't once you have read Chapter 3).

Why is it used?

- To differentiate between individuals or teams.
- To improve movement or performance, as in gait analysis and video analysis.
- To provide qualitative feedback.

Semi-quantitative analysis

What do we use for this?

- Mostly as for qualitative analysis plus some simple measurements, for example: joint ranges of motion; durations of sub-phases of the movement, such as the stance and support phases in running, and their ratios to the overall movement time; distances, such as stride length; joint angles at key times, such as knee angle at take-off for a jump; notation – goals scored, passes, etc.

Who uses this?

- Pretty much as for qualitative analysis; perhaps less used by teachers.

Why is it used?

- Pretty much as for qualitative analysis, but when comparisons are more important.
- For scaling aspects of a performance; for example, poor to excellent on, say, a five-point scale.

Quantitative analysis

What do we use for this?

- Image-based motion analysis, mostly using videography or automatic marker-tracking systems (see Chapter 4) plus, when occasion demands, force or pressure plates or insoles (see Chapter 5) and electromyography (see Chapter 6).
- Statistical modelling of movement technique or of movement patterns in games, artificial intelligence, computer simulation modelling.
- Software packages for quantitative biomechanical analysis (see Chapter 4).

Who uses this?

- Mainly researchers.

Why is it used?

- To aid performance comparisons.
- To predict injury risk.
- To provide quantitative feedback.

Qualitative vs quantitative analysis

- Qualitative analysis describes and analyses movements non-numerically, by seeing movements as 'patterns', while quantitative analysis describes and analyses movement numerically.
- Quantitative analysis can sometimes appear more objective because of its 'data'; however, the accuracy and reliability of such data can be very suspect, particularly when obtained in competition.
- Qualitative analysis is often more strongly rooted in a structured and multidisciplinary approach, whereas quantitative analysis can appear to lack a theoretical grounding and to be data driven.

Background to qualitative analysis

To be objective and scientific, qualitative analysis needs to use a structured approach, moving from preparation, through observation, evaluation–diagnosis, to intervention (and review) – this approach will be explained fully in Chapter 2. The movement analyst should involve the coach, or whoever commissioned the analysis, from the outset in a 'needs analysis' and keep them in the loop at all stages. Qualitative analysis requires applying basic biomechanical principles to the movement. We need to know what to observe; coaches have important knowledge and contributions to make here too.

Qualitative analysts need an excellent grasp of the movement techniques in a specific sport; coaches have great depth and breadth of that knowledge. Deterministic models (see Chapter 2) can give a theoretical basis to the analysis, which can otherwise become discursive. This modelling approach can be represented graphically so as to be coach friendly.

Good-quality digital video cameras are needed, with adequate frame rates and shutter speeds. This equipment is familiar to coaches and extra equipment is rarely necessary. Qualitative analysis should uncover the major faults in an unsuccessful performance by an individual or a team; it is the approach actually used by most coaches and teachers.

Strengths and weaknesses of qualitative analysis

Strengths

- No expensive equipment (basically, just digital video cameras).
- Field based not laboratory based, which enhances ecological validity.
- When done properly, it can be highly systematic.
- Movement patterns speak far more loudly than numbers – remember the cliché: a picture is worth a thousand words.
- Coach friendly.

Weaknesses

- Apparent lack of 'data' (but is this really such a weakness?).
- Need for considerable knowledge of movement by analysts.
- Reliability and objectivity are questionable and often difficult to assess; observer bias.

Background to quantitative analysis

Mathematical models based on biophysical laws can give a sound theoretical basis to the analysis, which can otherwise become data driven; most of these models are too far removed from coaching to be of practical use. Good quantitative analysts need a sound grasp of techniques involved in a specific activity, as do good qualitative analysts. However, not all quantitative analysis follows this principle, which might make much of the work dubious in a practical context.

A quantitative analyst needs to decide upfront on measurement techniques and methods to be used to obtain the information required. Careful attention should be paid to what to measure, the research design, data analysis, validity and reliability.

Strengths and weaknesses of quantitative analysis

Strengths

- Lots of biomechanical data (but is this really a strength?).
- Reliability and objectivity can be easily assessed, even if they rarely are.

Weaknesses

- Expensive equipment and software; the user requires many technical skills.
- Often laboratory and not field based, which reduces ecological validity.
- Apparent lack of a theoretical basis when done poorly, when it can seem data driven and non-systematic.
- Need for careful data management, as there is so much information available.
- Not coach friendly.

SUMMARY

We started this chapter by outlining a novel approach to sports biomechanics and establishing that our focus in this chapter would be the qualitative analysis of human movement patterns in sport. We defined movements in the sagittal, frontal and transverse planes. We then considered the constraints-led approach to studying human movements, and went on to look at examples of walking, running, jumping, throwing, striking and kicking, including the subdivision of these fundamental movements into phases. For each of these fundamental movements, we focused on describing the most important joint rotations for that movement; we saw that this approach helps us to compare movement patterns, for example between ages, sexes, footwear, skill levels and tasks. We then compared qualitative and quantitative analysis, looking at their background, uses, and strengths and weaknesses.

STUDY TASKS

1. Answer all of the multiple-choice questions for Chapter 1 in the Interactive eTextbook.
   Hint: Keep repeating this until you have answered all of the questions correctly.

2. Outline the phases into which running and walking are most simply divided and the key events that separate those phases. Give one important role of each phase for running. What biomechanical features are most important in distinguishing walking from running?
   Hint: You may wish to re-read the subsections on 'Walking' and 'Running', focusing on Figures 1.11 and 1.15, in particular, and watch the video clips of walking and running (from which those figures were taken) in the Interactive eTextbook before undertaking this task.

3. In the subsections on walking and running earlier in this chapter, I described the sagittal plane movements, focusing mainly on the period from touchdown of one foot to the next touchdown of the same foot. Repeat this for both walking and running, focusing instead on the period from toe-off of one foot to the next toe-off of the same foot.
   Hint: You may wish to re-read the subsections on 'Walking' and 'Running' and watch video clips of walking and running in the Interactive eTextbook before undertaking this task.

4. Name, and illustrate, the movements about the shoulder joint in all three planes, as might be observed, for example, in an overarm throwing or striking skill of your choice.
   Hint: You may wish to re-read the section on 'Defining human movements' and the subsection on 'Overarm throws', and watch several video clips of overarm throwing and striking skills in the Interactive eTextbook before undertaking this task.

5. Outline the three phases into which a throw, striking action or kick is usually divided. What is the main biomechanical function of each phase? Do these functions change with different types of throw, striking action or kick?
   Hint: You may wish to re-read the subsections on 'Throwing' and 'Striking and kicking' before undertaking this task.

6. Outline the advantages and disadvantages of qualitative and quantitative movement analysis and explain why and by whom one might be preferred over the other.
   Hint: You may wish to re-read Box 1.3, 'Comparison of qualitative and quantitative movement analysis' before undertaking this task.

7. Try to explain why either the height jumped in a standing vertical jump or the distance jumped in a standing long jump are affected by the use of the arms and by the use of a countermovement. In the relevant video sequences in the Interactive eTextbook, you can assess the relative long jump distance from the white tape markings on the floor, while the height jumped is probably more apparent from the front views of the jumps.

Hint: You may wish to re-read the subsection on 'Jumping' before undertaking this task. You are strongly advised to download the video sequences for either the five standing vertical jumps or the five standing long jumps for the young female from the Interactive eTextbook.

8 Tabulate the durations of the phases of the throwing, striking or kicking skills and performers noted. Choose the **three** of the five comparisons that most interest you. Comment briefly on your results.

   i) The action phase (from furthest back position of the ball until ball release) for a forehand and a backhand draw and a drive by a skilful and an inexperienced male lawn bowler.

   ii) The bound stride (that before the delivery stride) from take-off to back foot landing, the delivery stride from back foot to front foot landing, and the timing of ball release after front foot landing in the delivery stride for one ball by a female and one by a male cricket bowler.

   iii) The action phase (from furthest back position of the ball until ball release) for short, medium and long rugby line-out throws.

   iv) The preparation (from ball toss to lowest position of racket head behind the back), action (from end of preparation phase until impact) and recovery (considered here to be from impact until both feet touch the ground) phases of a first and a second serve in tennis.

   v) The preparation (from start to end of knee flexion) and action (start of knee extension to impact) phases of a rugby punt, drop kick and place kick.

   Hint: You may wish to re-read the subsections on 'Throwing' and 'Striking and kicking' as well as downloading and viewing the relevant video clips from the Interactive eTextbook before undertaking this task.

9 Note, and comment on, the main differences in structure and joint movements, particularly in the action phases, between the following throwing, striking or kicking skills. Choose the **three** of these five comparisons that most interest you.

   i) A basketball free throw, three-point throw and layout hook shot by a male player and a female player.

   ii) A netball chest pass, bounce pass and overhead pass.

   iii) A soccer shot, cross and pass.

   iv) A hockey shot, push pass and sweep pass.

   v) A forehand and a backhand volley in tennis.

   Hint: You may wish to re-read the subsections on 'Throwing' and 'Striking and kicking' as well as downloading and viewing the relevant video clips from the Interactive eTextbook before undertaking this task.

10 **Case study**. Download the walk-to-run transition sequence of video clips from the Interactive eTextbook.

   a) Answer the five multiple-choice questions for this study task in the Interactive eTextbook.

   b) For one stride at each of the five speeds in the sequence, calculate the following phase ratios by counting frames and dividing. Tabulate this information clearly and concisely. Summarise the information in section i) below using a suitable graph or chart.

  i) The percentage durations of the stance and swing phases to the overall stride time for the left and right legs separately.

  ii) The ratios of the durations of the single-support to double-support phases and of both these phases to the overall stride time for the two walking speeds (6.0 km/h and 8.0 km/h).

  iii) The ratios of the no-support to the single-support phases and of both these phases to the overall stride time for the three running speeds (8.6 km/h, 10.0 km/h and 12.6 km/h).

c) Briefly explain the changes in these ratios through the sequence, from the slower walking speed to the fastest running speed, in not more than 250 words.

Hint: You may wish to re-read the subsections on 'Walking' and 'Running' before undertaking this task as well as watching the five video clips very carefully.

SORTING AND LABELLING ACTIVITIES (INTERACTIVE ETEXTBOOK ONLY)

Q

Sorting activity.
Labelling activity.

FURTHER READING

Hay, J.C. (1993) *The Biomechanics of Sports Techniques* (4th edn), Englewood Cliffs, NJ: Prentice Hall. This well-regarded book by the late Dr James Hay, sometimes regarded as the founder of the discipline of sports biomechanics, was the first biomechanics text to influence my approach to the discipline when it was first published in 1973. He takes a typically mechanistic approach to biomechanics, but it is one of the easiest such texts for a student to follow. Read the sports chapters that interest you as these are the greatest strength of the book – has any other biomechanics author had such knowledge and insight into so many sports movements? A new, posthumous edition of this book is long overdue, something that the International Society of Biomechanics in Sports is looking into.

APPENDIX 1.1 PHASE ANALYSIS OF SPORTS MOVEMENTS

As noted in this chapter and in Chapter 2, phase analysis involves the breaking down of movements into phases. The phases have biomechanically distinct roles in the overall movement and each phase has easily identified phase boundaries, often called 'key events'. The duration of the phases can be determined – to the accuracy of the time resolution of the recording system – for comparison between and within performers (hence the other name, temporal analysis). Any phase analysis should start with a statement of the reason for performing the analysis, which should preferably be done in the preparation stage but can be delayed until later if video is recorded. The movement analyst then needs to specify phases, identify their boundaries and determine their distinctive biomechanical features. The examples below, in addition to that of the long jump in Chapter 2, should clarify various aspects of phase analysis.

Running – a more detailed phase analysis

In the section on running in this chapter, we divided the running cycle (for one foot) into two rather obvious phases, stance and swing, for which the key events are clearly touchdown and toe-off. The functions of these two phases can then be defined as follows: the stance phase absorbs impact, allows an active landing, maintains forward momentum and accelerates to toe-off; the swing phase allows recovery of the non-support leg and prepares for foot descent to hit the ground with an active landing. This two-phase schema results in overly complex biomechanics of the phases. An alternative, more attractive schema biomechanically, subdivides the movement into three sub-phases within each of the above stance and swing phases, as follows. Although this phase analysis is far more biomechanically sound, it is unlikely that the phase boundaries of the short duration foot-strike phase will be discernible from 25 or 30 Hz digital video recordings, an important practical drawback.

- Foot strike – starts at first foot contact with the ground (touchdown). This is a very short phase in which the foot should, ideally, hit the ground moving backwards. The main function of this phase is impact absorption.
- Mid-support – starts after the impact peak as limb length starts to shorten. This phase is characterised by relative shortening of the overall length of the support limb towards the centre of mass. The hips and knees flex (see also Figure 3.11(a), region a–b), the ankle dorsiflexes and the foot pronates. Its functions are maintenance of forward momentum, support of body weight and storage of elastic energy.
- Take-off – starts as limb length starts to increase, ends at toe-off. This phase involves relative lengthening of the overall limb length. The hips and knees extend (see also Figure 3.11(a), region c–d), the ankle plantar flexes and the foot supinates. Its functions are to accelerate the body forwards and upwards and to transfer energy from the powerful thigh muscles to the faster muscles of the calf.
- Follow-through – starts at toe-off. This phase is characterised by slowing of hip extension then start of hip flexion, both accompanied by, and the latter assisting, knee flexion (see also Figure 3.11(a), region d–e). It functions as a decelerating phase for the recovery leg.

- Forward swing – starts as the foot begins to move forward relative to the body. The hip flexes with the knee flexing or flexed (see also Figure 3.11(a), at f). Its main function is to coordinate the recovery leg movement to enhance the forwards–upwards reaction force from the ground, as this phase coincides with the take-off phase of the other leg (similar to the coordination of arm and leg movements in the vertical jump examples in this chapter). The phase also prepares for the next phase – foot descent.
- Foot descent – starts as the forward movement of the leg and foot stops, ends at first foot contact. The hip and knee extend (see also Figure 3.11(a), region g–a) after the arresting of the forward leg swing by the hamstring muscles; the gastrocnemius muscle at the back of the calf is pre-activated for landing. This phase's main function is to have the foot strike the ground in an active landing, to prevent braking of forward movement of the centre of mass.

Phase analysis of ballistic movements

Ballistic movements, which include throwing, striking and kicking skills, subdivide into three phases: preparation or backswing; action; recovery or follow through. In the tennis serve (see Figure 1.31), for example, the key events are:

- The start of the preparation phase (or backswing) – the initiation of ball toss.
- The end of the preparation phase which is also the start of the action phase – this is somewhat arbitrary, but often defined as the racket reaching its lowest point behind the server's back.
- The end of the action phase and start of recovery – impact of the racket and ball.
- The end of the recovery phase – also rather arbitrary and could be defined as the end of the serving arm's follow through or the start of the player's movement into the next stroke.

Here, the preparation phase has various important functions:

- It puts the body into an advantageous position for the action phase.
- It maximises the range of movement of the racket – it increases the acceleration path (see Appendix 2.1).
- It allows the larger segments to initiate the movement (see Appendix 2.1).
- It stretches the agonist muscles, increasing the output of the muscle spindle receptors, and allowing the storage of elastic energy (the stretch–shortening cycle, see Appendix 2.1).
- It increases the length of the muscles responsible for the action (called the prime movers or agonists, see Chapter 6) to that at which maximum tension is developed.
- It provides neural facilitation (through the Golgi tendon organs) by contraction of the group of muscles that may slow the movement in the recovery phase (the antagonists).

The important functions of the action phase are:

- Movements are initiated by the large muscle groups and continued by faster, smaller, more distal muscles of the limbs, increasing the speed throughout the movement as the segmental ranges of movement increase (see Appendix 2.1).
- The accuracy of the movement increases through the recruitment of muscles with progressively decreasing innervation ratio (see Appendix 2.1).
- The segmental forces are applied in the direction of movement and movements are initiated with minimum inertia as movement proceeds along the segment chain (see Appendix 2.1).

The recovery phase:

- Involves controlled deceleration of the movement by, usually, eccentric (lengthening) contraction of the appropriate antagonist muscles.
- May achieve a position of temporary balance, as at the end of a golf swing.
- For a learner, may require a conscious effort to overcome neural inhibition from the Golgi tendon organs, which is reinforced by antagonistic muscle spindle activity.

Although phase analysis is very helpful in identifying critical features of a movement and in building a deterministic model, it does have important limitations. The phase boundaries need to be easily observable, but there is some arbitrariness in specifying them, as in the tennis serve example above. The end of the backswing of the racket might conveniently define transition from the preparation to the action phase; however, at that instant, the legs and trunk are in their 'action' phase while the distal joints of the racket arm may still be in their 'preparation' phase. The extension of the three-phase ballistic model to other activities is unhelpful, although common. The biomechanical structure of other movements may require more than three phases, as in the following examples.

Phase analysis of more complex movements

Three examples are given below, focusing on the name and main functions of each phase only. You might want to view some videos of these activities on, for example, YouTube (www.youtube.com).

Phase analysis of the volleyball spike

This is probably best analysed in seven phases:

1 Run-in: generating controllable speed.
2 Landing: impact absorption.

3 Impulse drive: horizontal to vertical momentum transfer.
4 Airborne phase of preparation: as ballistic movements.
5 Hitting phase: as ballistic movements.
6 Airborne phase to landing – airborne recovery: as ballistic movements.
7 Landing: to absorb impact, control deceleration and prepare for next move.

Phases 4 to 6 are seen to follow the ballistic sequence within a more complex movement.

Phase analysis of the javelin throw

1 Run-up: generating controllable speed.
2 Crossover steps: 'withdrawal' of javelin to extend acceleration path; transfer from forwards to sideways action.
3 Delivery stride: the action phase; similar, in many ways, to that for ballistic movements.
4 Recovery – to avoid crossing foul line.

Historically, phase 2 would have been split into the withdrawal and one crossover step. Phases 2 to 4 follow the ballistic sequence within a more complex movement structure.

Phase analysis of front crawl swimming

Swimming can, conveniently, be broken down into the time spent starting, stroking and turning. Focusing only on the stroking part of this subdivision for the front crawl, we can identify the following phases for each stroke:

1 Initial 'press': smooth entry of the hand into the water.
2 Outward scull: propulsive force generation by the arm moving outwards and backwards through the water; this extends the acceleration path; the hand acts as a hydrofoil.
3 Inward scull: propulsive force generation by the arm moving inwards and backwards through the water; this extends the acceleration path; the hand acts as a hydrofoil.
4 Recovery: moving the arm through the air for the next stroke.

2 Qualitative biomechanical analysis of sports movements

Knowledge assumed
Ability to undertake simple analysis of videos of sports movements (Chapter 1)
Movements in sagittal, frontal and transverse planes (Chapter 1)
Fundamental movements, such as running, jumping, throwing, striking and kicking (Chapter 1)

INTRODUCTION

In the previous chapter, we considered human motion in sport and exercise as 'patterns of movement', and introduced key aspects of the qualitative and quantitative analysis of human movement patterns in sport. This chapter is designed to provide a contextual structure for carrying out qualitative movement analysis. The main approach to the qualitative analysis of movements in sport and exercise that I have adopted for this chapter is based on previous books on qualitative analysis of human movement (see Further Reading for more details) and many years of practical experience. This approach is very similar to that recommended by some professional agencies that represent sports biomechanists, or by agencies that hire sports biomechanists. The structured approach outlined here can be, and is, used by qualitative and quantitative movement analysts as a coherent framework for their work. It could beneficially be used even more widely. We will also look at some alternative approaches to qualitative analysis, particularly to the identification of the 'critical features' of various sports movements.

BOX 2.1 LEARNING OUTCOMES

After reading this chapter you should be able to:

- understand how qualitative biomechanical analysis fits within the multidisciplinary framework of qualitative movement analysis
- plan and undertake a qualitative video analysis of a sports movement of your choice
- develop critical insight into qualitative biomechanical analysis of movement in sport and exercise
- appreciate the need for a structured approach to qualitative movement analysis
- outline the principles of deterministic modelling and perform a qualitative analysis of a sports skill in detail, using a deterministic model
- appreciate how the use of a deterministic model can avoid some of the pitfalls of qualitative analysis
- outline other approaches to the identification of the critical features of a sports movement
- understand the roles, within qualitative analysis, of phase analysis of movements and the movement principles approach.

A STRUCTURED ANALYSIS FRAMEWORK

The real world of sports performance outside of academia – coaches, athletes and other practitioners – has generated an increasing demand for good qualitative movement analysts; this is our main focus in this chapter. The approach outlined in this section, and developed further in the four sections that follow, focuses on the systematic observation and introspective judgement of the quality of human movement to provide the best intervention to improve performance. This approach is necessarily interdisciplinary and integrated, involving motor development, motor learning and biomechanics, together with some aspects of physiology and psychology.

The various approaches to qualitative analysis used by movement analysts have focused on biomechanics, motor development or pedagogy, and have sometimes been cross-disciplinary. Previous work has included development approaches, for example, looking at whole-body developmental sequences, as in the four stages of acquiring throwing skills, or adopting a 'movement-component approach', focusing on the legs, arms or trunk. More recent developments have included logical decision trees, as in Figure 2.1. So far, at least, there have been few attempts to use the Expert System approach of Artificial Intelligence, which has been widely adopted in gait analysis and medical diagnostics.

In the various pedagogical approaches, the focus has varied. Sometimes, the observer has been recommended to attend to the temporal phases and spatial aspects of the movement. Other approaches have integrated various disciplines, considered the pre-observation, observation and post-observation stages of analysis, and introduced the concept of 'critical features'. Critical features are those components of a movement that make an essential contribution to successful performance of that skill; for a qualitative analysis, the critical features need to be observable.

The various biomechanical approaches have, typically, identified the critical features of a skill using 'biomechanical principles' – better called movement principles. These approaches include POSSUM – the purpose-observation system of studying and understanding movement. In this approach, the movement is classified by its purpose, as in Figure 2.2(a), which is associated with 'observable dimensions' of the movement that the observer evaluates. In the example of Figure 2.2(a), the focus is a projectile – the whole body of a sports performer or an object, such as a shot. If the purpose is

Figure 2.1 Simplified logical decision tree approach to qualitative classification of fast bowling technique.

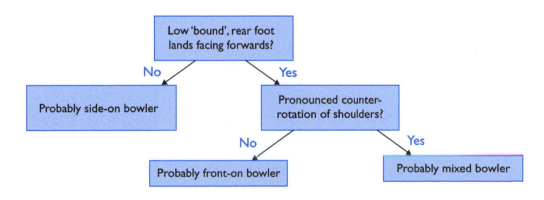

height, then the release or take-off is vertical; if the purpose is horizontal distance (range), the release is around 45° (but see Chapter 4 for further consideration of this point); if the purpose is minimising the time the projectile is in the air, the release is nearly horizontal. The focus of the observer can be on the whole body or specific body segments. This approach was extended around 10 core concepts of 'kinesiology', as in Figure 2.2(b). Other biomechanical approaches have also tended to be based on a list of movement principles, for example Figure 2.2(c). It is instructive to compare such sets of principles, such as those of Figure 2.2(b) and (c), and to note that they do not seem to correspond exactly. This led several movement analysts, including me, to develop three sub-classes of principles (see Appendix 2.1). The first of these – universal principles – apply to all sports movements. The second – partially general principles –

Figure 2.2 'Principles' approach to qualitative analysis (adapted from Knudson and Morrison, 2002; see Further Reading): Top left: (a) classifying movement by its purpose; Top right: (b) core concepts of kinesiology; Bottom left: (c) movement principles approach; Bottom right: (d) comprehensive approach to qualitative analysis (for outline of details of each stage, see Box 2.2).

apply to groups of sports movements, such as those in which the task constraints demand a focus on speed generation or on accuracy. Finally, there are principles applying to a specific skill, such as javelin throwing – these are specific principles.

The 'deterministic' or 'hierarchical' modelling approach, to which we will return later in the chapter, incorporates movement principles within a more structured framework, which should reduce the need to memorise lists of principles.

Nearly all of these approaches focus on qualitative analysis based on identifying errors in the movement and how to correct them. Whichever approach has been used, the tendency has been to focus on instantaneous events, such as a leg, arm or trunk angle at release of an implement. Such 'discrete' parameters often tell us little about the overall movement, the distinctive features of which are its wholeness and its coordination (or possible lack of coordination in novices). These discrete parameters are often more easy to observe (or measure) and analyse than continuous movement patterns; they will, therefore, be a major focus in this chapter. However, one of the aims of this book is to seek to rectify the lack of focus by sports biomechanists on movement coordination; we will return to this theme in Chapter 3. The most convincing approach to a structured qualitative analysis of sports movements, in my view, is that of Knudson and Morrison (2002; see Further Reading), which I have overviewed and extended in the next five sections, and which is represented diagrammatically in Figure 2.2(d); this approach is summarised in Box 2.2 and elaborated on in the next four sections.

BOX 2.2 STAGES IN A STRUCTURED APPROACH TO ANALYSIS OF HUMAN MOVEMENT IN SPORT

Preparation stage

- Conducting a 'needs analysis' with the people 'commissioning' the study – usually coaches or athletes – to ascertain what they want from it.
- Gathering all relevant knowledge of the sports activity.
- Establishing critical features of the movement and, possibly, their range of correctness; the latter moves us into semi-quantitative analysis (see Chapter 1).
- Developing a systematic observation strategy for the observation stage.
- Deciding on any other movement patterns (such as graphs; see Chapter 3) to be used in the analysis.
- Obtaining knowledge of relevant characteristics of the performers.
- Developing knowledge of effective instruction, including cue words and phrases, for the intervention stage.

Observation stage

- Implementing the systematic observation strategy developed in the preparation stage.
- Gathering information about the movement from the senses and from video recordings.

- Selecting the focus of observation, for example, on particular phases of the movement.
- Deciding where to observe – for example, in a controlled environment or an ecologically valid one.
- Deciding from where to observe the movement (in North America these are often called 'vantage points') – this usually means where to position the video cameras.
- Choosing the number of observations to be made, or trials to be recorded, bearing in mind that there is really no such thing as a representative trial.

Evaluation and diagnosis stage

- Evaluating the strengths and weaknesses of the performance.
- Deciding on the use of other movement patterns in addition to video images (see Chapter 3).
- Addressing the issues of validity and reliability, which are generally poor to moderate for a single analyst and poor across analysts; increased training of analyst and analysing more trials both help.
- Selecting the best intervention to improve performance; this involves judgement of the causes of poor performance. There are several approaches to prioritising the order in which weaknesses in performance might be tackled, based on features of the movement that:
  - relate to previous actions
  - are in a correct sequence
  - promise greatest improvement in performance or reduction in injury risk
  - proceed in order of difficulty of changing, from easiest to hardest
  - work from the base of support up.
- Considering various issues in movement evaluation and diagnosis and their implications:
  - variability of movement
  - movement errors
  - use of critical features or an 'ideal form' approach
  - analyst bias
  - lack of a coherent theoretical basis (this is not necessarily true).

Intervention stage

- Emphasising feedback to performers to improve the movement technique and performance.
- Addressing the many issues about how, when and where to provide feedback.
- Considering various issues about practice, which need to address motor control models, and about technique – or skills – training, and other aspects of training.
- Conducting the main review of the overall qualitative analysis process in the context of the needs analysis from the preparation stage – this does not preclude reviews at other stages of the process, as implied by the solid red arrows in Figure 2.2(d).

PREPARATION STAGE – IDENTIFYING CRITICAL FEATURES

As can be seen from Box 2.2, the preparation stage involves much gathering of knowledge, including the undertaking of a needs analysis, identifying critical features of the sports movement under investigation, and preparing for later stages in the analysis process. We will focus here mainly on the first two of these – gathering knowledge and, particularly, identifying the critical features of the movement.

Gathering knowledge

The gathering of relevant knowledge is dynamic and ongoing. A successful movement analyst needs knowledge, first and foremost, of the activity or movement, from which he or she will then develop the critical features of performance. Secondly, knowledge is needed of the performers; this includes the performers', and coaches' or therapists', needs, which should be identified through a 'needs analysis'. Although the preparation for later stages of the qualitative analysis process takes place, at least in terms of gathering relevant knowledge, in the preparation stage, these will be dealt with under later stages. Developing a systematic observation strategy is covered in the next section and developing an intervention strategy is dealt with in the section on the intervention stage. In Chapter 3, we will discuss the qualitative graphical movement and coordination patterns, in addition to video analysis, which can be used in the evaluation and diagnosis stage.

Your knowledge of the activity, as a movement analyst, should draw on many sport and exercise science disciplines. For example, as a primary Physical Education teacher, you would source knowledge mainly from the discipline of motor development; a secondary Physical Education teacher, by contrast, would probably focus more on an analysis of individual skills and techniques using, primarily, sports biomechanics. As a movement analyst working with novices, motor learning and practice would be major sources of information for you. On the other hand, a movement analyst working with good club-standard performers would probably focus on a biomechanically derived identification of critical features, and a movement analyst working with elite performers would concentrate on the critical features at that standard, and might use a more quantitative approach.

In all of our work as movement analysts, whether qualitative or quantitative, we should always seek to adhere to 'evidence-based' practice, which raises the question as to what evidence to gather and from where. A movement analyst has, in general, access to various sources of knowledge about the sports activity being studied. Some issues arise in using these sources, including the fragmentary nature of some sources and weighing conflicting evidence from various sources. Experience also influences success in using source material, and helps to deal with anecdotal evidence and, with care, personal bias. The gathering of valid knowledge of the sports activity under consideration is invaluable if done systematically, and one needs to keep practising the establishment of the critical features of the movement based on the knowledge gathered.

A warning here is appropriate: although the Internet is a fruitful source of information, in general there is little, if any, quality control over what appears there. Valid information is best sourced from such expert opinion, which can also be found in professional journals such as the *Sport and Exercise Scientist* (British Association of Sport and Exercise Sciences, UK; www.bases.org.uk) and sport-specific coaching journals (such as *Swimming Technique*, now an integral part of *Swimming World Magazine*; www.swimmingworldmagazine.com) – most of these sources are accessible though the Internet. The sports performers and their support staff included in any 'real-world' study are also a potential source of knowledge about their sport, as may be other coaches and performers involved; not all of their knowledge will normally be evidence based and some may be biased, so care is needed in using it. Problems associated with synthesising all of this knowledge include conflicts of opinion, a reliance on the 'elite athlete template' – what the most successful do must also be right for others – and incorrect notions about the critical features of the movement.

Scientific research should provide the most valid and accurate sources of information. Movement analysts need some research training, however, to interpret research findings: applied BSc or MSc degrees should provide such training in an applied context, while research PhDs often focus more on quantitative biomechanical analysis, which we will discuss in Chapters 4 to 6. The best sources of relevant, applied research are applied sports science research journals, such as *Sports Biomechanics* (www.tandf.co.uk/journals/rspb) published on behalf of the ISBS, and the best coaching journals, such as *New Studies in Athletics* (www.iaaf.org/development/new-studies-in-athletics). Sport-specific scientific review papers draw together knowledge from many sources and provide a valuable source of information for movement analysts, providing the reviews have an applied rather than a fundamental research focus. A fruitful source for such review papers has been the *Journal of Sports Sciences* (www.tandf.co.uk/journals/titles/02640414.asp). The main problem with scientific research as a source of information for the qualitative movement analyst might be called the validity conflict, between internal (research) validity and ecological (real-world) validity – in the laboratory or in the field.

It is not sufficient just to gather knowledge of the activity; it must also be theoretically focused and practically synthesised. Adopting a 'fundamental movement pattern' approach is now seen as flawed, because of its over-reliance on the motor program concept of cognitive motor control. The constraints-led approach, introduced briefly in Chapter 1, considers the movement 'space' (the set of all possible solutions to the specific movement task) as constrained by the task, environment and organism; this is the approach of ecological motor control, which is still evolving. The critical features approach, adopted in the next subsection, is probably the most widely used by movement analysts from a sports biomechanics perspective. The analyst needs to keep practising this approach, whose points are widely used in teaching and coaching. The movement criterion might be injury risk, movement effectiveness – defined as achievementof the movement goal – or efficiency – the economical use of metabolic energy; our focus here will be on improved performance. Analysts often specify a range of correctness of critical features; this range must be observable. One common error is not focusing sufficiently on devising cue words for use in correcting technique errors; error correction should be seen as the responsibility of the movement analysis team, which includes the coach and the movement analyst, not the coach alone.

Relevant knowledge of the performers will include their age, sex and standard of performance; physical abilities, such as fitness, strength and flexibility; injury status and history; and cognitive development, which relates to the feedback to be provided in the intervention stage. Also relevant here is knowledge of the particular sports activity as related to a specific performer, which may require knowledge from motor development and motor learning. An extremely important knowledge source is the 'needs' of the performers and their coaches or therapists; to address this properly requires a 'needs analysis' led by the movement analyst, based on the foregoing points and knowledge of the sports activity. This needs analysis (including, in the real world, a project costing to deliver what is needed) then has to be approved by the 'clients', before leading into the acquisition of other relevant knowledge, being translated into a systematic observation strategy, driving the evaluation and diagnosis, and providing the structure for the intervention.

The requisite knowledge for development of a systematic observation strategy (see also the next section) includes how to observe, based on the overall movement or its phases (see Appendix 1.1), the best observation (or vantage) points, and how many observations are needed. Aids to the development of this strategy include the use of videography and rating scales. It is advisable for all movement analysts to practise observation even when using video, particularly if movements are fast and complex. Furthermore, the analyst should develop pre-pilot and pilot protocols to ensure all problems are overcome before the 'big day'. The advice 'pilot, pilot, then pilot some more' is well founded.

Knowledge of effective instruction, feedback and intervention provide the appropriate information to translate critical features into intervention cues, couched in behavioural terms, which are appropriate to one's 'clients'. These should not be verbose – no more than six words – and figurative, not literal. Remember that analogies must be meaningful; advising that the backhand clear in badminton is like 'swiping a fly off the ceiling with a towel' has no meaning to someone who has never performed such an action or seen another person do it. The cues to be devised can be verbal, visual, aural or kinaesthetic, and may differ for various phases of a movement; for example, a javelin coach may see value in attending to the aural cues of footfall during the run-up, but would switch to other cues for the delivery phase. The movement analyst needs, therefore, to derive relevant cues for each movement phase, and should attend to: the cue structure (what the action is); its content (what does the action – the 'doers'); and cue qualification (how to gauge success). Special conditions may be added if more information is needed. Examples include: rotate (action) the hip and trunk (the doers); swing (action) the racket (doer) forwards (qualification).

Identifying critical features of a movement

Much of our work as movement analysts involves the study and evaluation of how sports skills are performed. To analyse the observed movement 'technique', we need to identify critical features of the movement. These features should be crucial to improving performance of a certain skill or reducing the injury risk in performing that skill, or sometimes both. For a qualitative biomechanical analyst, this means being able to observe those features of the movement; for the quantitative analyst, this requires measuring those features and, often, further mathematical analysis (see Chapters 4 to 6). Identification of these critical features is probably the most important task facing a qualitative biomechanical analyst, and we will look at several approaches to this task in this sub-section. None are foolproof but all are better in identifying these crucial elements of a skill than an unstructured approach. Sometimes it can be helpful to define a 'scale of correctness' for critical features, for example, poor = 1 to perfect = 5, or a 'range of correctness', such as 'wrist above elbow but below shoulder'. We will return to this theme later in the chapter.

The 'ideal performance' or 'elite athlete template' approach

This approach involves the use of an ideal (sometimes called a 'model') performance, often that of an elite performer, hence the alternative name. This approach has nothing to recommend it except, for a lazy analyst, its minimal need for creative thought. It assumes that the ideal or elite performance – and the movements used to produce it – can be applied to the person or persons for whom the analyst is performing his or her analysis. There is now wide agreement among movement analysts that there is no universal 'optimal performance model' for any sports movement pattern. Each performer brings a unique set of organismic constraints to a movement task; these determine which movements, out of the many possible solutions for the task under those constraints, are best for him or her. You are strongly advised to avoid this approach.

Movement principles approach

Categorising principles as general, partially general or specific (as in Box 2.3), while it does conform to the constraints-led approach (see below), does not provide a 'recipe' approach to identifying the critical features of a movement. I would caution against a mechanistic application of the movement principles approach. I would advise instead that you develop an awareness of the important movement principles (these are developed further in Appendix 2.1) that are used in devising a deterministic model of a given sports activity. Then you should proceed by the judicious use of the movement principles that conform to the constraints on the performance of that activity. The principles used should be specific to the sports activity, the performer and the constraints on the movement. An example of the use of movement principles within a deterministic modelling approach is given in the next subsection.

BOX 2.3 SUMMARY OF UNIVERSAL AND PARTIALLY GENERAL MOVEMENT PRINCIPLES

(See Appendix 2.1 for further details of universal and partially general movement principles.)

Universal principles

These should apply to all sports tasks:

- Use of the stretch–shortening cycle of muscle contraction.
- Minimisation of energy used to perform the task.
- Control of redundant degrees of freedom in the segmental chain.

Partially general principles

These apply to groups of sports tasks, such as those dominated, for example, by speed generation, accuracy, or balance:

- Sequential action (or sequential coordination) of muscles.
- Minimisation of inertia (increasing acceleration of movement).
- Impulse generation or absorption.
- Maximising the acceleration path.
- Stability.

Specific principles

These apply to the specific sports activity under consideration and are derived and used for the long jump in the next subsection.

Deterministic modelling

Principles of deterministic modelling

Deterministic models of sports activities, also known as 'hierarchical models', as they descend a hierarchical pyramid, can be easily drawn using SmartArt hierarchical models in Microsoft Word. They work best with sports that have an objective performance criterion – the outcome or result. This is often, in track and field athletics, for example, to go faster, higher or further. In such cases, we have a clear and objective performance criterion, such as race time, which we seek to minimise, or distance jumped or thrown, which we seek to maximise. Splitting a movement into phases, as we have done below for the long jump (see also Appendix 1.1), can not only aid the establishment of a deterministic model but also help the identification of critical features for each phase.

The next stage is to subdivide the performance criterion, where possible, as in the examples below (see also Figure 2.3). The crucial stage of identifying critical features then follows. Once this is done, and the model has been developed to the necessary level – which should arrive at observable critical features for a qualitative analysis or measurable ones for a quantitative analysis – it needs to be evaluated and its limitations noted. Generally, the critical features highlighted in the model will be biomechanical features or variables such as joint angles, or body segment parameters such as a skater's moment of inertia. Generally, it is advisable not to use ambiguities, such as 'timing' or 'flexibility' or even, perhaps, 'coordination'. If critical, these should be identified more precisely, such as specifying why hamstring flexibility is important because it improves the joint range of movement, or which joint movements need to be coordinated and how.

A model entry at one 'level' should be completely defined by those associated with it at the next level down, for example, those at the top level, 1 – this would be the performance criterion – by those at level 2. This association should either be a division – as in the link between levels 1 and 2 in the simple examples of a throw model and a swimming model in Figures 2.4 and 2.5 respectively – or a biomechanical relationship, as in the links between levels 2 and 3 in those two models. In the simple throw model Figure 2.4, the principle (or equations if you prefer) of projectile motion (this could be considered as a specific movement principle) link flight distance and the release parameters of the throw. In the swimming model, Figure 2.5, the swimming time (level 2) is linked to distance swum and swimming speed (level 3) by the simple movement relationship: mean speed equals distance swum divided by the time taken. A further movement relationship is found between levels 3 and 4, for which average speed equals average stroke length multiplied by stroke rate, a specific movement principle.

The difference between the use of movement principles within a deterministic model and simply using a 'recipe' list of movement principles is that, in the former approach, the principle flows from the model rather than being slavishly adopted from a list.

Figure 2.3 The various levels of a general deterministic model.

Level 1: Performance Criterion – the Result (e.g. time of race; distance or height of jump or throw; points awarded or deducted, e.g. in gymnastics).

Level 2: Subdivision of Performance Criterion (if possible; e.g. durations of phases of a race, or distances of phases of a jump or throw).

Level 3, 4, etc.: Critical Features – the Body Actions that Produce the Result.

Figure 2.4 Levels 1, 2 and 3 of a deterministic model of a throw. The release distance is the distance that the centre of mass of the thrown object is ahead of (or behind, with a negative value) the point from which the throw is measured, such as the stop board in a shot, discus or hammer throw. The landing distance is the distance the object lands ahead of its centre of mass; this will normally be zero, however for a javelin throw it will be the distance that the point of the javelin (to which the throw is measured) lands ahead of its centre of mass.

Figure 2.5 Levels 1 to 4 of a deterministic model of swimming.

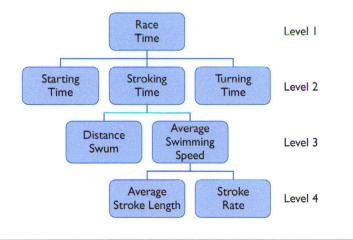

In addition, this modelling approach is easily adapted to alternative ways of identifying critical features, for example, through a constraints-led approach. Another advantage of deterministic models over lists of principles is that they help the movement analyst to spot 'blind alleys'; this is illustrated in the example below. A further advantage is that the development of the critical features arises from the model structure, which incorporates the relevant movement principles, so the critical features identified should, providing sufficient care has been taken, be just that – critical to the performance of the movement, rather than arbitrary.

A deterministic model for qualitative analysis of the long jump

The first step in developing a full deterministic model for qualitative analysis of the long jump is to define the performance criterion, which is very simple for this task, being the distance jumped. We will ignore here compliance with the rules of the event, which are task constraints in their own right, assuming the jumper analysed is able to conform to the rules. The next step – level 2 of our model, as in Figure 2.6 – is to ask if we can divide the distance jumped into other distances, which often relate to the phases of the movement. Here, it can be subdivided into the take-off distance, the flight distance and the landing distance (these are explained in Figure 2.7).

We have now completed level 2 of our long jump model and need to prioritise further development according to which of the three sub-distances is most important. Clearly, from Figure 2.7, the flight distance is by far the most important; this is the distance the jumper's centre of mass travels during the airborne, or flight, phase. This distance can be specified by a biomechanical relationship as it fits the principle of projectile motion.

Figure 2.6 Levels 1 and 2 of a long jump deterministic model – division of distance jumped into its three sub-distances.

Figure 2.7 Diagrammatic explanation of the three sub-distances of the long jump model: TOD = take-off distance; LD = landing distance. White circles denote the positions of the whole-body centre of mass of the jumper at take-off and landing.

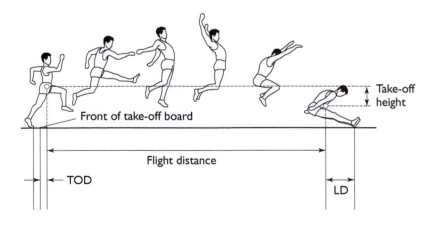

We have to make a choice at this stage. Do we represent the take-off parameters for the long jump similarly to those for the simple throw model of Figure 2.4; here, these would become the take-off speed, take-off angle and take-off height? Or do we use the alternative approach represented in Figure 2.8, in which we view the take-off velocity as being specified not by the take-off speed and angle but by the take-off horizontal and vertical velocity components? The latter approach is preferable for two reasons. First, while on the take-off board, a long jumper needs to generate vertical velocity while minimising the loss of horizontal velocity from the run-up; for the horizontal component, there tends to be an initial 'braking' force followed by an accelerating force. Secondly, muscles generate force, hence acceleration and velocity, not angle; take-off angle is the consequence of the ratio of the two velocity components, not the other way round. Level 3 of our deterministic model for the flight distance (Figure 2.9) also shows that this distance is affected by the aerodynamics of the jumper – the air resistance. This can be neglected for the long jump.

We now need to prioritise the development of level 3 of the model. Which of the take-off parameters is most important? We will choose to develop our model for the take-off horizontal velocity before that for the take-off vertical velocity, if for no

Figure 2.8 Take-off velocity components for long jump.

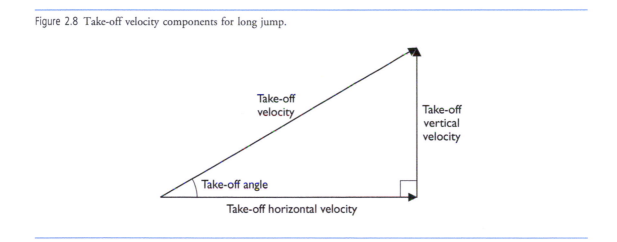

Figure 2.9 Level 3 of the long jump deterministic model – factors affecting the flight distance.

other reason than that the horizontal component is about 2.5 times greater than the vertical one. Level 4 for the take-off horizontal velocity is shown in Figure 2.10, in which the take-off horizontal velocity has been divided into the touchdown horizontal velocity (the horizontal velocity at board contact, or the run-up speed) and the horizontal velocity added (or lost) on the take-off board. The first of these gives us our first critical feature – the jumper must have a fast run-up; we need to develop an 'eye' for this as qualitative analysts, whereas a quantitative analyst would need to devise the best way of measuring this speed. The second component – horizontal velocity added on the board – is of little direct use, being unobservable (although measurable), so we need to develop it further, into level 5, using the appropriate biomechanical relationship.

The one relationship that springs to mind – because it is the simplest – is the impulse–momentum relationship (see Appendix 2.1 under 'Impulse generation or absorption'). This could be represented graphically by developing horizontal velocity added on the board (level 4a) as the take-off impulse and the athlete's body mass (at level 4b of the model). Take-off impulse, in turn, would depend at the next level down (level 4c) on the mean force and the time spent on the take-off board. However, for the long jump, this 'branch' of the model would be a blind alley. The reason is that it would suggest that the jumper needs to maximise both the mean force and the time on the board to improve performance. Given the fast run-up of good long jumpers, trying to extend the board contact time (about 120 ms) would be difficult at best; if feasible, it would have a negative effect on the mean force. Fortunately, we avoid this blind alley simply by being unable to observe the critical features based on the impulse–momentum relationship – impulse, mean force and time on the board; this is not always the case.

A better approach altogether for the long jump example is to use the work–energy relationship (see under 'Maximising the acceleration path' in Appendix 2.1). Here, the work done (mean force multiplied by the distance over which the force acts) is approximately (ignoring changes in potential energy) the change in the jumper's kinetic energy, which relates to the jumper's mass and change of velocity. This is shown in levels 4a–c of our model for take-off horizontal velocity in Figure 2.10. Although the mean force and the acceleration path of the jumper's centre of mass will not yet appear to be observable, we do have the right relationship, as the jumper correctly needs to try to maximise both of these factors. You should note the deceleration and acceleration sub-phases of the board contact phase implied in this model. The first sub-phase involves the mean horizontal 'braking' force and horizontal deceleration path of the whole-body centre of mass; the jumper should strive to minimise this sub-phase. This is followed by an acceleration sub-phase, in which the jumper should strive to maximise the mean horizontal acceleration force and horizontal acceleration path of the whole-body centre of mass. The model for the take-off vertical velocity (Figure 2.11) is simpler as it only involves an acceleration phase, assuming the vertical velocity at touchdown on the board is zero, which is very nearly the case.

Now all we have to do is develop observable features that capture these biomechanical entities. At this stage, to remove what are now superfluous details, so as to clarify the model, I have deleted level 4a (take-off horizontal velocity equals the horizontal velocity

Figure 2.10 Level 4 of the long jump deterministic model – factors affecting take-off horizontal velocity using work–energy relationship. See text for further explanation. CoM = whole-body centre of mass of jumper.

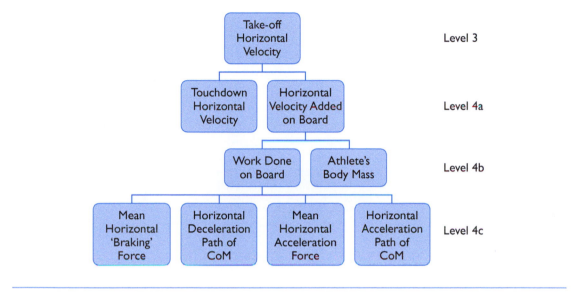

Figure 2.11 Level 4 of the long jump deterministic model – factors affecting take-off vertical velocity using work-energy relationship. CoM = whole body centre of mass of jumper.

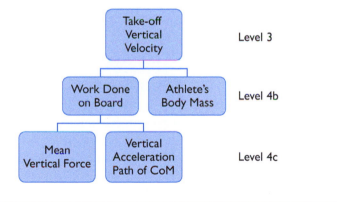

at touchdown plus the horizontal velocity added on the take-off board). I have also removed the 'work done on board' boxes of our long jump model (level 4b), as these are completely specified by the level below, and omitted the 'athlete's body mass' box (also level 4b), as this is rather trivial. As the take-off velocity is made up of the take-off horizontal and vertical velocities, we can combine these simplified figures, from Figures 2.10 and 2.11, into the final branch of our long jump model for take-off velocity (take-off vertical and horizontal velocity) of Figure 2.12.

Figure 2.12 Levels 3 to 6 of the long jump deterministic model for combined take-off horizontal and vertical velocity showing derivation of critical features (CF) 1 to 7. See text for further details. CoM = whole-body centre of mass of jumper.

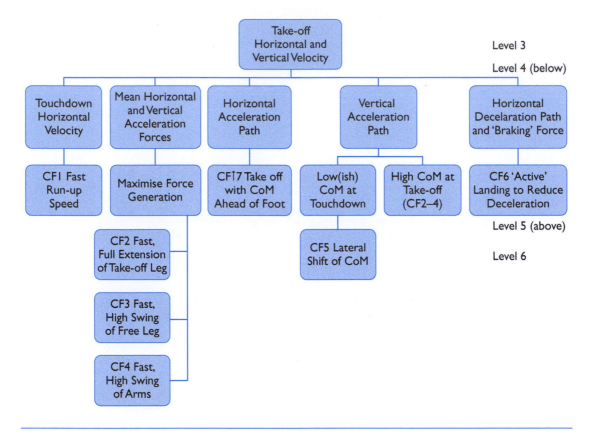

We now need to consider what observable, critical features of the movement contribute to the lowest level of each branch of this model. We depart slightly from slavish adherence to the principles of deterministic modelling at this stage but we must ensure that we can propose biomechanical, physiological or other scientific principles to justify these lower levels of the model. That approach avoids arbitrariness in developing the movement's critical features. We have already identified 'fast run-up speed' as a critical feature (CF1 in Figure 2.12) for this event. We have also noted that maximising the mean force and the acceleration path are desirable to maximise take-off velocity (but see below), so we now need only to translate these terms into things that can be observed. The mean forces are maximised by the jumper maximising force generation. This can be done in three ways: directly, by a fast and full extension of the take-off leg (CF2) increasing the force on the take-off board, and, indirectly, by a fast, high and coordinated swing of the free leg (CF3) and the two arms (CF4). These are demonstrated clearly by the diagram of the jumper in Figure 2.7.

Moving on to maximising the vertical acceleration path, we first note that this is expressed as the difference between the heights of the athlete's centre of mass at take-off and touchdown. The jumper can achieve a high centre of mass at take-off by a combination of critical features 2 to 4 (CF2–4). A 'lowish' centre of mass at touchdown might suggest a pronounced and deliberate flexing of the knee at touchdown. Knee flexion will occur to some extent, because of the force of impact – and this will help to reduce the transmission of impact forces through the body and thereby reduce injury risk. However, it would be a mistake for the jumper to try to increase this flexion – it would lower the centre of mass height at touchdown but would also have far more important, negative effects on the take-off speed. A mechanism that many good long jumpers tend to use to lower slightly the centre of mass at touchdown is a lateral pelvic tilt towards the take-off leg (CF5). This is clearly evident from a front-on view and illustrates two important points for a successful qualitative movement analysis: know your sport or event inside out and never view a sporting activity just from the side, even when it seems two dimensional.

Now let us consider the horizontal acceleration path. This is more tricky since, in the first part of board contact until the centre of mass has passed forward of the support foot, the horizontal velocity will tend to decelerate, not accelerate. The last thing the jumper would want to do is to plant the take-off foot too far ahead of the centre of mass, which would increase the deceleration of the centre of mass, another blind alley. Instead, the jumper minimises this distance by seeking an 'active' landing – one in which the foot of the take-off leg would be moving backwards relative to the take-off board at touchdown – to reduce the horizontal deceleration (CF6). Then, once the centre of mass has passed over the take-off foot, the jumper needs to lengthen, within reason, the acceleration path of the centre of mass up to take-off, which can be done by taking off with the centre of mass ahead of the foot (CF7). This also serves to minimise any tendency for the take-off distance to be negative. This is also excellently illustrated by the diagram of the jumper in Figure 2.7.

Well, we have finished with take-off velocity. The take-off height is the height of the whole-body centre of mass at take-off minus the height of the whole body centre of mass at landing in the sand pit (see Figure 2.7). The height at take-off (level 3 of the model, see Figure 2.9) depends mainly on critical features 2 to 4 (CF2–4, Figure 2.12). We still need to look at the landing component of the take-off height, which we will do in the next paragraph, as part of considering the two remaining sub-distances from level 2 (Figure 2.6) – the take-off and landing distances.

From Figure 2.7, it should be obvious that the take-off distance is the distance of the centre of mass in front of the take-off foot at take-off minus the distance of the take-off foot behind the front of the take-off board, from which the jump distance is measured. We have already considered how to increase the first of these distances (CF7, Figure 2.12), so we now note the need to plant the take-off foot as close to the front of the take-off board as possible (CF8, Figure 2.13) – this has implications for the control of the run-up, so we might wish to amend our first critical feature (CF1) to 'fast and controlled run-up'. The landing distance (Figure 2.7) is the distance of the centre of mass behind the feet at landing minus the distance that the point of contact of the jumper's body closest to the take-off board is behind where the feet land. That leads to Figure 2.14, which contains

Figure 2.13 Level 3 of a long jump deterministic model for take-off distance, showing derivation of critical features (CF) 7 and 8. CoM = whole-body centre of mass of jumper.

Figure 2.14 Levels 3 to 5 of a long jump deterministic model for landing distance, showing derivation of critical features (CF) 9 to 11. See text for further details. CoM = whole-body centre of mass of jumper.

our last three critical features. First, from the observation that the athlete should land with his or her centre of mass behind the feet, and low to increase take-off height, we derive the need to land with 'hips flexed and knees extended' (CF9), which is evident from Figure 2.7. To reduce any loss of landing distance from touching the sand behind the landing point for the feet, we note simply 'don't touch sand behind landing point' (CF10). The final critical feature is less obvious and emphasises two important points: the need to be aware of the movement principles relevant to the activity analysed and the need to have a thorough knowledge of that activity. The forces acting on the jumper from the take-off board generate 'angular momentum' that tends to rotate the jumper forwards during flight. If uncontrolled, this would cause an early landing in the pit, which is why tucking or piking during flight would be counterproductive. Instead, the jumper needs either to minimise forward rotation by adopting an extended 'hang' position, as in Figure 2.7, or, for longer jumpers, to transfer this angular momentum from the trunk to the limbs using, a 'hitch-kick' technique ('running in the air'), leading to our last critical feature, 'use hitch kick or hang' (CF11).

Well, we've got there, although it may have seemed a long journey. It is worthwhile, because we finish up with confidence in our critical features based on the rigour of the deterministic modelling process, which is impossible to achieve from the copying of an 'ideal' or 'model' performance, very difficult to achieve merely from a list of movement principles, and not always clear from other approaches. Also, as already noted, the process highlights blind alleys, helping us to avoid them, and provides a well-structured approach for identifying critical features.

Identifying critical features when there is a subjective performance criterion or more than one performance criterion

In sports involving a subjective judgement, such as gymnastics, diving and figure skating, we may approach identifying a performance criterion differently, although a deterministic modelling approach is still possible. The score awarded by the judges will not depend upon a single performance factor, whether objective or subjective, but on guidelines established by the sport. Consider a women's artistic gymnastics vault. What is the performance criterion? Clearly, it is the judges' score. Can we model this deterministically: can the score be subdivided? Yes, first into the scores by the 'A' Judges and 'B' Judges. A Judges mostly look at the vault difficulty and related aspects. B Judges address technical faults – execution and artistry – and apply deductions. Generally, we'd focus on the latter as they relate more to vaulting technique.

On the other hand, a better approach would be to use the judging guidelines of the sport, which are based mainly on technical elements of the skills involved. These should largely have been developed from movement principles applicable to movements within that sport, so this approach has much to recommend it. In other words, we would use the criteria for awarding and deducting points, here Article 8 of the International Gymnastics Federation (FIG) Code of Points (CoP) for Women's Artistic Gymnastics (WAG; available on the FIG website, www.fig-gymnastics.com). Table 2.1 shows some score deductions. We then have a movement phase approach. It is relevant to ask, are these technical points observable? For judges, clearly the answer is yes. Furthermore, in the context of later chapters, they are also generally measureable.

Some sports, such as ski jumping, combine objective (distance) and subjective (style) criteria – the former lends itself to being modelled deterministically, unlike the latter. So how do we proceed when the performance criterion is:

- A combination of objective and subjective criteria, as for ski jumping? Model each separately, emphasising the most important first; for ski jumping, this would be the distance jumped.

Table 2.1 Part of faults table and points deductions (0.1, 0.3 or 0.5) for women's artistic gymnastics vault (see www. fig-gymnastics.com).

FAULTS	POINTS DEDUCTED		
	0.1	0.3	0.5
First flight phase			
Incomplete longitudinal (LA) turn	≤45°	≤90°	>90°
Poor technique			
- Hip angle	x	x	
- Arch	x	x	
- Legs separated	x	x	
- Knees bent	x	x	x
Repulsion phase			
Poor technique			
- Staggered/alternate hand placement	x	x	
- Shoulder angle	x	x	
- Failure to pass through vertical	x	x	
Bent arms	x	x	x
Prescribed LA turn begun too early	x	x	x
Second flight phase			
Height	x	x	x
and so on . . .			

- A combination of subjective criteria, as in gymnastics – A Judges' specific score, B Judges' specific score, and general points? Look at each separately, choosing the most critical first, as discussed above.
- A combination of objective criteria – for example, for fast bowling in cricket, speed and accuracy (the latter can be modelled as the distance off line or the angle off line)? Model each separately, emphasising the most important first.

OBSERVATION STAGE – OBSERVING RELIABLY

As should be evident from Box 2.2, the observation stage primarily involves implementing the observation strategy devised in the preparation stage, and videographing the performers involved in the study. I use the term 'videographing', or video recording, advisedly: first, considerable skill is needed to observe fast movements in sport reliably by eye alone and, second, good high-definition digital video cameras are now readily available and inexpensive. It is also worth noting that, although much of our emphasis is on obtaining visual records of the movements that we are going to analyse, information from our other senses can be useful – the sound of footfall patterns, for example, in a javelin run-up.

We need to record sports movements as they are fast, and the human eye cannot resolve movements that occur in less than 0.25 s. Two important benefits of videography are that the performers can observe their own movements in slow motion and frame by frame, and that it makes qualitative analysis much easier. However, there are some potential drawbacks. Performers might be aware of the cameras and, consciously or subconsciously, change movement patterns (the Hawthorne effect). Also, there are ethical considerations about video recording, particularly with minors and the intellectually disadvantaged. Our systematic observation strategy should have addressed both what to focus on and how to record and observe the movements of interest. Clearly, we should focus on the critical features of the movement identified in the preparation stage; if the performance model that we have used is robust, then these should all be relevant. We also need to decide on the environment in which to videograph, the best camera locations within that environment and how many trials of the movement to record for analysis.

The other main issues in videography for qualitative analysis are as follows. We need to attend to the choice of camera shutter speed, where to conduct the study, the camera locations and whether the cameras are to be stationary (usually mounted on tripods) or moved (panned or tilted) to follow the analysed movements. We need to decide how many trials to record, when relevant. We need to assess whether to use additional lighting, which must be adequate for the shutter speed and frame rate. The frame rate is normally fixed, for 'domestic-quality' video cameras (or camcorders), at 25 frames per second in Europe (PAL) and approximately 30 frames per second in North America (NTSC). The unit hertz (Hz) is normally used for events per second but is confusing for video cameras, for which it could mean frame rates or field rates. The background should be plain and uncluttered to help objective observation, but this is not always feasible, particularly when videographing in competitions. Participant preparation needs careful attention – briefing, clothing, habituation and debriefing. We need to optimise the size of the performer on the image – the bigger the better – but this might require zooming the camera lens (assuming that the camera has a zoom lens) while also panning and tilting it during filming. Finally, we need to consider checks for reliability (within, or intra-, observer) and objectivity (among, or inter-, observers) in any study.

So, let us now look at these points in a little more detail. The shutter speed is the time that the camera shutter stays open for each 'picture' that the camera records. If too slow the picture will blur; if too fast for the lighting conditions, the picture may be too dark. A guide to the slowest satisfactory shutter speeds is given in Table 2.2; not all digital video cameras for the domestic market will have the fastest of these shutter speeds (the ones with the larger numbers in the denominator). You should treat with caution the 'sports mode' option that some cheaper camcorders offer instead of a range of specified shutter speeds.

Normal video camera frame rates, also known as sampling rates, of 25 or 30 Hz are far from satisfactory for the fastest activities in Table 2.2. Even the 50 fields per second (PAL), or approximately 60 fields per second (NTSC), that can be obtained by

Table 2.2 Recommended slowest camera shutter speeds for various activities.

ACTIVITY	SLOWEST SHUTTER SPEED (S)
Walking	1/50
Sit to stand	1/50
Bowling	1/50
Basketball	1/100
Vertical jump	1/100
Jogging	1/100 to 1/200
Sprinting	1/200 to 1/500
Baseball pitching	1/500 to 1/1000
Cricket fast bowling	1/500 to 1/1000
Batting (baseball or cricket)	1/500 to 1/1000
Soccer kicking	1/500 to 1/1000
Tennis	1/500 to 1/1000
Golf	1/1000 or faster

'splitting' each frame into its two constituent fields for interlacing cameras is not ideal for fast movements. Furthermore, not all video analysis software can separate out the two fields from which each interlaced frame is made up. Most movement analysts do not have routine access to high-speed video cameras with sampling rates up to thousands of frames per second. If a needs analysis showed a clear requirement for high frame rate cameras, then this should be factored into the project costing in the preparation stage.

When deciding where to conduct the study, we have to balance an environment in which we have control over extraneous factors, such as lighting and background, with one that is similar to that in which the movement is normally performed; the latter ensures ecological validity. Normally, the latter dominates for qualitative analysis, but the decision may be affected by the skill of the performers, whether the activities being recorded are open or closed skills, and videographic issues. When selecting camera vantage points, the movement analyst has to address from where he or she would want to view these activities for qualitative analysis, with how many cameras and whether the cameras need to be stationary.

The decision of how many trials, or performances, to record is very important for the reliability of qualitative analysis. However, that decision is not always made by the movement analyst. For example, if you were recording from a game, say of football, for notational analysis, you only have control over how many games you will record. If recording for analysis of a performer's movement technique in competition, the number of recordable trials is probably fixed at, for example, six throws in the finals of a discus competition, the heats plus the finals of swimming events, and as many attempts as the jumper needs in the high jump until three failures. If recording out of competition, we need to decide how many observations we need; generally, within reason, the more the better. Because of movement variability, there is no such thing as a representative trial even for stereotyped closed skills. The more trials we record, the more likely our results are to be valid. Various rules of thumb have proposed between 5 and 20 trials as a minimum requirement; 10, if you can record that many, is often highly satisfactory. A very important consideration is the number of trials you can reasonably expect your sports performer to undertake in the time available. For maximal effort activities, fatigue and injury risk need to be carefully evaluated.

Finally, we need to ensure that, in this stage, we attend to issues that affect our ability to assess, and improve, intra- and inter-analyst reliability. Reliability is consistency in ratings by one analyst; so we need to be able to check this over several days. Objectivity is consistency in ratings across several analysts, so we need enough analysts to be able to check this; clearly, this will be affected by how well trained the analysts are. Our assessments of objectivity and reliability can be improved by identifying critical features, and how and in which order they will be evaluated; developing specific rating scales; analyst training and practice; and increasing the number of analysts or trials. However, it remains true that one of the main disadvantages of qualitative analysis is establishing its reliability.

EVALUATION AND DIAGNOSIS STAGE – WHAT'S WRONG?

The hard work for this stage should already have been completed during the preparation stage – the identification of the critical features of the movement. The observation stage should then have allowed us to collect the video footage that we need, as qualitative movement analysts, to evaluate these critical features in the performances that have been recorded. This stage also prepares us for the intervention stage. Often, in the evaluation and diagnosis stage – probably the most intellectually difficult of the four-stage process – you will start by describing the movement and progress to analysing it; trying to analyse a movement before you have thoroughly and scientifically described it can be fraught with difficulties. In this context, it should be noted that the work we do in this stage can do more harm than good; that is, we could reduce performance or increase injury risk, particularly if we have not identified and prioritised the correct critical features. This overall stage could be called the 'analysis' stage; however, there are two separate aspects to this stage (though they often overlap). The first task is to evaluate strengths and weaknesses of performance – to establish what the symptoms are. The second aspect is to diagnose which weaknesses to tackle and how – to diagnose the symptoms and prepare to treat the condition.

Evaluation of performance

To evaluate performance we effectively need to compare the observed performances with some model of good form. However, as there is no general optimal performance model, we need a model that is appropriate for the performers being evaluated – the model needs 'individual specificity'. For most good qualitative analysis, this clearly requires prior identification of the movement's critical features in the preparation stage, often by the use of a deterministic model. Furthermore, a ranking of the 'correctness' of the identified critical features on some scale or within some band of correctness can be very helpful; for example, 'joint range of motion: inadequate, within good range, excessive'; or 'excellent 5 . . . OK 3 . . . very poor 1'. Correctness scales may be essentially subjective, which is useful when no semi-quantitative assessment is observationally possible; 'a fast, high swing of the arms' could provide an example for the long jump model. This could be assessed as: 'fast', 'quite fast', 'quite slow' or 'slow'. If length and angle measurements are possible, as they are in most software packages for qualitative biomechanical analysis, or if such variables can be observed accurately within a particular range, then semi-quantitative scales can be developed. In a kick for distance, for example, we might rank the knee angle at the end of the preparation (backswing) phase (from 1 – very poor to 5 – excellent) as, say: >130° (1), 110–130° (2), 90–110° (3), 70–90° (4), <70° (5). I have used a similar ranking of the height of the free leg at take-off in the long jump based on thigh angle in the Siliconcoach 'wizard' later in this chapter (see Figure 2.17). Careful attention to construction of ranking scales can save much time and effort later, as well as aiding the assessment of observer reliability.

As well as needing a model that is individual specific, other difficulties arise in the evaluation of performance. The first of these relates to within-performer movement and performance variability; as we noted in relation to the observation stage above, this can only be accounted for by recording multiple trials. Identifying the source of movement errors can also be problematic as they can arise from: body position or movement timing (biomechanical); conditioning (physiological); the performer evaluating environmental cues (perceptual-motor); or motivational factors (psychological). All of these factors could be important, for example, in a run-out in cricket (see Study Task 4). These factors support the need for movement analysts to be able to draw on a range of disciplinary skills and knowledge. In the real world of sport, movement analysts are usually most effective when they work as part of a multidisciplinary team of experts but this is often financially prohibitive. Analyst bias, reliability and objectivity also present problems. Bias can be reduced by the use of 'correctness' criteria. Assessing reliability and objectivity requires multiple trials and analysts respectively; the latter is often a luxury, the former is vital.

Diagnosis of movement errors

Perhaps the major issues in the evaluation and diagnosis stage relate to the lack of a consistent rationale for diagnosing movement errors: our 'critical features' approach is best, providing that we can identify and prioritise the correct critical features. As only one intervention at any time is best (in the intervention stage), we need to focus diagnostically on one correction at a time. This raises the question of how to decide the order in which to tackle movement errors in the intervention stage, if we have identified that more than one aspect, or critical feature, of the movement requires correction. One of five approaches is generally used, depending on the activity, the skill of the performer and other circumstances.

The first approach focuses on 'what came before'; here, we try to establish if an error in a particular action arose from previous actions. This is most often used in sports in which actions follow in sequence. For example, an error leading to a volley played out of court or into the net by the server in tennis may be traced back to a poor serve rather than a poor volley; we would then focus our attention on the serve rather than the volley. The second approach, somewhat related to the first conceptually, looks at the sequence of actions through the phases of a movement, focusing on earlier phases first, as in the long jump example above. For example, in our long jump model, landing problems are often due to poor generation of rotation on the take-off board or control of it in the air, so our first focus would be on what went wrong on take-off or in the air. These two approaches are conceptually attractive, as problems usually arise before they are spotted. I would normally recommend starting with one of these two approaches.

The third and perhaps the most conceptually obvious approach involves prioritising for attention in the intervention stage those critical features that maximise performance improvement. To use the long jump model again, if a long jumper is not jumping far, speed is overwhelmingly the most important factor; so what critical feature would we prioritise to maximise performance? Run-up speed, obviously. However, in many cases, it is not at all easy to know what would maximise improvement in performance; furthermore, we often need also to balance short-term and long-term considerations.

A fourth and seemingly attractive approach, in terms of successful outcomes, is to seek to make the easiest corrections first. In other words, if several movement faults have been identified, we first tackle the one that will be easiest for the athlete to correct. This approach is impeccably logical from a motor skills viewpoint, if movement errors seem unrelated and cannot otherwise be ranked. However, there is little, if any, clear support for its efficacy in improving performance.

Finally, for activities in which balance is crucial, such as gymnastics and weightlifting, we might prioritise from the base of support upwards – in other words, we look for errors close to the point of balance contact with the environment. This would be the ground in weightlifting and could be the ground or, say, the beam or vaulting box in gymnastics. You might like to consider whether this approach would work best in a sport such as target shooting.

INTERVENTION STAGE – PUTTING THINGS RIGHT

We come now to the final stage of our four-stage process of qualitative analysis – the intervention stage, in which we have the opportunity to correct movement errors, or put things right. Before getting this far, the movement analyst must first have conducted a means analysis with the performer and his or her coach or therapist, identified the critical features relevant to the question to be answered, and prepared how feedback will be provided, including, for example, intervention cues. Second, the movement analyst will have obtained relevant video footage and any other movement patterns (see Chapter 3 for discussion of the latter). Finally, the movement analyst will have analysed the video and movement patterns and prioritised the critical features to be addressed.

The main focus in this final stage is on feedback of information to address the requirements of the needs analysis. If the previous three stages have been done badly, nothing in the intervention stage will sort matters out. On the other hand, provision of inappropriate feedback can jeopardise even good work done in the previous stages.

You should note that the intervention stage involves the movement analyst's administration of feedback, corrections or other changes in the environment to improve performance. Intervention is more comprehensive than just providing feedback, instruction or error correction. It can provide positive reinforcement, help in performance modelling, guide modifications to practice and prescriptions for training, and help to adjust equipment for optimal performance. You should also be aware that there is not enough documented evidence of successful interventions to improve performance over time.

Augmented feedback

The information that we feed back augments that available to performers from their senses; it is referred to as augmented feedback. Augmented feedback can be in the form of knowledge of results (KR) – the outcome – or knowledge of performance (KP) – the movement process. The movement analyst must address what information is fed back, how this is done and when (this should have been partly addressed in the preparation stage of the movement analysis process). It should be self-evident that the feedback used should involve the right information at the right time and in an easily understood format; the speed of feedback and its presentation and interpretation are all important. However, there is often a great deal of information available, and it is not clear what should be provided or how. The frequent calls for rapid feedback and more feedback from both coaches and scientists often do not pay heed to the effects, if any, of feedback, nor to how and when it is best presented.

The main goal in providing feedback is to correct a 'fault' so as to improve performance (or to reduce the risk of injury). The intention of providing feedback to enhance performance is not to improve performance for the rest of the training session, or whenever feedback is provided, which immediate feedback can achieve, but to retain that performance improvement for the next competition. We need, therefore, to look critically at the retention phase of the overall feedback process. The provision of feedback needs to address relevant motor learning theories. Although many of these theories have been developed for discrete laboratory tasks and have not been adequately tested on real-world tasks, such as sport, they do provide some evidence to which sports biomechanists should attend.

Methods for providing augmented feedback include verbal feedback; use of verbal and other cues; visual models; manual or mechanical guidance; and modifying the task, practice or conditioning (see also Knudson and Morrison, 2002, in Further Reading). In giving verbal and other sensory feedback, we need to provide appropriate information – to translate critical features into intervention cues in behavioural terms, appropriate to the group with whom we are working. Cues can be verbal, visual, aural or kinaesthetic and we need to derive relevant cues for each critical feature that we intend to address in our intervention strategy. Verbal cues should be no more than six words and figurative, not literal. We must use analogies that are meaningful. As we noted in the section on the preparation stage, the structure of a verbal cue should be: action; content (what does the action); qualification (how to gauge success); special conditions (if more information is needed). Examples would be: rotate hip and trunk; swing racket forwards relative to the ground. The latter example would seem preferable as it focuses externally (racket) rather than internally (hip and trunk). Not all of these methods are equally effective in particular circumstances.

Video feedback is now routinely provided on competition performance or performance in training sessions. Unfortunately, much of this feedback is unstructured, often it lacks a valid model against which to compare current performance and it rarely includes an objective evaluation of its utility in improving performance. Sometimes video feedback is provided simply by replaying video footage to the athlete and his or her coach immediately after performance. The use of software packages for qualitative biomechanical analysis (see the next section), such as Siliconcoach, Dartfish and Kinovea, allows video feedback of two or more performances simultaneously for comparison. This 'dual-screen' or 'multi-screen' option is very useful for comparing, for instance, successful and unsuccessful performances by one athlete. However, these options should be used very cautiously when comparing two different athletes, when one is often used as a 'model' of what the other should be doing. As we have previously noted, use of an inappropriate model of performance can be counterproductive and can increase injury risk. Video feedback works best when it is supported by a valid underlying model of performance, as discussed in the next subsection.

There are, of course, other reasons for providing biomechanical feedback to coaches and athletes other than to remedy movement deficiencies to improve performance, on which this section focuses. Feedback may be provided, for example, to fulfil an educational role. Some forms of feedback may be immediate (within seconds or minutes, usually after each trial), for example running speed measurements from photocells or simply replaying a video recording of a performance. Medium-term feedback, after several days or weeks, may be more appropriate when seeking to change a movement technique permanently, for example using detailed qualitative or quantitative video analysis and statistical modelling. Some aspects of modification of movements may require longer-term research studies, carried out over months or even years, to provide the necessary scientific basis for a correct performance model; quantitative analysis (Chapters 4 to 6) would often be relevant in this context.

The implicit assumption, in many publications about the use of feedback, that any feedback is inherently good is not totally supported. It is important not to give too much feedback – providing more information does not always improve performance and may cause confusion, particularly if the information presented offers no clear solution to the problem identified; this may be true for complex kinetic variables, such as the forces on bicycle pedals or oars. Practitioners are not always receptive to feedback, particularly if it is not obviously relevant to improving performance. Despite these points, and the view that information feedback is the single most important variable (excluding practice) for skill learning and modification, too few studies have directly addressed the provision of augmented feedback to athletes and coaches of information from biomechanics research into sports movements.

As an example of how movement analysts and coaches have got feedback wrong, let us look at how views of the generation of front crawl propulsive force have changed over the years – the wrong view often led to the provision of the wrong feedback to swimmers. In the early 1970s, the predominant view was that the hand behaved as a paddle, pushing the water back – this led to coaches instructing swimmers to pull the hand back below the body in a straight line. By the mid-1970s to the 1980s, swimmers' hands had been shown, through cinematography, to make an S-pattern through the water, in an outward-inward-outward sculling pattern. The hand was now envisaged as a hydrofoil, using lift and drag forces (see Chapter 5) to generate propulsion. Coaches now emphasized to their swimmers the need to develop a 'feel' for the water and to use sideways sculling movements. By the mid-1990s, these observed sideways movements had been shown to be due to body roll; the pattern of the hand relative to the swimmer's frame of reference – his or her body – consisted of an outward-inward scull, confounding the previous view, which had adopted a frame of reference fixed in the camera or swimming pool.

Models of performance and their use in providing feedback

To make meaningful statements about the movement technique of an athlete and how to improve it, a model is needed against which we can compare that movement technique and which will help in improving it. Important requirements for movement analysts are, therefore, to be able to construct and use 'performance models' of the sports activities we analyse and choose the most appropriate model for our purposes. The effectiveness of any feedback will depend not only on observing or measuring an athlete's current performance, but also on identifying that athlete's 'target', or 'model', performance.

Earlier in this chapter, we discussed the use of deterministic models of performance in the context of the four-stage process of qualitative biomechanical analysis. We noted that to improve performance we need a model against which to compare an athlete's current movement technique. Deterministic models can well serve that purpose for the qualitative analyst. An important question is how these models can best be used in the intervention stage of the movement analysis process to compare an athlete's model performance with his or her current performance.

If providing knowledge of performance, then we definitely need a model against which we can assess current performance. There is no general agreement about how we establish a model performance or movement pattern. However, such models can function in comparing and improving movement techniques, developing training and aiding communication. I emphasise that there is no such thing as a general optimal performance model, so any model must be individual-specific. From a qualitative analysis viewpoint, the correct set of critical features, appropriately presented, can provide such a model.

Our model performance could take the form of a live demonstration. These have their use in the field, to show an athlete how to perform or modify their movements. However, they can be subjective, depending very much on the coach or whoever provides the demonstration. Furthermore, they require far deeper information about the movement technique to be known by the coach if this approach is not to degenerate into simply copying the movements of a more successful performer. Their lack of individual specificity is their major drawback. Historically, the 'textbook' movement technique often served as the model against which others were evaluated. Such models are often hard to digest, particularly where complex movements are involved, and often contain too much information. Examples can be found in almost all coaching texts in which sports movement techniques are described in detail. These models have little practical use in the process of identifying and eradicating movement faults. Again, they lack individual specificity.

To summarise, useful feedback to improve the performance of an athlete generally requires a target performance against which an athlete's current performance can be compared. The most appropriate performance model should be used (natural language is the least useful). The model should seek to manage detail and establish clarity. The structure of the model should be carefully considered. Some evidence supports the idea that the best feedback involves the presentation of the target and current movement techniques in the same form, for example both as computer graphic displays.

Information feedback and motor learning

Several issues about feedback from a motor learning perspective revolve around the questions: What is best? When is best? How is best? We have considered the first of these earlier in this section (for an overview, see Bartlett and Bussey, 2012, in Further Reading). Immediate feedback is not necessarily best, as demonstrated by some of the literature on motor learning. For discrete laboratory and several sport-specific tasks, summary feedback (of results) after several trials has often been found to be better than immediate feedback for the retention stage of skill learning, which is the important stage – we want our performers to perform better the next day or week, rather than straight after feedback has been provided. However, it is still not clear if this applies to sport skills in general. Furthermore, some evidence is contradictory; for example, no difference was found for learning modifications to pedalling technique by inexperienced cyclists, when they were provided with feedback from force pedals.

We might ask if the 'picture' about when to provide feedback, and how much to provide, changes if we accept the 'constraints-led' view of ecological motor control. That viewpoint sees augmented feedback as directing the performer's search for solutions to a specific sports task that satisfy the constraints imposed on him or her. Researchers from this paradigm have suggested that an external focus of attention, on movement effects, is better than an internal one on movement dynamics. An emphasis on task outcomes allows learners to search for a task solution and does not interfere with the self-organisational processes of movement dynamics. These views have been supported by research in slalom skiing, the forehand drive in tennis, the golf pitch shot and the basketball free throw. There is evidence that 'less is more' – in other words, that better performance is achieved with less frequent augmented feedback, for example in learning the lofted pass in soccer. Again, it is, however, unclear if these results generalise to all stages of skill acquisition. If a focus of attention on movement effects is better than one on movement dynamics in correcting movement faults in skilled performers, we must be careful to tailor our feedback accordingly. This could be held to support the qualitative analysis approach, rather than the complexities of quantitative modelling of performance.

Finally, how is best? Well, probably, as simply as possible, using qualitative information that is easy to assimilate, preferably provided graphically and with appropriate cues, perhaps supported with some semi-quantitative data, such as phase durations, ranges of movement or correctness scores. We should avoid complex quantitative data – if we do provide quantitative feedback, it should be graphical rather than numerical. Any feedback needs to be concise. It is very beneficial if we can compare good and bad performances, as we can with qualitative video analysis packages such as those discussed in the next section. Finally, it is advantageous if feedback can be provided in a take-away format, using DVDs or other electronic storage devices.

The review

The final task of the intervention stage is to review the success of the project. This should be done independently, at least in the first instance, by the movement analyst and the 'clients'. The former should evaluate the whole four-stage process in the context of the needs analysis carried out in the preparation stage. The analyst and practitioners should then come together to discuss how improvements could be made in future intervention studies. It is worth noting in this context that very few studies have addressed the efficacy of interventions by movement analysts. Although this is very difficult to establish, far too little attention is paid to addressing this important issue; after all, what is the point of the intervention stage if it doesn't have some proven benefit to performers?

SOFTWARE PACKAGES FOR QUALITATIVE BIOMECHANICAL ANALYSIS

Most qualitative biomechanical analysts will have access to a software package for qualitative biomechanical analysis, such as Dartfish (www.dartfish.com), Siliconcoach (www.siliconcoach.com) or Kinovea (www.kinovea.org). These offer many options that can help the analyst to pinpoint weaknesses in performance. As I mainly use Siliconcoach – it was developed by graduates from the School of Physical Education at the University of Otago and was one of the best of these packages – and Kinovea, which can be downloaded with no charge from their website, the examples below will be based on these packages.

It is worth noting that such software packages come at various prices, so it is important to ensure that you know what you need and what is on offer. All of them capture digital video recordings and allow still and slow motion replay and the capture of still

Figure 2.15 Annotated upper arm and thigh angles to the horizontal on still video frames of a very successful lawn bowler at the end of the preparation phase for: Top (a) a draw, in which the aim is to place the ball as close as possible to the target ball (the jack); Bottom (b) a drive, in which the aim is to remove opponents' balls from the vicinity of the jack. The drive is much faster than the draw. Produced using Kinovea.

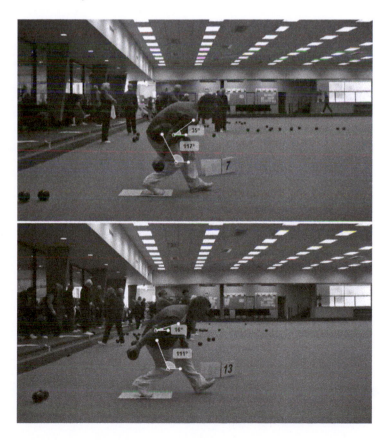

images. All allow the viewing of two (Kinovea) or more (Siliconcoach, Dartfish) video sequences on the same screen. Similarly, two or more still images can be displayed and saved on the same screen. These options are useful, for example, for looking at two views of the same action, such as a golf shot, or differences between different variants of the same basic movement technique, such as the draw and drive shots in lawn bowling (Figure 2.15), or a successful and unsuccessful performance – or more and less successful performances (Figure 2.16). Some of these packages allow the viewing of two performances superimposed on one image, usually by matching the backgrounds, which can also allow the use of moving cameras. The use of any of these dual-screen or multi-screen options to compare different performers should be treated with great caution. Different individuals bring their own organismic constraints to a sports task, which interact with the constraints of the task and those of the environment to evolve unique solutions to the task. Seeking to copy others has not been proven to improve performance and can lead to an increased risk of injury. However, one justifiable use of such comparisons is when the view of one performer is used as an exemplar of one or more critical features of a deterministic model, such as the long jump take-off example of Figure 2.17 where one such exemplar image is shown in the long jump 'wizard'.

Figure 2.16 Simple line annotations to show the heights reached by the top of the head at the peak of the jump in standing vertical jumps: Left (a) a squat jump; Right (b) a countermovement jump with the performer's preferred arm action. Produced using Kinovea.

Most software packages for qualitative biomechanical analysis also allow simple line drawing to highlight, for example, a specific aspect of the movement (as in Figure 2.16). All of these packages provide simple measurement of angles (as in Figure 2.15) and lengths. Some also allow the calculation of speed and other derived variables; the sampling rate of the video footage or out-of-plane movements may compromise the accuracy of these calculations, however. Video examples of the use of Siliconcoach by students in qualitative movement analysis are available in the Interactive eTextbook, covering: barbell back squat, front leg axe kick in Taekwondo, hiking in Laser dinghy sailing, hockey hit, tennis serve.

One of my favourite options in Siliconcoach was the ReportPak Wizard Editor, which allowed highly structured templates of correct movement technique, known as

Figure 2.17 Siliconcoach wizard for long jump, based on the deterministic model developed in this chapter. The first level of indentation contains the 'aspects' of the jump – either phases of the movement (such as run-up and flight) or key events (such as board contact and take-off). The second level of indentation contains the 'details' of the jump – the 11 critical features. The 'Value' (column 2) is based on one of several options. Yes (or no) is fairly self-explanatory – it is correct, hence the tick in the next ('Movement') column. The other three 'values' are based on 'look-up tables' – 'Thigh at 75 degrees or more to the horizontal' is deemed 'Optimal' for a 'Fast, high swing of the free leg', hence the tick in the next column (the other options in the look-up table for this critical feature are: 'Thigh at 60–75 degrees to the horizontal, which is deemed 'Insufficient' and 'Thigh at <60 degrees to the horizontal', which is deemed 'Wrong'). 'Too far back' is deemed 'Insufficient' for 'Contact near front of board', hence the minus sign in the next column ('Very close to front of board' is deemed 'Optimal' and 'Over front edge – foul jump' is 'Wrong'). The other options in these look-up tables, which are not visible in the wizard, make them simple scales of correctness. The 'Priority' column would be completed by the movement analyst to prioritise the critical features that need attention for the 'client' athlete. The take-off aspect has been highlighted, hence the Exemplar Image of take-off, room for the analyst to add his or her Client Image, and the Aspect Notes about the board contact phase and the key event of take-off, which are, of course, closely related. The analyst would probably add Help notes for the athlete or coach.

'wizards', to be developed and used. This option allowed the wizard editor to convert deterministic models, such as the one we developed earlier in this chapter for the long jump, into a wizard format that could be used by a movement analyst (see Figure 2.17) and then put into a report format for the coach. Sadly, from my perspective, this option has now been phased out for a more text-based approach. You should note how several 'look-up' tables in the wizard use correctness scales or rankings, which I introduced in the section above on evaluation and diagnosis.

SUMMARY

In this chapter, we considered how qualitative biomechanical analysis of movement is part of a multidisciplinary approach to movement analysis. We looked at several structured approaches to qualitative analysis of movement, all of which have, at their core, the identification of critical features of the movement studied. We identified four stages in a structured approach to movement analysis, considered the main aspects of each stage and noted that the value of each stage depends on how well the previous stages have been implemented. We saw that the most crucial step in the whole approach is identifying the critical features of a movement, and we looked at several ways of doing this, but found that none is foolproof. We worked through a detailed example of the best approach, using deterministic models, and considered the 'movement principles' approach and the role of phase analysis of movement. We then looked at the observation stage and some of the points that must be addressed for it to be successfully executed. We then considered various issues that need to be considered in the evaluation and diagnosis stage, including several ways to prioritise aspects of the movement to be addressed in the intervention stage, which was our next concern. Finally, we briefly overviewed some of the features of software packages for qualitative biomechanical analysis.

STUDY TASKS

Q

1   Answer all of the multiple-choice questions for Chapter 2 in the Interactive eTextbook.
    Hint: Keep repeating this until you have answered all of the questions correctly.
2   For each of the bullet points for the four stages of our structured approach to qualitative movement analysis in Box 2.2, explain, in one or two sentences only, the main matters to be attended to. Do this only for the 'first-level' bullet points that are not cross-referenced to another chapter (such as 'Gathering all relevant knowledge of the sports activity').
    Hint: You may wish to refer to the stage-specific sections of the chapter if you are struggling with this task.

3   Identify the movement phases into which the long jump can be divided, specify the boundaries of each phase (the key events) and outline the main functions of each phase (between one and three functions for each phase). Which three of the critical features in Figures 2.12 to 2.14 would most probably have the greatest effect on performance?

Hint: You may wish to refer to the deterministic model of the long jump above and to Appendix 2.1 before undertaking this task.

4   Biomechanical, physiological, perceptual-motor and psychological errors could all contribute to a batter being run out in cricket. Give a couple of examples of errors that would fall into each of these four categories.

Hint: You may wish to watch a few cricket run-outs on YouTube (www.youtube.com) or other websites before undertaking this task.

5   Show, diagrammatically, the two main rules to be used in moving down one level in deterministic modelling.

Hint: You may wish to re-read the subsection 'Principles of deterministic modelling' before undertaking this task.

6   For one of the following sports activities, a movement phase approach to each of which is outlined in Appendix 1.1, identify the most important phase from a performance perspective and then derive, and display diagrammatically, levels 1 to 3 of a deterministic model for that phase: stroking in swimming, the volleyball spike, and the javelin throw.

Hint: Before undertaking this task, you should read Appendix 1.1; you may also wish to re-read the subsection 'Principles of deterministic modelling' and those parts of the subsection 'A deterministic model for qualitative analysis of the long jump' that deal with levels 1 to 3 of that model. You may also find useful aids in Chow and Knudson (2011) – see Further Reading.

For the next three study tasks, you will need to choose a sports activity – other than the long jump – in which you are interested and with which you are very familiar. This need not be the same activity for each of these tasks, but you will see more continuity – and you will be closer to the approach movement analysts use in the world of sports analysis – if you do stick to the same movement throughout these three tasks. I strongly advise you to select an activity with an objective, rather than a subjective, performance criterion, or that is referred to in Chow and Knudson (2011; see in the Further Reading section). Also, specify the age, sex and performance standard of the performer whom you will consider in the three study tasks below. Assume that a needs analysis with the performer's coach, or the performer, has highlighted your need to identify the main factors that contribute to success in the chosen sports activity.

7   Identify and list all the sources that you could use to gather evidence-based information about a chosen movement. Summarise, in not more than 1000 words, the main features of the movement that you would use in a qualitative analysis of your chosen performer. From Appendix 2.1, identify the universal and partially general movement principles that are most and those that are least

applicable to your chosen activity; include also two activity-specific movement principles.

Hint: You are advised to re-read the long jump model above, read carefully the sources of information you use, and pay careful attention to the points in Appendix 2.1 and Box 2.3.

8   Use a deterministic model to identify about six observable critical features for performance of your chosen activity (for this study task, the activity should, to save you unnecessary effort, be the same as the one you use for Study Task 10 below). You will need to develop fully, and represent diagrammatically, levels 1 and 2 of the model, but you should not need to follow every branch down through further levels (as we did in the long jump example above) – you should focus on developing the boxes in level 2 that most affect performance.

Hint: You are advised to re-read the subsection on the long jump model above and, when developing your deterministic model, to pay careful attention to the relevant principles that relate to your chosen activity.

9   Devise a systematic observation strategy for your chosen activity, including recording location, number of cameras, their positions, any auxiliary lighting, camera shutter speed, performer preparation and the required number of trials. Set out an instruction sheet for conducting an initial pilot study. Outline, briefly, how you might assure validity, reliability and objectivity while minimising observer bias.

Hint: Before undertaking this task, you may wish to re-read the section 'Observation stage – observing reliably' and, if necessary, read Chapter 5 in Knudson and Morrison (2002) – see Further Reading.

10 **Case study**. Choose a throwing, striking or kicking activity in which you are interested. This could, but need not, be the same activity that you chose for Study Task 8 above. You need to obtain video footage for this study task. If you do not have access to a video camera or suitable video clips, then you are welcome to use any of the videos listed below in the Interactive eTextbook.

This case study must involve a comparison of two (or more) trials, conditions (for example, before and after a short coaching intervention), different types of action – such as a first and second serve in tennis – or people (remember that the last of these must be done with great care!). A list of 21 video clips available in the Interactive eTextbook is shown at the end of this section (but note that they do not allow all of the above comparisons to be made).

You also need access to a software package for qualitative biomechanical analysis; if you do not already have access to one, then download Kinovea from www.kinovea.org and familiarise yourself with its use. Use the qualitative analysis package to load the videos that you are going to analyse. Select video frames that give a good view of the various critical features of the movement. Make graphical and text annotations on those video frames to highlight differences between the trials, conditions, actions or people that you have chosen (see Figures 2.15 and 2.16 for simple examples, and the video clips from Siliconcoach in the Interactive eTextbook). Save the annotated video frames. Prepare a report, of no more than 1000 words and ten figures, for the person or people involved in your study. This report should include:

   i) A brief rationale for the study in one or two sentences: this is entirely up to you.

  ii) The six or so critical features on which you focused, and why they were chosen (you can start developing the critical features from Figure 2.4 and proceed down the levels similarly to our long jump model).

 iii) For each of the critical features, a 'look-up' table, or a semi-quantitative scale of observable points to assess whether the critical feature is being performed well, or not. Examples are provided in Figure 2.17 for the long jump.

 iv) The annotated video frames (see Figures 2.15 and 2.16 for simple examples, and the video clips from Siliconcoach in the Interactive eTextbook).

  v) A short written section explaining the main points from the annotated video images, in the context of the rationale for the study.

Hint: Before undertaking this task, you should obtain the relevant video footage and familiarise yourself thoroughly with the qualitative analysis software that you will use. You should study carefully the video clips from Siliconcoach in the Interactive eTextbook, particularly those for the front leg axe kick in Taekwondo, the hockey hit and the tennis serve.

Available video clips in Interactive eTextbook:

Basketball free throw
Basketball layup
Basketball three-point shot
Hockey hit
Hockey push pass
Hockey sweep pass
Lawn bowls draw (forehand)
Lawn bowls drive
Netball chest pass
Netball bounce pass
Netball overhead pass
Rugby line-out throw: short
Rugby line-out throw: medium
Rugby line-out throw: long
Soccer penalty
Soccer cross
Soccer pass
Tennis backhand volley
Tennis forehand volley
Tennis first serve
Tennis second serve

SORTING AND LABELLING ACTIVITIES (INTERACTIVE ETEXTBOOK ONLY)

Q **Sorting activity**.
Labelling activity.

FURTHER READING

Bartlett, R.M. and Bussey, M. (2012) *Sports Biomechanics: Reducing Injury Risk and Improving Sports Performance*, London: Routledge. Chapter 8 addresses intervention to improve performance mostly from a sports biomechanics perspective in more detail than this chapter, including some intervention case studies.

Chow, J.W. and Knudson, D.V. (2011) Use of deterministic models in sports and exercise biomechanics research. *Sports Biomechanics*, 10, 219–233. Although this journal article focuses mostly on the use of deterministic models in quantitative research, it provides many references to sources that contain deterministic models of various sports activities, which should be of interest to you as further examples of this approach; some will also help with your study tasks.

Hughes, M.D. and Franks, I.M. (2004) *Notational Analysis of Sport*, London: Routledge. Although written mainly from a notational analysis viewpoint, Chapters 1 to 3 contain valuable information about performance-enhancing augmented feedback.

Knudson, D.V. and Morrison, C.S. (2002) *Qualitative Analysis of Human Movement*, Champaign, IL: Human Kinetics. The first edition of this book was for many years one of the few real gems in the Human Kinetics list of sports science texts; the second edition continues that tradition. However, the authors have not yet welcomed a wider interpretation of qualitative movement analysis and a crucial (perhaps the crucial) 'critical feature' of skilled human movement – coordination – receives only one page reference in the index. The structured approach to movement analysis outlined in this chapter is covered in far more detail in Part II of Knudson and Morrison, while Part I sets the scene nicely and Part III outlines applications of their approach, with many diagrammatic examples. Highly recommended and well written.

Kreighbaum, E. and Barthels, K.M. (1996) *Biomechanics: A Qualitative Approach for Studying Human Movement*, New York: Macmillan. I find the approach taken by these authors overly mechanics based; such an approach has turned so many students off sports biomechanics over the years. However, Chapters 13 to 16 still have much to recommend them, even 18 years later.

APPENDIX 2.1 UNIVERSAL AND PARTIALLY GENERAL MOVEMENT (BIOMECHANICAL) PRINCIPLES

Universal principles – these should apply to all (or most) sports activities or tasks

- Use of the stretch–shortening cycle of muscle contraction.
  Also referred to as the use of pre-stretch; in performing many sports activities, a body segment often initially moves in the opposite direction from the one intended. This

initial countermovement is often necessary simply to allow the subsequent movement to occur. Other benefits arise from the increased acceleration path, initiation of the stretch reflex, storage of elastic energy and stretching the muscle to optimal length for forceful contraction – relating to the muscle's length–tension curve. This principle appears to be universal for movements requiring force or speed or to minimise energy consumption.

- Minimisation of energy used to perform the task.
  Some evidence supports this as an adaptive mechanism in skill acquisition, for example, the reduction in unnecessary movements during the learning of throwing skills. The many multi-joint muscles in the body support the importance of energy efficiency as an evolutionary principle. However, little evidence exists to support this as a universal principle for sports tasks involving speed or force generation.

- Control of redundant degrees of freedom in the segmental chain.
  This is also known as the principle of minimum task complexity. The chain of body segments proceeds from the most proximal to the most distal. Coordination of that chain becomes more complex as the number of degrees of freedom – the possible axes of rotation plus directions of linear motion at each joint – increases. A simple segment chain from shoulder girdle to the fingers contains at least 17 degrees of freedom. Obviously many of these need to be 'controlled' to permit movement replication. For example, in a basketball set shot players may keep their elbow well into the body to reduce the redundant degrees of freedom. The forces need to be applied in the required direction of motion. This principle explains why skilled movements look so simple.

Partially general principles – these apply to groups of sports activities or tasks, such as those dominated by speed generation

- Sequential action (or sequential coordination) of muscles.
  This principle – also referred to as the summation of internal forces, serial organisation or the transfer of angular momentum along the segment chain – is most important in activities requiring speed or force, such as discus throwing. It involves the recruitment of body segments into the movement in a sequential coordination pattern. Movements are generally initiated by the large muscle groups, which produce force to overcome the inertia of the whole body plus any sports implement. The sequence is continued by the faster muscles of the extremities, which not only have a larger range of movement and speed but also improved accuracy, owing to the smaller number of muscle fibres innervated by each motor neuron (the innervation ratio). In sequential coordination, proximal segments move ahead of distal ones, which ensures that muscles are stretched to develop tension when they contract; the principle appears to break down for internal–external rotation of the upper arm and pronation–supination of the forearm, which occur out of sequence in, for example, the tennis serve.
- Minimisation of inertia (increasing acceleration of movement).

This is most important in endurance and speed activities. Movements at any joint should be initiated with the distal joints in a position that minimises the moment of inertia, to maximise rotational acceleration. For example, in the recovery phase of sprinting, the hip is flexed with the knee also flexed; this configuration has a far lower moment of inertia than one with an extended or semi-flexed knee. This principle relates to the generation and transfer of angular momentum (see Chapter 5), which are affected by changes in the moment of inertia.

- Impulse generation or absorption.

This principle is mainly important in force and speed activities. It relates to the impulse–momentum relationship (see also Chapter 5): impulse equals the change of momentum, which equals the average force multiplied by the time the force acts. This shows that a large impulse is needed to produce a large change of momentum; this requires a large average force or a long time of action. In impulse generation, the former must predominate because of the explosive, short duration of many sports movements, such as a high jump take-off, which requires power, or the rapid performance of work (see below). In absorbing momentum, as when catching a cricket ball, the time is increased by 'giving' with the ball to reduce the mean impact force, preventing bruising or fracture and increasing success.

- Maximising the acceleration path.

This principle arises from the work–energy relationship, which shows that a large change in mechanical energy requires a large average force or the maximising of the distance over which we apply force. This is an important principle in events requiring speed and force, for example a shot-putter makes full use of the width of the throwing circle.

- Stability.

A wide base of support is needed for stability; this applies not only for static activities but also for dynamic ones in which sudden changes in the momentum vector occur.

3 More on sports movement patterns – the geometry of motion

Knowledge assumed
Ability to undertake simple analysis of videos of sports movements (Chapter 1)
Familiarity with graphs of one variable plotted as a function of a second variable, often time
Ability to visualise the slope and curvature of a line

INTRODUCTION

Much of our work as sports biomechanists involves the study and evaluation of how sports skills are performed. To analyse the observed movement 'technique', we need to identify important features of that technique. For a qualitative biomechanical analyst, this means being able to observe those features of the movement; for the quantitative analyst, this requires measuring those features and, often, further mathematical analysis. As I explained in Chapter 1, the increasing demand from the real world of sport and exercise outside of academia – coaches, athletes and other practitioners – has generated an increasing demand for good qualitative movement analysts; this is, again, our main focus in this chapter.

In Chapter 1, we considered human motion in sport and exercise as 'patterns of movement'. This chapter is designed to extend your understanding of the 'geometry' of movement in sport and exercise. We will outline some questions that determine what other movement patterns may be of use to a qualitative movement analyst, to supplement his or her analysis of video. The branch of biomechanics that deals with the geometry of movement without reference to the forces causing the movement is often called 'kinematics', although we will generally avoid this technical term.

BOX 3.1 LEARNING OUTCOMES

After reading this chapter you should be able to:

- explain the various movement patterns that can be used by qualitative (and, indeed, quantitative) movement analysts to provide additional information that is not directly observable from video recordings
- be able to interpret graphical patterns of one movement variable (position, velocity or acceleration) in terms of the other two from the shapes of the patterns
- define linear, rotational and general motion
- understand the physical model appropriate to each type of motion and appreciate the uses and limitations of each model
- appreciate the importance of linear and angular motion in sport and exercise
- understand several ways to study coordination between pairs of joints, to sketch and describe some example coordination patterns, and to appreciate the uses, advantages and drawbacks of each in studying the coordination of sports movements.

MOVEMENT PATTERNS REVISITED

In Chapter 1, we focused on video sequences as the basic representation of movement patterns in sport. We noted, however, that these sequences are complex, because they contain so much information. It is often beneficial for the qualitative movement analyst to look at simpler, if less familiar, representations of movement patterns. In this chapter, we will explore the various movement and coordination patterns that a movement analyst can use, at his or her discretion, to supplement, though not to replace, qualitative video analysis. The patterns that we will consider are all – even if this is not immediately obvious to you at this stage because of their unfamiliarity – far simpler than video recordings because they focus on specific aspects of a movement; this simplicity underpins their usefulness to movement analysts. These movement and coordination patterns – I sometimes call them 'movement analysis supplements' – are particularly relevant when we ask the question that kept arising in the section on fundamental movements in Chapter 1, 'How are these movements coordinated to produce the desired outcome?'

To access the movement and coordination patterns that are the focus of this chapter, a qualitative movement analyst needs to be able to measure distances and joint angles, even though their analysis of them may be almost entirely qualitative. Distances and two-dimensional (planar) joint angles can both be easily measured from software packages for qualitative biomechanical analysis, such as those discussed in Chapter 2; most qualitative movement analysts will us these routinely in their work. Because the angles measured in these packages are usually planar, the focus in this chapter will be on data in the sagittal plane. (I have to admit here that more accurate data can usually be obtained from a software package designed for quantitative analysis; we will consider these in Chapter 4). The chapter will also focus on the qualitative (with some semi-quantitative) analysis of the movement and coordination patterns that we will discuss. I feel strongly that even quantitative analysts need to be able to describe and to analyse movement and coordination patterns qualitatively, if they are to understand them fully; the numbers are really just the 'icing on the cake'.

The movement and coordination patterns that we will look at in this chapter are all graphs. Graphs can be of several types, of which the most useful for the qualitative movement analyst are position or angle time series and several coordination patterns – angle–angle diagrams, continuous relative phase (obtained from phase planes) and cross-correlation functions. Time series are simply graphs of one movement variable, such as joint angle, as it changes over time during the course of the movement. We will summarise how angle–time graphs can be analysed qualitatively – focusing on their geometry, or shape, not on numerical values. Several time series can be plotted on the same graph. We will look at the various coordination patterns very much from a qualitative analytical perspective. All of these graphs will be discussed in detail in later sections.

Both movement and coordination graphs can add substantially to our understanding of a movement and help us to assess ways in which changes might be made to improve performance. Because different individuals find unique solutions to the demands of a sports task, under the various constraints of that task, the environment and their own organism, intra-individual studies are usually more productive than inter-individual ones in shedding light on how movements might be improved. We might, for example, compare different speeds of locomotion, or different stroke rates in rowing, or track an athlete recovering from injury. This approach deserves attention from qualitative biomechanical analysts rather than just from researchers.

FUNDAMENTALS OF MOVEMENT

Motion in sport can be linear, rotational or, more generally, a combination of both. Each type of motion is associated with a physical model of the sports performer or sports object being studied. The behaviour of this physical model can be represented by mathematical equations, which constitute a mathematical model of the object or performer. These mathematical models can then be used to investigate how the object or performer moves.

Figure 3.1 Curvilinear motion.

Linear motion and the centre of mass – the 'point' model

Linear motion is movement in which all parts of the body travel the same distance in the same time in the same direction. If two points on the body are joined by a straight line then, in successive positions, this straight line will remain parallel to its initial orientation. Linear motion is often subdivided into rectilinear motion, which is one-dimensional, as for a puck travelling across an ice rink, or curvilinear, which can be two- or three-dimensional, as for the centre of mass of a shot when in the air or the centre of mass of a ski jumper. It is important to note that, although in curvilinear motion the centre of mass – like the skis in Figure 3.1 – follows a curved path, no rotation about the centre of mass is involved.

The overall linear motion of a sports performer or object, such as a shot, can be specified by the motion of a single point. This imaginary point, which has the same mass as the performer or object, is known as the centre of mass. The mass of the performer is evenly distributed about this point. The motion of the centre of mass of an object, including the sports performer, totally specifies the linear motion of the object as a whole, even if the object's overall motion is more general. Linear motion ignores any rotation about the centre of mass, which means that it only tells us about part, often only a very small part, of the movement pattern we are studying. Linear motion is sometimes known as 'translation', but we will use 'linear motion' throughout this book.

Rotation and rigid bodies – the 'rigid body' model

Rotation, or angular motion, is motion in which all parts of an object travel through the same angle in the same time in the same direction about the axis of rotation. The movement of a body segment about a joint, as in Figure 3.2, is motion of this type. An object

Figure 3.2 Angular motion.

that retains its geometrical shape, for example a cricket bat, can be studied in this way and is known as a rigid body. Human body segments, such as the thigh and forearm, are often considered to be close enough approximations to rigid bodies to be treated as such. The complete human body is not a rigid body, but there are sports techniques, as in diving and gymnastics, in which a body position is held temporarily, as in a tuck or pike. During that period, the performer will behave as if he or she were a rigid body and can be described as a quasi-rigid body. In most sport activities, the human performer does not behave as one rigid body. We then need to use the following model.

General motion and the human performer – the 'multi-segmental' model

Most human movements involve combinations of rotation and linear motion, for example the cross-country skier shown in Figure 3.3.

Such complex motions can be represented by a linked, multi-segment model of the performer, where each of the body segments is treated as a rigid body. The rigid bodies are connected at the joints between body segments. Such movement patterns can be

Figure 3.3 General motion.

very difficult to analyse, but simpler representations of the structure of the movement can be very helpful, as we shall see.

LINEAR MOTION AND THE CENTRE OF MASS

A sprint coach might wish to know how long it takes one of his or her novice athletes to reach maximum horizontal velocity, often referred to as running speed, and what happens thereafter, when running a 100 m race. To do this, we would need to record the position of the athlete's centre of mass – we will return to how we can do this in Chapter 4 – at equal intervals of time – we can do the latter using a video camera. Let us assume for now that the movements of a particular point that we mark on the pelvis closely approximate those of the centre of mass; we could obtain the positions of this point from biomechanical software packages for qualitative video analysis, such as Siliconcoach (www.siliconcoach.com), Dartfish (www.dartfish.com) and Kinovea (www.kinovea.org). This example is a curvilinear movement, but we make it rectilinear by ignoring the vertical movements of the sprinter and focusing only on the horizontal ones. Our geometrical pattern in this case represents the horizontal path taken by the centre of mass during the time of the race and might look something like Figure 3.4, a pattern of the centre of mass movement – its horizontal displacement – over time.

It is often said that a picture is worth a thousand words, so let us see what we can deduce from the movement pattern of Figure 3.4, which, as we noted above, is known as a 'time series', because we are looking at the pattern over time. But first, a few important terms.

Figure 3.4 Hypothetical horizontal displacement of the centre of mass with time for a novice sprinter.

The time-series graph, which is a special kind of movement pattern, of Figure 3.4 is called a displacement–time graph, which, for all important purposes, is the same as a position–time graph. The rate of change of displacement or position with time is known as velocity; the rate of change of velocity with time is called acceleration. We can find important information about velocities and accelerations from a displacement–time graph qualitatively, without recourse to any mathematics, if we accept two extremely important relationships:

- The velocity can be obtained from the gradient – or slope – of a displacement–time graph. Likewise acceleration can be obtained from the slope of a velocity–time graph if we have one.
- The acceleration can be obtained from the curvature of a displacement–time graph.

So, from our displacement–time graph, we can qualitatively describe two further movement patterns; we can specify important features of the velocity–time pattern and the acceleration–time pattern. As we will now see, this qualitative information will answer fully the questions that our hypothetical sprint coach posed.

The gradient – or slope – of a line should be intuitive. All you need to do is to consider 'walking' along the graph from left to right:

- If you are going uphill, the gradient, that is the velocity, is positive. This happens throughout Figure 3.4.
- If you are going downhill, the gradient and velocity are negative.
- Where the direction changes from uphill to downhill, the gradient and velocity are zero, and the gradient and velocity change from positive to negative.
- Likewise, where the direction changes from downhill to uphill, the gradient and velocity are zero and the gradient and velocity change from negative to positive.

This doesn't, perhaps, seem to help much with our coach's questions.

Curvature is probably less intuitive, so let us define two types of curvature as in Figure 3.5, which we can call 'valley-type' and 'hill-type' curvature; we will also use the terms 'positive' and 'negative' curvature. Positive curvature is what you would see looking at a simple curved valley from the side and negative curvature corresponds to the side view of a simple curved hill. Let us walk along the graph in Figure 3.4 again, seeking this time to indicate curvature not gradient. At the start of the race, the curvature is positive (valley-type); it changes at about 60 per cent of the race time to negative. And what is the gradient doing there? It changes from becoming steeper to becoming less steep; in other words, the velocity stops increasing and starts decreasing (Figure 3.6). Our coach's novice performer takes 60 per cent of the race to reach maximum speed and then starts to slow down; we have answered our coach's question. This pattern is not, I must admit, typical for a good sprinter, who would probably maintain a constant speed from about 30 m to 90 m, before slowing slightly, but it does provide a simple example of qualitatively interpreting curvature. To summarise:

- When the curvature is positive, the acceleration is positive, and the gradient and velocity are increasing; this is why we called valley-type curvature positive.
- When the curvature is negative, so is the acceleration, and the gradient and velocity are decreasing; this is why we called hill-type curvature negative.
- Where the curvature and acceleration change from negative to positive, the acceleration is instantaneously zero; the velocity stops decreasing and starts increasing.
- Where the curvature and acceleration change from positive to negative (at 60 per cent of the race time in Figure 3.4), the acceleration is instantaneously zero (see Figure 3.6); the velocity stops increasing and starts decreasing.

Figure 3.5 Top: positive (valley-type) curvature; Bottom: negative (hill-type) curvature.

Positive curvature

Negative curvature

Figure 3.6 Hypothetical centre of mass displacement (continuous black curve), velocity (dashed black curve) and acceleration (red curve) variation with per cent race time for a novice sprinter.

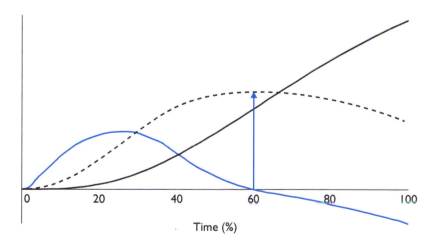

Time (%)

For an elite sprinter, we might find a straight portion on the horizontal displacement–time graph where the curvature was zero. The curvature would change from positive to zero at the start of that portion of the graph and from zero to negative at its end. The acceleration during that portion of the graph would be zero and the gradient, the velocity, would be constant.

When you have the above information about what the changes in gradient and curvature on a displacement–time graph represent for velocity and acceleration then, with experience, you will find that you can roughly – and non-numerically – sketch the velocity and acceleration patterns to obtain further movement patterns for qualitative analysis. All quantitative analysis packages will do this too, and provide more accurate velocity and acceleration patterns; these can also be analysed qualitatively through their shape as well as quantitatively.

THE GEOMETRY OF ANGULAR MOTION

In the previous section, we considered linear motion – the movement patterns of a point. The sports performer or sports object can be represented as a point situated at the centre of mass. The linear motion of this point is defined independently of any rotation taking place around it. The centre of mass generally serves as the best, and sometimes the only, point about which rotations should be considered to occur. All human motion, however, involves rotation, or angular motion, for example the movement of a body segment about its proximal joint. An understanding of angular motion is crucial for the movement analyst seeking to understand, and improve, an athlete's performance.

Angular motion is far more complex than linear motion. The rules that apply to the rotation of a rigid body can be directly applied to an object such as a cricket bat or, as an approximation, to body segments. They can also be applied to a non-rigid body, which, instantaneously, is behaving as though it were rigid, such as a diver holding a fully extended body position or a gymnast holding a tuck. Such systems are classified as quasi-rigid bodies. Applications of the laws of rotational motion to non-rigid bodies, such as the complicated kinematic chains of segments that are the reality in most human movements, have to be made with considerable care. The theory of the rotation of even rigid bodies in the general case is complicated and many problems in this category have not yet been solved.

The movement variables in angular motion are defined similarly to those for linear motion. Angular displacement is the change in the orientation of a line segment. In two-dimensional motion, also known as planar motion, as it takes place in a two-dimensional plane, this will be the angle between the initial and final orientations regardless of the path taken. Angular velocity and acceleration are, respectively, the rates of change with time of angular displacement and angular velocity. The segment or joint angles used in biomechanics can be absolute or relative. An absolute angle is the angle of a body segment to an absolute line in space, usually a horizontal line pointing to the right or a vertical line. Relative angles are the angles between two adjacent segments, in other words, joint angles. In general, I prefer to use joint rather than segment angles as muscles, which generate motion, span joints, attaching to two (or more) segments. It is sometimes convenient, or improves accuracy, to define absolute angles of the trunk, upper arm and thigh. Joint angles provide us with the most important examples of angular motion, first when we look at the change of the angle over time (as in this section) and then at other combinations of variables (as in the next section). Joint angle patterns are, in general, far more important than linear motion patterns and they open the way to so many fascinating human movement patterns.

The angle–time pattern of Figure 3.7, a time-series pattern, shows how the flexion–extension angle of the knee changes with time over one stride of treadmill running for a particular runner and speed. We can learn a lot about this pattern by studying its geometry – the gradient or slope (the two terms are essentially the same in this context) and curvature of the graph – as we move through time from left to right. As this analysis focuses on the qualitative aspects, rather than the numbers, you need to be aware of the joint angle convention used. Here we adopt the convention that we touched on in Chapter 1 and that is used by many (although not all) sports biomechanists in two-dimensional analysis: a fully extended knee would be a larger angle (about 180°) than a flexed knee – the angle increases upwards in the figure. Different conventions are used by some biomechanists and in most three-dimensional motion analyses, so be wary!

Before you read on, satisfy yourself that you can:

- Identify where the knee is flexing and where it is extending in Figure 3.7(a).
- Determine the gradient of the graph in each region of the overall pattern; clue – would you be going uphill or downhill walking along the pattern?
- Identify the curvature of the various regions of the pattern – are they positive ('valley-type') or negative ('hill-type')? Refer to Figure 3.5 if you have forgotten.

Check your answers with Figures 3.7(b) and (c). The gradient changes at the black vertical lines in Figure 3.7(b), from positive to negative or from negative to positive; the gradient is instantaneously zero at the vertical lines. The gradient of the angle time series is important as it gives us the angular velocity (here, of the knee), which, with our angle convention, is positive for extension and negative for flexion. The curvature changes, again from positive to negative or vice versa, at the red vertical lines in Figure 3.7(c); the curvature is instantaneously zero at those vertical lines. The curvature of the angle time series is important as it gives us the angular acceleration. The regions of flexion and extension (Figure 3.7(b)) and those of positive and negative curvature (Figure 3.7(c)) are also shown. Study these patterns very carefully and ensure that you understand them fully before carrying on. If you were wrong, go back to Figure 3.7(a) and try to ascertain where and why you went wrong.

Figure 3.8 is a combination of Figures 3.7(a) to (c). I have added the angular velocity (continuous red curve) and angular acceleration (dashed red curve) patterns to Figure 3.7(a). Angular velocity – the continuous red curve – is positive when the knee is extending and

Figure 3.7 Variation of knee angle with time for a specific individual in treadmill running. Top: (a) angle time series only; Middle: (b) regions of flexion and extension (negative and positive gradient); Bottom: (c) regions of positive and negative curvature. Note that these patterns will vary somewhat with running speed and between individuals.

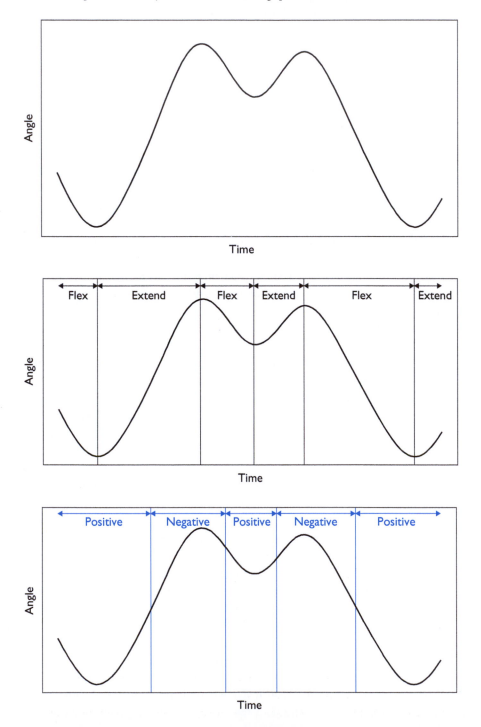

Figure 3.8 Variation of knee angle (continuous black curve), angular velocity (continuous red curve) and angular acceleration (dashed red curve) with time in treadmill running obtained from Figure 3.7. Vertical black lines separate positive (extension) and negative (flexion) angular velocity (gradient) and vertical red lines separate positive and negative angular acceleration (curvature). The data have been 'normalised' to fit the range −1 to +1.

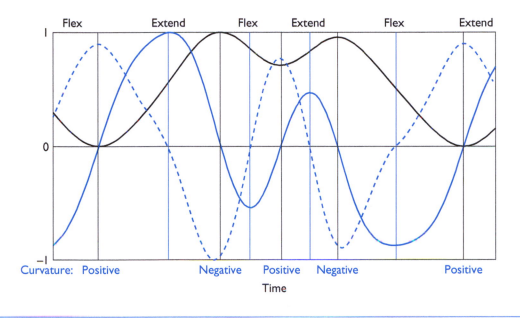

negative when it is flexing. The horizontal line marked 0 shows where the angular velocity or acceleration is zero; values below this line are negative, those above are positive. The angular acceleration – the dashed red curve – is positive, corresponding to positive (valley-type) curvature of the knee angle curve, when it is driving the knee from a flexed to an extended position; we can call this an extending acceleration. The angular acceleration is negative, corresponding to negative (hill-type) curvature of the knee angle curve, when it is driving the knee from an extended to a flexed position; we can call this a flexing acceleration. Trace through the entire patterns of Figure 3.8 until you thoroughly understand them and can explain them to your fellow students; this is a very important step towards becoming a good movement analyst.

You should note that the angular velocity and angular acceleration curves in Figure 3.8 have been calculated from the knee angle data; however, with experience, it is possible to sketch their shape quite accurately from qualitative analysis of the angle–time curve. The curves in Figure 3.8 have been 'normalised' to fit the range 0 to 1 for knee angle, and by setting the largest magnitude of the variable to −1 (if the largest magnitude was negative) or to +1 (if the largest magnitude was positive), while preserving the 0 value, for angular velocity and angular acceleration.

Another noteworthy geometric feature of Figure 3.8 is the sequence of the three movement patterns: an extending (positive) angular acceleration, caused by muscle tension, occurs before the angular velocity changes from flexing (negative) to extending (positive). The resulting sequence of peaks (or troughs) is: angular acceleration; angular velocity; angle. Also notable is the inverse phase relationship between the angle and angular acceleration patterns: one is increasing while the other is decreasing; this is typical of cyclic movements, but not always so apparent in movement patterns in discrete sports skills, such as jumping and throwing.

THE COORDINATION OF JOINT ROTATIONS

Before looking at how we interpret qualitatively graphical representations of coordination, let us begin by considering what we mean by this important term 'coordination'. In Chapter 1, we saw how well-coordinated arm movements can improve the height achieved in a standing vertical jump. So, we could study coordination of arm movements with vertical ground reaction forces for such jumps, but this would be a very ambitious starting point. In Chapter 2, when considering movement principles, one of the universal principles we noted was 'control of redundant degrees of freedom in the segmental chain'. This is one statement of what movement coordination involves. A rather longer definition, which elaborates on the one in the previous sentence, introduces the idea of 'coordinative structures'. This viewpoint sees the acquisition of coordination as constraining the degrees of freedom into coordinative structures, which are functional relationships between important anatomical parts of a performer's body, to perform a specific activity. An example would be groups of muscles or joints temporarily functioning as coherent units to achieve a specific goal, such as hitting or catching a ball. As muscles act around joints, this explanation leads us to look at joints and their interrelationships to gain an initial insight into how sports movements are coordinated.

In the following subsections we will look at the qualitative analysis of several different coordination patterns. Angle–angle diagrams are graphs of one joint angle as a function of another. The focus is on how one angle changes with changes in a second angle; in other words we focus on how the two angles 'co-vary' rather than how they each evolve with time. Angle–angle diagrams are used extensively in the study of movement coordination. The phase planes used in studying human movement coordination are normally graphs of the angular velocity of one joint as a function of the angle of that same joint. The focus is on the so-called 'coordination dynamics' of that joint. Phase planes are also used extensively in the study of movement coordination and from them we can derive graphs of continuous relative phase as a function of time. Cross-correlation functions look at how the correlation coefficient between two time series, such as joint angles, changes as one time series lags behind the other. All of these graphs will be discussed in detail in the following subsections. The focus is on interpreting these graphs qualitatively (and semi-quantitatively); developing such interpretive skills is important to appreciating how coordination patterns can then be used to try to improve sports performance.

Angle–angle diagrams

In the previous section, we looked at joint angles as a function of time – a time series. However, time series involving several angles, as in Figure 3.9, can be difficult to interpret for coordination. An alternative is to plot angles against each other – these are called angle–angle diagrams; we could plot three angles in this way to form a three-dimensional plot, but this is rarely done.

Figure 3.9 Hip (red continuous curve), knee (black continuous curve) and ankle (red dashed curve) angle time series for three strides of treadmill locomotion. Top: (a) walking; Bottom: (b) running. Black vertical line indicates touchdown and red vertical line indicates toe-off.

Time

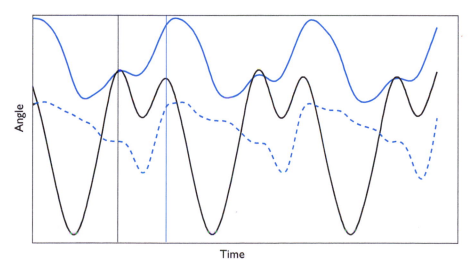
Time

Several forms of coordination can be brought to light through angle–angle diagrams. Some of these relate to the differences between synchronous and sequential coordination that we touched upon in the sections on jumping and throwing in Chapter 1. In synchronous – or simultaneous – coordination, joints move more or less together. These synchronous movements may be 'in-phase' coordination, as when the hips and knees flex during the downward phase of a standing vertical jump (SVJ) and extend during the upward phase (this is shown in Figure 3.10(e), which is similar in many respects to in-phase turning-point coordination in Figure 3.10(b), except that the SVJ is a discrete movement so has a turning-point coordination change only at the bottom of the lowering phase). Another example is the synchronous extension of the hips and the knees during the drive phase of rowing (see Figure 3.14). If the two angles change at the same rate, a linear relationship, such as that of Figure 3.10(a), would result; this is rarely seen in human movements in sport. More often, the joints will show in-phase 'turning point' coordination, as in Figures 3.10(b) and (e). The synchronous movements may also be out of phase: this occurs when one joint flexes and another extends in the sagittal plane, or when one joint abducts while another adducts in the frontal plane: we then have 'anti-phase' or 'out-of-phase' coordination. An example is the action phase of a darts throw in which the upper arm abducts while the wrist adducts from a partially abducted position at the start of the phase (the elbow extends at the same time, also in synchrony but in a different plane of motion). Linear anti-phase coordination is shown in Figure 3.10(c) – again, this is rarely found in human movements in sports – and anti-phase turning-point coordination in Figure 3.10(d).

Figure 3.10(f) shows 'phase offset' or 'decoupled' coordination. In this type of coordination, the two joints change their relative roles during a cycle of a movement, switching between in-phase and anti-phase coordination. Reading from point 'A' anticlockwise, both angles flex in-phase, until 'B', then Angle 2 continues to flex while Angle 1 extends (anti-phase). From 'C' to 'D', both angles extend in-phase and, finally, Angle 1 flexes from 'D' to 'A' while Angle 2 continues to extend (anti-phase). Finally, we have sequential coordination, to which we will return later in this section. Coordination in actual human movements is often more complex than these basic patterns, as for the hip–knee angle–angle diagram for one running stride in Figure 3.11. Please note that the diagram has been slightly 'massaged' so that it forms a continuous loop, which is rarely the case owing to movement variability and measurement errors, as shown in Figure 3.12. Please also be careful to distinguish between the use of the word 'phase' as in phases of a movement, here of a running stride, and in relation to in-phase and anti-phase coordination.

Reading around Figure 3.11, starting at the lower right-hand spike at 'a', which corresponds roughly to touchdown, or heel strike, and progressing anticlockwise, the pattern is as follows: at the start of the stance phase, the hip and knee both flex until 'b'; then, briefly, the knee continues to flex while the hip extends to 'c'. From 'c' to 'd' the two joints extend in phase. From 'd', which is roughly at toe-off, another brief period until 'e' sees the knee flex while the hip extends at the start of the swing phase. From 'e' until 'f' both joints flex in phase during the next part of the swing phase, after which

Figure 3.10 Basic types of coordination. In-phase – Top left: (a) linear; Top right: (b) turning-point coordination. Anti-phase – Middle left: (c) linear; Middle right: (d) turning-point coordination. Bottom left: (e) hip and knee angle coordination in a standing vertical jump with countermovement – compare this with (b). Bottom right: (f) phase offset or decoupled coordination.

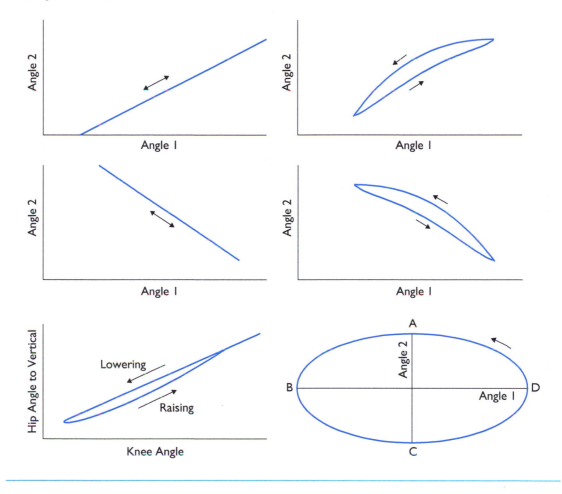

the knee extends while the hip continues to flex until 'g'; both joints then extend in phase until around touchdown. You should now try to repeat this description of joint movements for the same running stride but looking at the ankle–knee and ankle–hip joint couplings, in Figures 3.11(b) and (c) (see Study Task 5).

The study of movement coordination is crucial for movement analysts, both qualitative and quantitative. Angle–angle diagrams have both advantages and disadvantages. Their advantages include that we don't have to flip between angle–time graphs (such as those of Figure 3.9) to see how angles co-vary, and that we can pair joint angles of interest easily to show how they co-vary. These graphs show coordination patterns qualitatively, which can facilitate comparisons, for example, between individuals or for one individual during rehabilitation from an injury. They also show all of the fine details of

Figure 3.11 Angle–angle diagrams for one 'ideal' treadmill running stride. Top: (a) hip–knee coupling; Middle: (b) ankle–knee coupling; Bottom: (c) ankle–hip coupling.

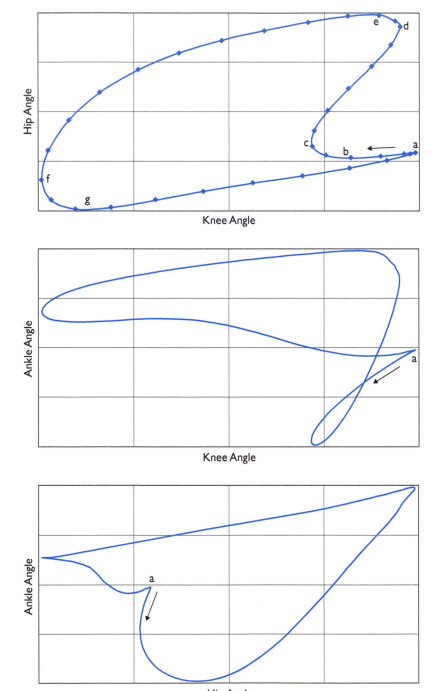

Figure 3.12 Angle–angle diagrams for three strides in treadmill running. Top: (a) hip–knee coupling; Bottom: (b) ankle–knee coupling.

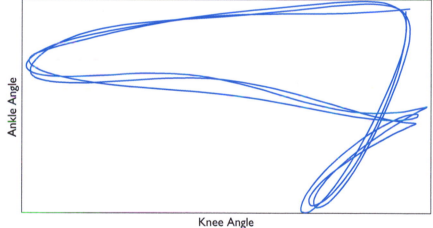

how the two joints change coordination during the movement, as in Figure 3.11(a). We can also compare patterns between, for example, running and walking. Many attempts have been made to quantify angle–angle diagrams; such a reduction of a rich qualitative pattern to a few numbers seems bizarre to me and ignores the saying 'a picture is worth a thousand words'. Few attempts have been made to distinguish patterns qualitatively; one of the very few is known as 'topological equivalence'. Two shapes are topologically equivalent if one can just be stretched – albeit by different amounts in different places – to form the other; two shapes are not topologically equivalent if one has to be 'folded' rather than just stretched to form the other. Simplistically, this means that if the shapes have different numbers of loops, they are not topologically equivalent; they are then qualitatively rather than just quantitatively different, as for the ankle–knee but not the hip–knee or ankle–hip couplings when comparing the running angle–angle diagrams in Figure 3.11 with those for walking in Figure 3.13.

An important point to make here, and it applies to other coordination patterns too, is that of inter-individual differences. Consider, for example, Figure 3.14, which shows hip–knee angle–angle diagrams for four rowers performing a race trial on a rowing ergometer. Figures 3.14(a) and (b) are for two club standard rowers and Figures 3.14(c) and (d) are for two high performance rowers. It should be perfectly clear that there is no 'club' or 'elite' template here. All four rowers show a coordination pattern that is close to synchronised in-phase turning-point coordination; but this is not strictly true for the rowers in Figures 3.14 (a) and (d), for whom the top right loop close to the finish of the drive has a region where the knee flexes while the hip extends, an anti-phase pattern. The patterns for the two club rowers clearly differ, with one (club rower 1) having the broader part of the loop at the top right of the curve, the finish of the drive (Figure 3.14(a)), while the other (club rower 2) has the broader part of the loop at the bottom left, the start of the drive, or the 'catch' (Figure 3.14(b)). Both have two loops in their pattern, although these may not be immediately obvious from the figures: Figure 3.14(a) has a small second loop at the bottom left and Figure 3.14(b) at the top right of the angle–angle pattern. They are topologically equivalent but still different. The patterns for the two high performance rowers also differ. The rower represented by Figure 3.14(c) (high performance rower 1) has a single loop pattern, with the loop being broader at the start of the drive, whereas the rower in Figure 3.14(d) (high performance rower 2) has the broader part of the loop at the finish of the drive. The two patterns are also not topologically equivalent, with high performance rower 2 having a clear two-loop pattern in contrast to the single-loop pattern of high performance rower 1. If we compare across performance standards, we note the general shapes of the hip–knee angle–angle diagrams for club rower 1 and high performance rower 2 are similar; they are also topologically equivalent, as both have two loops. The general shapes of club rower 2 and high performance rower 1 are also similar in having the broader part of the loop at the start of the drive; however, they are not topologically equivalent. Each of these four rowers has evolved a hip–knee coordination pattern that 'matches' their organismic constraints to those of the task and environment; none of these patterns is inherently 'right' or 'wrong'. Coordination profiling, over multiple trials, has been proposed as a comprehensive way of highlighting coordination differences or similarities between individuals (see, for example, Button et al., 2006 in 'Further reading').

Disadvantages of angle–angle diagrams include their unfamiliarity compared to time series. Also, it is not always obvious from the diagram which way round the figure proceeds – clockwise or anticlockwise – or where key events, such as toe-off and touchdown in walking and running, occur; the latter is also true to some extent for time series. Some criticism can be made of the loss of time as a variable, although marking the data, or time, points, as in Figure 3.11(a), adds some indication of how the angles change with time. We do, however, lose access to time-series shape patterns – the slope equals angular velocity, the curvature equals angular acceleration; such relationships do not apply to angle–angle diagrams. To obtain that information, we need to study the time-series data from which our angle–angle diagram was plotted.

Figure 3.13 Angle–angle diagrams for one treadmill walking stride. Top: (a) hip–knee coupling. Middle: (b) ankle–knee coupling. Bottom: (c) ankle–hip coupling.

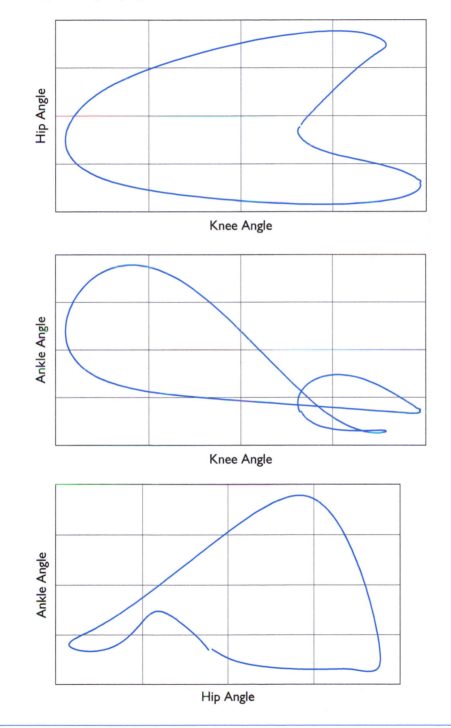

Figure 3.14 Hip–knee angle–angle diagrams for four rowers early in a 5-min race trial on a rowing ergometer, one 'stroke' only shown on each. Top left: (a) and Top right: (b) club standard rowers; Bottom left: (c) and Bottom right: (d) high performance rowers. The 'catch' is at the bottom left of each angle–angle diagram and the 'finish' near the top right. The angles are all normalised to the range −1 to +1.

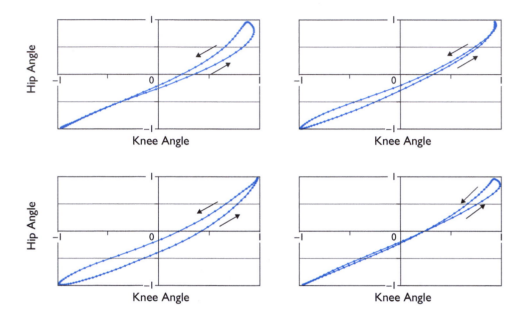

Phase planes

Perhaps the main criticism of angle–angle diagrams is that while they show how coordination between the two joints changes (by detailed analysis as above) they do not tell us why these changes take place. To try to do that, we need a different approach. Phase planes are based on the notion that any system, such as a body segment or joint, can be graphed as diagrams of two variables; for the phase planes used in human movement analysis, these variables are usually joint angle (sometimes segment absolute angle) and angular velocity. Although the relevance of a phase plane for a single joint to coordination between joints may seem hard to fathom, phase planes turn out to be pivotal for our understanding of movement coordination, as will be evident later in this section.

Example phase planes, for the hip (Figure 3.15(a)) and the knee (Figure 3.15(b)) joints in a treadmill running stride, are shown in Figure 3.15. Their description – although not their analysis – is 'child's play' compared to both angle time series and angle–angle diagrams. First, let us ask whether the phase plane progresses clockwise

Figure 3.15 Non-centred and non-normalised phase planes for one treadmill running stride. Top: (a) hip joint; Bottom: (b) knee joint.

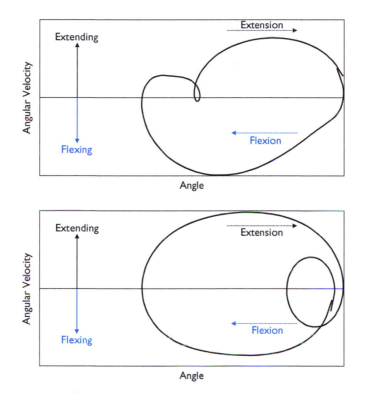

or anticlockwise with time around its loop – it must do one or the other. Because, in the sports biomechanics for two-dimensional analysis used in this book, we define flexion as a decrease in joint angle and extension as an increase, then flexion must be from right to left and extension from left to right along the horizontal axes in Figure 3.15. Similarly, as we saw in the previous section on time series, a flexion velocity is negative and an extension velocity is positive; so, flexion must be below the horizontal axes (zero angular velocity lines) in Figure 3.15 and extension above them. The phase planes of Figure 3.15 must, therefore, progress clockwise with time. Why? Well, let us assume the opposite – they progress anticlockwise with time. In this case, in Figure 3.15 (a), the hip joint would be flexing – from right to left – while its angular velocity was positive (above the zero line) indicating extension. We have proved a contradiction: the phase plane cannot progress anticlockwise with time. Therefore, it must progress clockwise with time; now the hip has positive angular velocity (above the zero line) while it is extending – from left to right – so all is well with the world.

Figure 3.16 Centred and normalised phase planes for one treadmill walking stride.

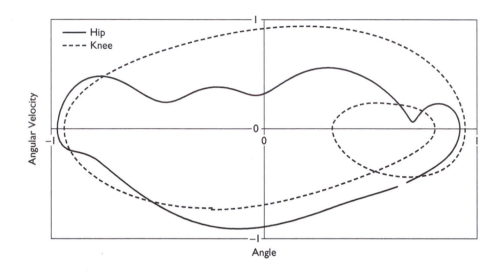

It is also worth noting that the phase planes for the hip angle in the examples of treadmill walking and running are not topologically equivalent (compare the continuous line in Figure 3.16 with Figure 3.15(a)); the phase plane for running has two loops while that for walking has only one. However, the example knee phase planes for treadmill running and walking are topologically equivalent as they both have two loops (as seen in the dashed line in Figure 3.16 and Figure 3.15(b)).

Continuous relative phase

The value of phase planes should start to become more evident when we define the so-called 'phase angle', as shown for the example of treadmill running in Figure 3.17. I have changed the graph so that it is 'centred' on its mean value, for reasons that need not concern us in this book. If we now subtract the phase angle – defined anti-clockwise from the right horizontal – for one joint from that for a second joint at the same instant, we define a variable known as relative phase. Here, we subtract the knee phase angle from that for the hip, rp = pah – pak (this is the usual way of doing such things – subtracting the distal joint phase angle from that for the proximal joint). We can do this for every data point (or time instant) in the phase plane (here defined by the running cycle) to arrive at values of relative phase as a function of time, which can then be graphed and is known as 'continuous relative phase'.

A graph of continuous relative phase as a function of time for this example of treadmill running by a particular individual at his preferred running speed is shown in Figure 3.18. Continuous relative phase is simply another coordination 'pattern',

Figure 3.17 Superimposed phase planes for the hip (red line) and knee (black line) joints in one treadmill running stride plus definition of their phase angles (pah and pak) and the relative phase angle (rp).

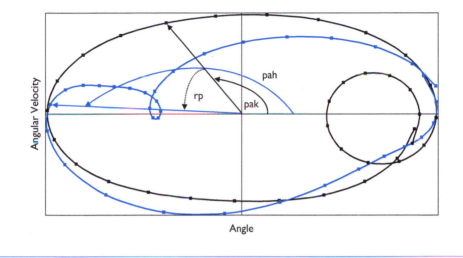

Figure 3.18 Continuous relative phase for the hip–knee angle coupling for one treadmill running stride, derived from Figure 3.17. The dashed vertical arrow indicates toe-off and the continuous vertical arrow indicates touchdown.

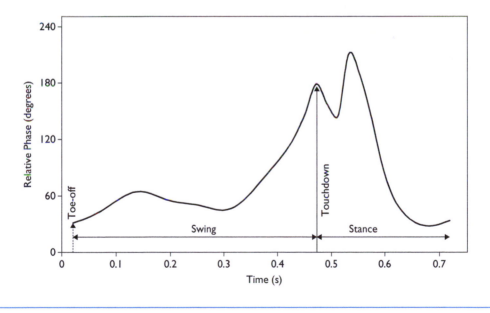

although more difficult to interpret than angle–angle diagrams. In Figure 3.18, for example, we see that the knee 'lags' the hip in 'phase space' (rp < 180°) except just after touchdown: the relative phase angle is around 30 to 60° for much of the swing phase (after toe-off) and changes to around 180° at touchdown, then fluctuates about that value at the start of the

Figure 3.19 Continuous relative phase for the hip–knee angle coupling for one treadmill walking stride, derived from Figure 3.16. The dashed vertical arrow indicates toe-off and the continuous vertical arrow indicates touchdown.

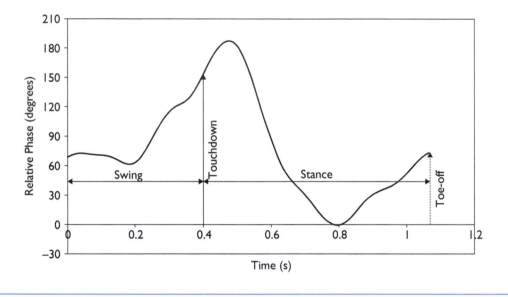

stance phase before returning to around 30 to 60° before toe-off. The change from 30 to 60°, to 180° or vice versa precedes (or 'announces') the change from swing to stance or vice versa, which can be interpreted as a preparatory or anticipatory change.

So what, you might be tempted to say? Well, relative phase has been found to be the 'collective variable' (or the 'order parameter') that best expresses coordination changes between two entities (two joints in our example) in a wide range of biological phenomena, including human movement. Examples in human movement include the transitions between walking and running, and bimanual coordination changes. For a further discussion of these and other biological examples of the use of relative phase (such as firefly synchronised flashing and lamprey swimming) see Kelso (1995) in the Further Reading section. So, relative phase is very important in understanding coordination! The concept of collective variables is very important in the study of coordination dynamics. Relative phase 'collects' together four variables – two joint angles plus the angular velocities of the same two joints.

The limitations of continuous relative phase (CRP) are, first, that it can only be used to study the coordination between two entities – normally two joints in human movement – and most sports movements involve far more than two joints. Second, phase angles can cross the 0 to 360° discontinuity, because the angle is plotted as a linear variable yet it is a circular one (the angles 0°, 360° and 720° are identical). This can lead to discontinuities in the CRP graph, unless plotted on the surface of a cylinder – not an easy task in a textbook. This leads to the possible need for the use of circular statistics to analyse data. The use of CRP assumes, for any statistical tests, that the datasets are sinusoidal – or very nearly so (this is mostly fairly true for cyclic movements) – and 'stationary' – that is, the statistical description of the dataset is invariant with time, which will not be true, for example, if impacts are involved. However, CRP is a continuous, rich measure, which shows up as a pattern that can be qualitatively compared with others. For example, note the similarities and the differences between the continuous relative phase patterns for running (Figure 3.18) and walking (Figure 3.19). An important similarity, touched on above, is that the change in CRP from one region to another precedes the change of movement phase, from swing to stance or vice versa. Differences include the lower minimum relative phase angle in the stance phase for walking and the lack of a double peak around 180° for walking, which has only a single peak. More detailed analysis of these CRP patterns is beyond the scope of this book.

For completeness, although it is not a movement pattern, but a discrete measure, Discrete Relative Phase is usually, but not always, measured as the difference between the largest and smallest angles on the CRP graph. For a cyclic activity, such as running or rowing, this would be during one stride or stroke. An additional discrete measure sometimes used in studying coordination is the time as a percentage of the cycle time (e.g. stride time or stroke time) between the largest and smallest (or vice versa) values of relative phase on the CRP graph.

Cross-correlation functions

Here, we will consider another graphical representation of coordination between joints – cross-correlation functions – and look at the strengths and weaknesses of this approach. I will begin by revising (or introducing, if you have not come across them before) Pearson product moment correlations, the basis of cross-correlation functions. Correlation tests are used when we suspect (hopefully based on some theory) that two variables are meaningfully interrelated. A correlation is a statistical technique to help us ascertain the extent of such a relationship. Correlations (expressed by correlation coefficients, r) vary from +1 through 0 to −1 (the line, if there is one, associating the two variables is called the regression line): +1 is a perfect positive correlation; −1 is a perfect negative (inverse) correlation; 0 indicates that the two variables are uncorrelated. Most r values are not 1 or 0.

Cross-correlations are similar to Pearson product moment correlations, but involve correlating variables (often angles) from two time series. They can be easily implemented by the function PEARSON in Microsoft Excel; e.g. = PEARSON(D2:D102, E2:E102); where the data for one angle are in cells D2 to D102 and for the second angle in cells E2 to E102 (see also Study Task 9). The term 'cross-correlation' is used to denote correlations between two different time series compared to 'auto-correlation' of one time series with itself. Cross-correlating two angle time series may obscure real relationships, if one angle 'leads' or 'lags' the other; in other words, if peaks and troughs are offset in time. If the time lag is removed, relationships may be

Figure 3.20 Indication of change of correlation coefficient with time lag. Top left: (a) cosine and sine series; Top right: (b) cosine series and sine series with one time lag removed; Bottom left: (c) cosine series and sine series with three time lags removed; Bottom right: (d) resulting cross correlation function plotted against removed time lag.

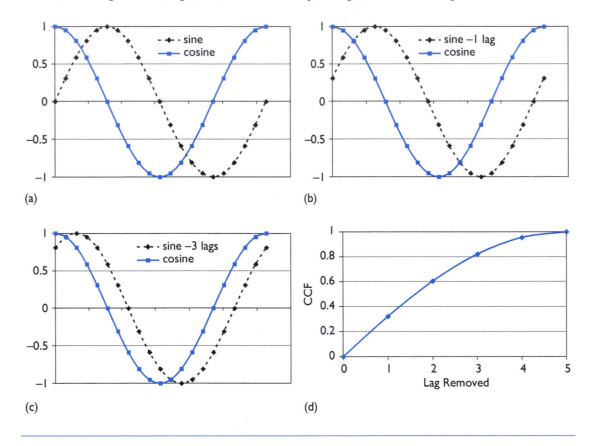

revealed. As an example, consider simple cosine and sine series as in Figure 3.20(a) ($r = 0$). The sine series lags the cosine series, here by 5 data points; for example, the cosine series reaches the value +1 five data points before the sine series does. If we now remove 1 lag (Figure 3.20(b)), $r = 0.32$; 2 lags, $r = 0.61$; remove 3 lags (Figure 3.20(c)), $r = 0.82$: 4 lags, $r = 0.96$; remove 5 lags and the two curves now overlie, so $r = 1$. If we now plot the correlation coefficients as a function of time lag for one time series against the other, showing the strength of the correlation at different lags, we obtain the cross-correlation function (CCF, Figure 3.20(d)).

Now let us consider the hip and knee angle time series for treadmill walking, for which we looked at the angle–angle diagram in Figure 3.9(a) above, and plot correlation coefficients for various time lags for one angle time series against the other, showing the strength of the correlation at different lags. The resulting cross-correlation functions can show, for example, that joints can be coordinated but out of phase, as in Figure 3.21. Here we have $r = 0.76$ at a lead of the hip over the knee of 17% of the stride time and $r = -0.75$ at 77%; by contrast, the original time series had $r \sim 0.2$, highly uncorrelated and, superficially, seemingly uncoordinated. Cross-correlations between suitable joint angles or angular velocities can also show proximal-to-distal joint sequencing in, for example, throwing.

Conjugate cross-correlations consider coordination between three or more variables, such as the angles of the hip, knee and ankle in our example of treadmill walking (Figure 3.22), by plotting and analysing cross-correlation functions of the hip and knee, the knee and ankle, and the hip and ankle. Without going into this in too much detail, it is clear that the cross-correlation functions of the hip and knee and the hip and ankle are inverted. The cross-correlation function of the knee and ankle

Figure 3.21 Cross-correlation function for the hip and knee angles in treadmill walking for a specific individual at preferred walking speed.

Figure 3.22 Conjugate cross-correlation functions between the hip and knee, knee and ankle, and hip and ankle angles in treadmill walking for a specific individual at preferred walking speed.

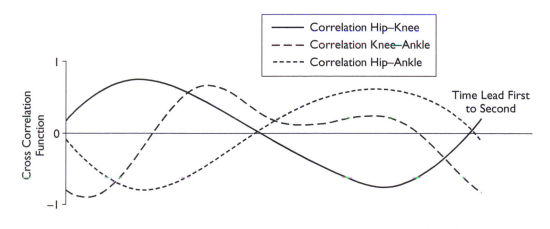

is entirely different in shape and in the time leads, or lags, to its largest positive and negative correlation coefficients.

Cross-correlation functions can reveal aspects of coordination not apparent in the other approaches that we have considered in this section; for example, they show whether one joint lags behind another. This is particularly useful in studying proximal-to-distal sequential coordination, as in most throws for distance; the comparisons need to be pairwise (two joints at a time), a limitation of this approach. Although the calculation of cross-correlation functions might seem to be 'quantitative', the interpretation of them here is essentially qualitative, or semi-quantitative if we include the time lags and correlation coefficients. The cross-correlation function patterns are easy to interpret, although some people find the underlying concepts somewhat difficult. If we are only interested in calculating correlations, then the only underlying assumption is that the two variables are linearly related. It should be obvious that there must be a meaningful relationship between the two variables to be correlated, otherwise erroneous results will be obtained. Human movement dynamics are not, however, normally linear, but this is not an insurmountable difficulty as we can, for example, logarithmically transform the data. If we wish to test hypotheses, for example about the statistical significance of the correlation coefficient, the same assumptions must be met as for Pearson product moment correlations; this would definitely take us into quantitative analysis, which is beyond the scope of this chapter.

SUMMARY

In this chapter the principles of kinematics – the geometry of movement – which are important for the study of human movement in sport and exercise were covered. Our focus was very strongly on movement patterns and their qualitative interpretation. We considered the types of motion and the model appropriate to each. Several other forms of movement and coordination patterns (all of them graphs) were introduced, explained and explored. The importance of being able to interpret graphs of linear or angular displacement and to infer from these the geometry of the velocity and acceleration patterns was stressed. We looked at three ways of assessing coordination between two joints, using angle–angle diagrams and – through phase planes – relative phase, and cross-correlation functions; we briefly touched on the uses, strengths and weaknesses of each of these approaches.

STUDY TASKS

Q

1 Answer all of the multiple-choice questions for Chapter 3 in the Interactive eTextbook.
   Hint: Keep repeating this until you have answered all of the questions correctly.

2 Draw sketch diagrams from your own sports activities to show the three types of motion – linear, angular and general – and the model appropriate to each. List the uses and limitations of each model.
Hint: You may wish to re-read the section on 'Fundamentals of movement' before undertaking this task.

3 Download a knee angle–time graph for walking from the Interactive eTextbook. From this, and using the relationships between the gradients and curvatures of the graph, sketch the appropriate angular velocity and acceleration graphs. Remember that you move along the graph from left to right, going uphill and downhill noting the changes in gradient and curvature.
Hint: If you are struggling with this task, you may wish to re-read the section on 'The geometry of angular motion'; once you have completed this task, compare your answers with those in the Interactive eTextbook.

4 Repeat Study Task 3 for the hip angle in walking, which you can download from the Interactive eTextbook. Keep repeating this for other datasets, until you are able to sketch the angular velocity and acceleration graphs without reference to either the figures in the section on 'The geometry of angular motion' or the answers.
I must stress that analysis of such movement patterns is an essential skill for all movement analysts, whether they approach such a pattern qualitatively or quantitatively. Although these time-series movement patterns are less familiar to you than videos of sports movements, they are far simpler, so persevere with this. Then persevere some more: it will pay great dividends if you become any kind of movement analyst.
Hint: If you are struggling with this task, you may wish to re-read the section on 'The geometry of angular motion'; once you have completed this task, compare your answers for the hip with those in the Interactive eTextbook.

5 Describe the coordination sequences of the ankle–knee and ankle–hip joint couplings in Figures 3.11(b) and (c). Indicate the points on the figures that correspond to coordination changes (similar to points a–g in Figure 3.11(a)). Indicate also whether the joints are in-phase or anti-phase in each region of the diagram (for example, regions a–b and g–a in Figure 3.11(a) are in phase) – assume for this purpose that ankle plantar flexion is in phase with knee and hip extension. Note that the points in Figures 3.11(b) and (c) at which coordination changes will not necessarily be the same as those in Figure 3.11(a), however point 'a' and an anticlockwise progression are common to all three figures.
Hint: You should study in detail the description of Figure 3.11(a) in the subsection on 'Angle–angle diagrams' before undertaking this task.

6 Describe the coordination sequences of the ankle–knee and ankle–hip joint couplings for walking in Figures 3.13(b) and (c). Indicate the points on the figures that correspond to coordination changes (similar to points a–g in Figure 3.11(a)). Indicate also whether the joints are in-phase or anti-phase in each region of the diagram (for example, regions a–b and g–a in Figure 3.11(a) are in phase) – assume for this purpose that ankle plantar flexion is in phase with knee and hip extension.

Note that toe-off in walking does not occur at a point of near maximal knee extension as in running, so you will need to establish carefully where in Figure 3.13 toe-off and touchdown occur; the diagram, as for Figure 3.11, evolves anticlockwise.

Hint: You should study some videos of walking (there are several in the Interactive eTextbook) and revisit in detail the description of Figure 3.11(a) in the subsection on Angle–angle diagrams' before undertaking this task.

For Study Tasks 7 to 9, download and save the walking-to-running Excel file from the Interactive eTextbook. Successful completion of these study tasks is absolutely crucial if you want to become a competent movement analyst, so do persevere.

7   The hip, knee and ankle time-series graphs have been plotted in the data file for Speed 1 (Slower Walking). By selecting the appropriate columns from the relevant Excel worksheets, plot time-series graphs for the hip, knee and ankle angles for Speed 2 (Faster Walking), Speed 4 (Slower Running) and Speed 5 (Faster Running). Note briefly any observable differences between the movement patterns for walking and running.

Hint: You may wish to re-read the section on 'The geometry of angular motion' and to consult the examples in the Interactive eTextbook before undertaking this task.

8   The hip–knee and ankle–knee angle–angle diagrams have been plotted in the data file for Speed 1 (Slower Walking). By selecting the appropriate columns from the relevant Excel worksheets, plot angle–angle diagrams for the hip–knee and ankle–knee couplings for Speed 2 (Faster Walking), Speed 4 (Slower Running) and Speed 5 (Faster Running). Note briefly any observable differences between the angle–angle diagrams for walking and running.

Hint: You may wish to re-read the subsection on 'Angle–angle diagrams' and to consult the examples in the Interactive eTextbook before undertaking this task.

9   The hip, knee and ankle phase planes and the cross-correlation functions between the hip and knee, hip and ankle and knee and ankle (three curves) have been plotted in the data file for Speed 1 (Slower Walking). Again, by selecting the appropriate columns from the relevant Excel worksheets:

a) Plot phase planes (angular velocity versus angle) for the hip, knee and ankle for Speed 2 (Faster Walking), Speed 4 (Slower Running) and Speed 5 (Faster Running).

b) Plot cross-correlation functions for the hip and knee, hip and ankle and knee and ankle angles for Speed 2 (Faster Walking), Speed 4 (Slower Running) and Speed 5 (Faster Running).

For both these types of coordination pattern, note briefly any observable differences between the patterns for walking and running.

Hint: You may wish to re-read the section on 'The coordination of joint rotations' and to consult the examples in the Interactive eTextbook before undertaking this task.

10 **Case study**.

a) Answer the five multiple-choice questions for this study task in the Interactive eTextbook.

b) Based on the differences you have noted in Study Tasks 7 to 9, explain, in not more than 1000 words, whether and how each of the types of movement and coordination pattern that you looked at in those study tasks helps you to identify any qualitative differences between walking and running. Illustrate your answer with up to eight figures.

Hint: You may wish to re-read the sections on 'The geometry of angular motion' and 'The coordination of joint rotations' before undertaking this task.

SORTING AND LABELLING ACTIVITIES (INTERACTIVE ETEXTBOOK ONLY)

Sorting activity.
Labelling activity.

FURTHER READING

Button, C., Davids, K. and Schöllhorn, W. (2006). Coordination profiling of movement systems, in K. Davids, S. Bennett, and K. Newell (eds) *Movement System Variability*, Champaign, IL: Human Kinetics. The book looks at various issues in movement coordination and movement variability, mostly from a motor control perspective. Chapter 7 focuses on profiling movement coordination, and has more of a biomechanical 'flavour' than most of the other chapters; it also introduces the somewhat advanced topic of the study of multi-joint coordination using artificial neural networks. The chapter (like the rest of the book) is not 'easy going', but it is well worth reading, and draws on examples from throwing and catching skills.

Kelso, J.A.S. (1995) *Dynamic Patterns: The Self-Organization of Brain and Behavior, Cambridge, MS*: MIT Press; (Chapter 1: How Nature Handles Complexity; Most of you will not find this 'plain sailing' either, but again not because of any mathematics – there are no equations in this chapter – rather because of the novelty of much of the material. Stick with it; you too might be inspired by Scott Kelso's approach, and his subtle humour.

APPENDIX 3.1 FURTHER EXPLORATION OF ANGLE–TIME PATTERNS

Here, we find that the points on the angle time series at which interesting things happened in Figures 3.7 and 3.8 have names. At points A to E in Figure 3.23, the gradient of

Figure 3.23 Variation of knee angle with time in treadmill running; further explanation of angle–time patterns.

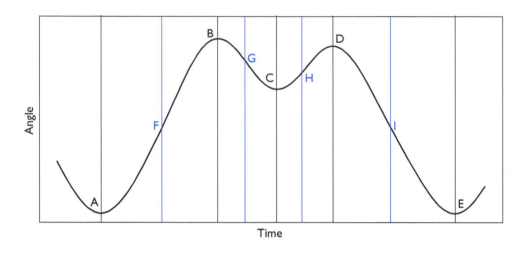

the tangent to the curve is zero as the tangent is horizontal. The rate of change of angle with respect to time at these points is therefore zero; that is, the angular velocity is zero. The point at which this happens is called a 'stationary point', which may be any one of three types; two of these are evident in A and B in Figure 3.23. These two points are known as 'turning points'. These are stationary points at which the gradient of the angle curve – the angular velocity – changes sign from positive to negative or vice versa. The third point of this type is far more rarely encountered. Points F to I in Figure 3.23 are known as 'points of inflexion', as they are points where the pattern changes its direction of curvature – from positive to negative or vice versa. We return to these later.

Local minimums

A turning point such as A, C or E in Figure 3.23 is known as a 'local minimum', for which two conditions are necessary:

- The angle at that point must be less than its value at any nearby point; it is not necessarily the overall or 'global minimum' value, hence the use of the term 'local'.
- The gradient of the angle curve, the angular velocity, must change from a negative value (when the angle is decreasing) to a positive value (when the angle is increasing); hence, the angular acceleration is positive.

For an angle–time graph, the above can be summarised as follows: a local minimum angle (A, C or E) corresponds to a condition of zero angular velocity – changing from a negative to a positive value – and a positive acceleration.

Local maximums

A turning point such as B or D in Figure 3.23 is known as a 'local maximum', for which two conditions are necessary:

- The angle at that point must be greater than its value at any nearby point.
- The gradient of the angle curve, the angular velocity, must change from a positive to a negative value; hence the angular acceleration is negative.

For an angle–time graph, a local maximum angle (B or D) corresponds to a condition of zero angular velocity – changing from positive to negative – and a negative acceleration.

Points of inflexion

To interpret these, consider the positive and negative curvatures of the angle time series of Figure 3.23 and the point at which they meet. If the curvature is positive, the gradient of the angle curve and, therefore, the angular velocity, is increasing. The acceleration must, therefore, be positive for this portion of the curve. For an angle–time curve, a positive curvature is a region of positive acceleration, reflecting an increasing angular velocity. If the curvature is negative, so is the acceleration, and the gradient of the angle–time curve – the angular velocity – is decreasing. The points of inflexion, F to I, in Figure 3.23 indicate instances of zero acceleration.

Stationary points of inflexion

A point of inflexion at which the gradient of the tangent happens to be zero fulfils the conditions of a stationary point, which is why it is called a stationary point of inflexion. It does not fulfil the extra condition required for a turning point, that the gradient changes sign. These are rarely encountered by human movement analysts.

4 Quantitative motion analysis in sports biomechanics

Knowledge assumed
Familiarity with use of digital
camcorders (Chapter 2)
Position–velocity–acceleration
relationships (Chapter 3)
Qualitative analysis of sports
movements (Chapter 2)
Coordination diagrams
(Chapter 3)
Basic algebra and trigonometry
Familiarity with basic
differential calculus and vector
algebra would be useful but is
not essential

INTRODUCTION

In this chapter (and the next two) we will focus on the quantitative analysis of sports movements. This chapter concentrates on what is often called by biomechanists 'motion analysis' (perhaps, more correctly, 'image-based motion analysis', but this is rather cumbersome). Implicit in the term 'motion analysis', as used in biomechanics, is that it involves quantitative analysis, and I will use 'motion analysis' in this way in this chapter; however, when it helps to add clarity, I will also use the term 'quantitative motion analysis', although the two are essentially synonymous. Motion analysis basically involves motion capture, or motion tracking, followed by analysis of the tracked motion. In this chapter, we will mostly explore the use of video analysis – videography – in the study of sports movements, including the equipment and methods used, experimental procedures and data processing (you, the reader, should also note that the term 'videography' is used outside of biomechanics to mean just the process of motion capture, with no reference to later analysis of the tracked motion, so be wary). Videography is by far the most likely method of motion analysis that an undergraduate student will come across. I will also provide an introduction to another method of motion analysis, using automatic marker-tracking systems. The increasing computer control of our main data collection equipment in sports biomechanics, along with much more accessible and user-friendly software, has lessened our need for repetitive and tedious mathematical calculations. Basic mathematical skills can, however, enable us to assess more critically factors that affect the accuracy of our experimental data. Such skills can also improve our understanding of sports performance; two cases in which this is very clear are introduced towards the end of this chapter – the first is projectile motion, and the second examines how rotation of a body generates linear velocities and accelerations. Symbolic representations are used in this chapter (some people, mistakenly, call this mathematics), but mathematical derivations are avoided.

BOX 4.1 LEARNING OUTCOMES

After reading this chapter you should be able to:

- understand the importance of videography in the study of sports movements
- undertake a quantitative video analysis of a sports movement
- understand the important features of video equipment for recording movements in sport
- outline the advantages and limitations of two- and three-dimensional recording of sports movements
- list the possible sources of error in recorded movement data
- describe and implement experimental procedures that would minimise measurement inaccuracy in a study of an essentially two-dimensional movement

---

- appreciate how these procedures can be extended and modified to record a three-dimensional movement
- achieve a basic knowledge of on-line motion analysis systems, which automatically track markers
- understand how 'noise' can be (partially) removed from videographic data
- appreciate the need for accurate body segment inertia parameter data, and some ways in which these can be obtained
- understand some of the effects of random errors (called 'noise') on data accuracy in sports biomechanics
- explain the differences between vectors and scalars
- calculate the maximum vertical displacement, flight time, range and optimum projection angle of a simple projectile for specified values of the three projection parameters
- understand simple rotation kinematics, including vector multiplication, and the calculation of linear velocities and accelerations caused by rotation.

BACKGROUND TO QUANTITATIVE MOTION ANALYSIS

Approaches used

Quantitative biomechanical analysts, like qualitative biomechanical analysts, are mainly interested in improving performance and reducing injury risk. They use a mixture of experimental and theoretical approaches to seek answers to such questions as: What is the best running technique to minimise energy expenditure? How should the sequence of body movements be coordinated in a javelin throw to maximise the distance thrown? Why are lumbar spine injuries so common among fast bowlers in cricket? Various issues in experimental (or research) design in sports biomechanics to address these and other questions are discussed in this chapter (for further elaboration of some of these research design issues, see Mullineaux, 2008; see Further Reading).

As we noted in Chapter 1, we can identify two fundamentally different approaches to experimental movement analysis in sport – qualitative analysis and quantitative analysis; the latter requires detailed measurement and evaluation of the measured data. Earlier chapters in this book had a strong bias towards qualitative analysis, whereas this chapter, along with Chapters 5 and 6, focuses mostly on quantitative analysis.

The quantitative experimental approach often takes one of two forms, usually referred to as the cross-sectional and longitudinal approaches. A cross-sectional study, for example, might evaluate a sports movement by comparing the techniques of different sports performers recorded at a particular competition. This can lead to a better overall understanding of the biomechanics of the skill studied and can help in diagnosis of faults in technique. An alternative cross-sectional approach, which is less frequently used, is to compare several trials of the same individual, for example a series of high jumps by one athlete in a competition or in a training session. This is done to identify the performance variables that correlate with success for that athlete. In a longitudinal study, the same person, or group, is analysed over a longer time to improve their performance; this probably involves providing feedback and modifying their movement patterns. Both the cross-sectional and the longitudinal approaches are relevant to the sports biomechanist, although conclusions drawn from a cross-sectional study of several athletes cannot be generalised to a single athlete or vice versa.

Movement analysts now use single-individual designs far more than in the past, recognising that group designs often obscure differences between individuals in the group and, indeed, the group mean may not apply to any single individual. After all, most athletes are mainly interested in factors that affect their own performance or might be an injury risk for them. In a case study, a single person may be analysed on one or just a few occasions; this approach is often used when assessing an injured athlete. A single-individual design usually involves studying that person across time; multiple single-individual designs study individual members of a group of performers across time. This also gives the analyst a chance to use a group design simultaneously with the multiple single-individual study. In such studies, it has been recommended that, for reasonable statistical power, 20 trials per person should be analysed for a group of five performers; for a group of 10 performers, 10 trials each; for a group of 20, five trials each. As we noted in Chapter 2, a very important consideration is the number of trials you can reasonably expect your sports performer to undertake in the time available. For maximal effort activities, fatigue and injury risk need to be carefully evaluated.

An experimental study should, to give it a theoretical underpinning, be used in conjunction with a theoretical approach, such as the use of deterministic models or some other way of identifying key factors in the movement (as in Chapter 2), or more advanced movement modelling techniques, such as computer simulation modelling or the use of artificial neural networks, which are beyond the scope of this book.

Motion capture

The main method currently used for recording and studying sports movements is digital videography. Cinematography – using cine film cameras – is now rarely used; the same almost applies to the use of 'analogue' video cameras; neither will be considered further in this chapter. On-line motion analysis systems, which automatically track markers mounted on the skin, are now commonly used in sports biomechanics research laboratories. These systems are many times more expensive than video analysis systems and are technically far more complicated, and some systems cannot be used in bright sunlight. Few students in the earlier years of their study will obtain hands-on experience of such motion analysis systems. However, because they are now routinely used in sports biomechanics research laboratories, one type of on-line motion analysis system – the one most commonly used in sports biomechanics – is introduced in this chapter (these systems are covered in more detail in Milner, 2008; see Further Reading).

A great strength of videography is that it enables the investigator to record sports movements not only in a controlled laboratory setting, but also in competition. It also minimises any possible interference with the performer. Indeed, performers can be 'videoed' without their knowledge, although this does raise serious ethical issues that would normally be addressed by your Institutional Research Ethics Committee.

Quantitative motion analysis will often involve the biomechanist having to 'digitise' a lot of data. This process of 'coordinate digitisation' involves identifying body landmarks, used to aid the estimation of joint axes of rotation, and recording their position. In videography at sports competitions, in which markers placed on the skin cannot be used, this is usually done by the investigator manually digitising the required points using a computer mouse or similar pointing device. Some software packages for quantitative biomechanical analysis of video can track markers placed on the skin of a sports performer, saving the investigator much time. In my experience, this automatic tracking option is far less reliable than on-line motion analysis systems, which are introduced later in this chapter; operator intervention is routinely necessary for complex sports movements. (These systems could be described as off-line systems with on-line capability.) On-line motion analysis systems, more accurately, I think, called automatic marker-tracking systems, as the latter name implies track markers automatically; the markers are also tracked in three-dimensional space. Even with these systems, operator intervention may still be needed if too few cameras can see a marker during some part of the movement. Whichever way coordinate digitising is performed, the linear coordinates of each digitised point are recorded and stored in computer memory.

What quantitative analysts measure

After digitising a movement sequence, linear and angular positions and displacements can be calculated and presented as a function of time – a time series (e.g. Figure 3.7). Some additional data processing will normally be performed to obtain displacements of the centre of mass of the performer's whole body (see Chapter 5). Velocities and accelerations will also probably be obtained from the displacement data (e.g. Figure 3.8). As well as these time-series movement patterns, coordination diagrams, such as angle–angle diagrams (e.g. Figures 3.11 and 3.13), phase planes (e.g. Figure 3.16), continuous relative phase (e.g. Figures 3.18 and 3.19) and cross-correlation functions (e.g. Figure 3.21) can also be obtained. Quantitative analysts often want to quantify such graphs, in contrast to the qualitative analyst, whose focus will be on their shape (topography). It should also be noted that these graphs are usually obtained from software packages for quantitative biomechanical analysis, even if they are analysed qualitatively, as in Chapter 3.

Quantitative motion analysts may also identify values of some variables at important instants in the movement to allow inter- or intra-performer comparisons (they could be measurable critical features; see Chapter 2). These values, often called performance parameters or variables, are usually defined at the key events that separate the phases of sports movements, such as foot strike in running, release of a discus or bar release in gymnastics. They are discrete measures that, although they can be very important for that performer, do not possess the richness of movement information contained in time-series graphs or coordination diagrams.

Computer visualisation, or animation, of the movement may also be possible. Simple computer visualisation is often available in video analysis software in the form of stick figure sequences, as in Figure 4.1. These are quick and easy to produce but can have ambiguities with respect to whether limbs are in front of or behind the body. In three-dimensional analysis, this can be partially overcome by filling in the body and using hidden line removal (as in Figure 4.1). Full solid-body modelling (Figure 4.2) is even more effective in this respect, but computationally somewhat time consuming. Solid-body models can also be made more realistic or dramatic through the use of animation software (for some example animation sequences of sports movements, see the Interactive eTextbook).

Calculating forces and torques (inverse dynamics)

As well as kinematic variables – specifically joint angles, angular velocities and angular accelerations – quantitative analysts also study the 'kinetics' of the movement – forces, torques and so on. This often involves the calculation of kinetic variables for joints and body segments to try to understand the underlying processes that give rise to the observed movement patterns. The method of 'inverse dynamics' is used to calculate net joint forces and moments from kinematic data, usually in combination with external force measurements from, for example, a force platform (see Chapter 5). The method of inverse dynamics is valuable in sports biomechanics research for providing an insight into the musculoskeletal dynamics that generate the observed characteristics of sports movements; we won't consider this advanced topic further in this book (readers interested in a simple introduction to the topic should see Bartlett and Bussey, 2012, listed in Further Reading). Many calculations are needed to determine net joint forces and moments, and an assessment of the measurement and data processing errors involved is important (see Challis, 2008, listed in Further Reading).

Figure 4.1 Computer visualisation of stick figures of a skier. Top: (a) front view; Middle: (b) side view; Bottom: (c) view from above.

Figure 4.2 Solid-body model of a cricket fast bowler.

VIDEOGRAPHY

Video camera and camcorders

Video technology has advanced rapidly in the third millennium. Digital video equipment has, by and large, replaced analogue video equipment; digital camcorders (a **cam**era re**corder** in which the camera and recorder are combined) have become commonplace. High definition video (HDV) is replacing standard definition video (SDV). Sports biomechanics has, unsurprisingly, been strongly influenced by these developments, which have brought sports biomechanists many benefits, but a few headaches too. One important reason for digital videography becoming so prominently used in quantitative motion analysis is that some digital video cameras can download directly to a computer without the need to record to an intermediate medium, such as a video cassette. Although some camcorders still use video cassettes, many use an internal flash memory, hard drive or SD (secure digital) card. For quantitative motion analysis, camcorder storage is an interim point between motion capture and transfer of the digital video images to a computer, where the images are stored and displayed on the computer monitor for coordinate digitising, and further data processing and analysis.

Camera sampling frequencies

Digital video recording is a sampling process; at each instance of 'sampling', an image is captured, over a short time (known, misleadingly, as the 'shutter speed'; see below) in a two-dimensional array of 'picture cells' or 'pixels'. The number of images recorded per second is usually called, in biomechanics, the 'sampling frequency' (or 'sampling rate'). Video technology uses the term 'frame rate' to refer to the number of video frames recorded per second; the two terms 'frame rate' and 'sampling frequency' are not necessary synonymous, as we shall see shortly.

As we noted in Chapter 2, most inexpensive video cameras and camcorders capture 25 frames of video per second for the PAL system, used in most of the world, and 30 frames per second for the NTSC system, used mostly in North America and Japan. Cameras that use interlaced scanning have two 'fields' that make up a video frame – in the PAL system, the fields are 0.02 s apart in time; one field contains the odd-numbered horizontal scan lines of pixels, and the other contains the even-numbered scan lines. Some computer software packages, including most of those used for quantitative motion analysis, can split an interlaced video frame into its two constituent fields, effectively doubling the sampling frequency to 50 Hz (or 60 Hz for the NTSC system), which is very important for the quantitative analysis of sports movements. However, there is a price to pay – one of our video headaches: each field has only half the vertical resolution of a frame (see below). Few sports movements – walking and, to some extent, swimming might be considered exceptions – are suitable for quantitative analysis at a sampling frequency of only 25 Hz. The 50 Hz option extends the range of sports that are suitable for quantitative biomechanical analysis to include, for example, running, the slower jumps and throws, and many gymnastic skills. (It should be noted, in passing, that the sampling rate cannot be doubled in this way, for technical reasons that need not concern us, for progressive scanning digital video cameras; they are not, therefore, a good option for quantitative motion analysis in sports biomechanics.) The limited sampling frequency is one of the two main drawbacks to the use of inexpensive PAL or NTSC digital video cameras or camcorders for quantitative analysis of sports movements. Fast human movements in sport often need sampling frequencies in the range 100 to 500 Hz; such cameras are commercially available but are more expensive than digital camcorders. The Basler 602FM digital video camera, for example, captures at 100 Hz but, with accessories and software, it is at least several times more expensive than a HD digital video camcorder; also, its resolution is only 640 × 480, it is monochrome, it records directly to a computer (via a Firewire port), which reduces its portability compared to a camcorder, and there is no viewfinder on the camera. The study of impacts between sports objects, such as bats and balls, requires even higher frame rates, typically up to 2000 Hz; these cameras are even more expensive and have their own limitations.

Image resolution

The image resolution has been the other of the two main drawbacks to the use of inexpensive PAL or NTSC digital video cameras or camcorders for quantitative motion analysis. The image resolution constrains, at least to some extent, the accuracy to which points on the image, such as anatomical landmarks, can be located. Standard definition PAL digital video (SDV) scans 720 horizontal lines of pixels per video frame with 576 pixels in each horizontal line; this resolution is rather low for the quantitative analysis of human movement in sport, particularly if each frame is split into two fields to increase the sampling frequency. It should be noted that some software packages for quantitative video analysis (or, if you prefer, video analysis systems) use interpolation of the position of the digitising cursor between pixels as a way around this problem. High definition video (HDV) comes in various specifications. Common ones have either 720 or 1080 horizontal scan lines of pixels with, respectively, 1280 or 1920 pixels per scan line. This is certainly an improvement on SDV. However, at the time of writing this book, not all software packages for quantitative biomechanical analysis can import and analyse all of the various formats (or codecs) used in HDV. Users of such software – and readers of this book – need to be aware of such limitations.

Other issues

Improvements in video technology in recent years have also included the increased availability of electronically shuttered digital video cameras. In these cameras, electronic signals are applied to the light sensor to control the time over which the incoming light is detected; this time is usually referred to, somewhat misleadingly, as the 'shutter speed'. It is essential to use cameras that have fast enough shutter speeds to obtain good quality, unblurred pictures. It is important that the camera used offers a range of shutter speeds, to suit the activity being recorded. A setting of 1/1000 s is normally adequate even for fast sports movements (see also Table 2.2); slower movements can tolerate a slower shutter speed. Be wary of the 'sports mode' function on some cheaper digital camcorders, as the shutter speed to which this setting corresponds is often not specified, and, therefore, unknown.

A further drawback to the use of most inexpensive digital video camcorders for quantitative motion analysis is that they cannot be 'genlocked' to allow the shutter openings of cameras to be synchronised when using more than one camera to record movement, as in three-dimensional studies. A few more expensive digital camcorders (e.g. the Canon XL H1 HDV 1080i) do allow genlocking, which makes them worth considering for three-dimensional analysis. Without a genlock capability, cameras can take pictures up to half a field (or 0.01 s) or a frame (0.02 s) apart; in quantitative motion analysis, this discrepancy must be corrected in the analysis software if data accuracy is not to be compromised. Digital video cameras that are fully under computer software control, such as the Basler 602FM mentioned above, can be genlocked. Some biomechanical video analysis packages (such as Simi Motion) provide shutter synchronisation for cameras controlled by their software.

Although digital camcorders are convenient and inexpensive, they often do not have interchangeable lenses, which can be useful. The quality of lenses on cheaper camcorders may result in image distortion, particularly at wide-angle settings on zoom lenses; this can lead to increased errors in digitised coordinates. Modern, solid-state digital video cameras detect the image using an array of light sensors precisely etched into silicon and are claimed to have zero geometric distortion; this is not true of the lenses, though.

Another important limitation of videography has been the vast amount of manual coordinate digitisation that has often been required for quantitative analysis. This is particularly the case when a three-dimensional analysis is undertaken, as at least two images have to be digitised for each field or frame to be analysed; it remains true in sports competitions, in which the placement of markers on the skin of competitors is not usually feasible. To overcome this drawback, specialised on-line motion-analysis systems that automatically track markers placed on the body have been developed; these systems include Vicon (www.vicon.com). These are introduced later in this chapter.

BOX 4.2 TWO-DIMENSIONAL OR THREE-DIMENSIONAL MOTION ANALYSIS?

An early decision that must be made in any quantitative video analysis of a sports movement is whether a two-dimensional or three-dimensional analysis is required. Both have advantages and disadvantages, as summarised below.

Two-dimensional motion analysis:

- Is simpler and cheaper, as fewer cameras and less other equipment are needed.
- Requires movements to be in a pre-selected plane (the plane of movement or plane of performance). It can yield acceptable results for essentially planar movements but it ignores movements out of the chosen plane. This can be important even for an event that might appear essentially two dimensional, such as the long jump. Segment movements outside of the selected plane will result in inaccurate measurement of associated joint angles.
- Is conceptually easier to relate to; this makes two-dimensional motion analysis a good starting point for aspiring quantitative biomechanical analysts, despite its many limitations.
- Requires less digitising time and has fewer methodological problems, such as the transformation of coordinates from the video image to the 'real-world' movement plane.

Three-dimensional recording and analysis:

- Involves more complex experimental procedures.
- Can show the body's true three-dimensional movements; no human movement in sport is truly two dimensional.
- Requires more equipment and is, therefore, more expensive.
- Has increased computational complexity associated with the reconstruction of the three-dimensional movement-space (or 'real-world') coordinates from the video images, and

requires software time synchronisation of the data from cameras that are not physically time synchronised (or genlocked), which is the case for most digital video cameras and camcorders.

- Allows angles between body segments to be calculated accurately, without viewing distortions. It also allows the calculation of other angles which cannot, in many cases, be easily obtained from a single camera view. One example is the horizontal plane angle between the line joining the hip joints and the line joining the shoulder joints, which can be visualised from above even if the two cameras were horizontal.
- Raises the problem of which convention to use for segment orientation angles, which two-dimensional analysis sidesteps.
- Enables the reconstruction of simulated views of the performance (e.g. Figure 4.1) other than those seen by the cameras, an extremely useful aid to movement analysis and evaluation.

Sources of error in videography

The purpose of recording human movement in sport can be formally stated as: to obtain a record that will enable the accurate measurement of the position of the centre of rotation of each of the moving body segments and of the time lapse between successive pictures. The following problems and sources of error can be identified in two-dimensional videography of sports movements:

- The three dimensionality of the position of joint centres of rotation requires the two-dimensional analysis of movements recorded from one camera to be done with care.
- Any non-coincidence of the movement plane (the plane of performance) and the plane perpendicular to the optical axis of the camera (the photographic plane) is a source of error if calibration is performed with a simple scaling object in the plane of motion.
- Perspective and parallax errors need attention. Perspective error is the apparent discrepancy in length between two objects of equal length, such as left and right limbs, when one of the limbs is closer to the camera than the other (the problem is evident in Figure 4.3(a) but not in the zoomed-in image in Figure 4.3(b)). It occurs for movements away from the photographic plane. The term is also sometimes used to refer to the error in recorded length for a limb or body segment which is at an angle to the photographic plane and, therefore, appears to be shorter than it really is. Associated with this error is that caused by viewing away from the optical axis, such that, across the movement plane, the view is not always side-on (this can be seen, for example, in the still frame sequences of Figures 1.11 and 1.15, which

Figure 4.3 Perspective error. Left: (a) two rods of identical length, held shoulder-width apart, appear to be of different lengths when photographed from a close range of 2 m; Right: (b) the same rods photographed from 9 m using a telephoto zoom lens are seen to be the same length.

were recorded, because of space limitations, with a wide-angle lens setting). This is sometimes referred to as parallax error. The combined result of these optical errors is that limbs nearer to the camera appear bigger and appear to travel further than those further away. This causes errors in the digitised coordinates.

- Lens distortions may be a source of error, particularly at wide-angle settings on inexpensive zoom lenses.
- Locations of joint axes of rotation are only estimates, based on the positions of superficial skin markers or identification of anatomical landmarks. Use of skin markers may help but can also hinder the movement analyst, as these markers move with respect to the underlying bone and to one another. The digitising of such markers, or estimating the positions of axes of rotation without their use, is probably the major source of random error ('noise') in recorded joint coordinates. A study that highlighted this point is considered later in this chapter. Locating joint axes of rotation is particularly difficult when the joint is obscured by other body parts or by clothing.

- Other possible sources of error include blurring of the image, camera vibration and digitising errors – related to image resolution and human operator errors, and computer round-off errors.

For three-dimensional analysis, there are other potential error sources, although several of those described above are partly or wholly overcome:

- Relating the two-dimensional video image coordinates to the three-dimensional movement-space ('real-world') coordinates may be a source of error. Use of an array of calibration points, such as a calibration object (see Figure 4.4(b) in the next section) is probably the most common method. Errors within the calibration volume can be accurately assessed, while those outside that volume will be larger and more difficult to assess. Errors will increase with the ratio of the size of the movement space to that of the image.
- All the calibration points must be clearly visible on the images from both cameras; they must also have three-dimensional coordinates that are accurately known.
- Placement of cameras must relate to the algorithm chosen for reconstruction of the movement-space coordinates. Errors will be caused by deviations from this requirement.

In summary, digitised coordinate data will be contaminated with measurement inaccuracies or errors. These will be random (noise), systematic, or both. All obvious systematic errors, such as those caused by lens distortion and errors in calibration objects, should be identified and removed, for example by calibration or software corrections. Any remaining sources of systematic error will then be very small or of low frequency and will, therefore, have little effect on velocities and accelerations. The remaining random noise in the displacement data, expressed as relative errors, has been estimated as within 1 per cent for a point in the photographic plane for two-dimensional videography and within 2 per cent for a point in the calibration volume for three-dimensional videography. Random errors must be minimised at source by good experimental procedures. Any remaining noise should be removed, as far as possible, from the digitised data before further data processing. These two aspects will be covered in the next two sections. Also, consideration needs to be given to the estimation of errors in digitised coordinate data and their effects on the accuracy of variables calculated from those coordinates; this will be considered briefly later in this chapter.

EXPERIMENTAL VIDEOGRAPHY PROCEDURES

Two-dimensional recording procedures

The following steps have often been considered necessary to minimise errors recorded during two-dimensional videography, thereby improving data accuracy. These steps are particularly useful for students who are unfamiliar with the use of videography. These

Figure 4.4 Typical calibration objects. Left: (a) 'chequerboard' of 100 mm squares often used for two-dimensional image calibration; Middle: (b) calibration frame often used for three-dimensional videography; Right: (c) calibration wand used in the Vicon automatic marker-tracking system.

procedures also allow a simple linear transformation from image to movement-plane coordinates using simple scale information recorded in the field of view.

- The camera should be mounted on a stationary, rigid tripod pointing towards the centre of the movement plane; no panning or tilting of the camera should be used.
- The camera should be sited as far from the action as possible to reduce perspective error (this is clearly evident in Figure 4.3). A telephoto zoom lens should be used to bring the performer's image to the required size.
- The focal length of the lens should be carefully adjusted to focus the image. This is best done, for zoom lenses, by zooming in on the performer, focusing and then zooming out to the required field of view. The field of view should be adjusted to coincide with the area that is to be recorded. This maximises the size of the performer on the projected image and increases the accuracy of digitising.
- Once the field of view has been set, the focal length of the lens must be kept constant – this means that the auto-focus option available on most digital video camcorders must be switched off, so that focusing is under manual control.
- The movement plane should be perpendicular to the optical axis of the camera. This requires careful attention and can be done in various ways, including the use of laser levelling devices, spirit levels, plumb lines and right-angled (3–4–5) triangles. If the movement takes place in a vertical movement plane on a level horizontal surface, this requirement means that the optical axis of the camera must be both horizontal and at 90° to the vertical movement plane.

Figure 4.5 Possible camera placements for movement such as long jump.

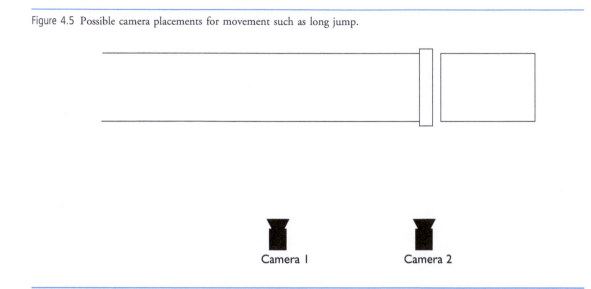

Camera 1   Camera 2

- Horizontal and vertical length scales – two one-metre rules are often adequate – and a vertical reference, for example a plumb line, must be included in the field of view. The length scales must be positioned in the plane of motion. Their lengths should be at least that required to give a scaling error, when digitised, of no more than 0.5 per cent of the field of view. Other means of performing scaling include the use of objects resembling chequerboards (Figure 4.4(a)) – if large enough, these allow calibration and accuracy checks across the whole field of view. This is rarely practical if filming in sports competitions, and is unnecessary providing strict experimental procedures are adopted throughout. Once in the correct position, the calibration object is captured on a short video clip; this is sometimes done both before and after video recording of the movements to be studied.
- The background should be as uncluttered as possible, plain and non-reflective. In a laboratory study, contrasting performer–background colours can be helpful.
- For particularly long movements, such as the long and triple jumps, consideration should be given to using two or more cameras to cover the filming area (Figure 4.5); with cameras and camcorders with no genlock capability, another method for event synchronisation will be needed, as discussed below.
- The use of colour contrast markers on appropriate body landmarks is usually recommended (see also Box 6.2). For two-dimensional analysis, these are usually placed to correspond to an axis through the appropriate joint centre, as seen from the camera, when the performer is standing in a specific position and posture: these markers are sometimes referred to (somewhat misleadingly) as 'joint centre' markers. The use of such markers is not normally possible in competition, and has some potential disadvantages when digitising (see below). If using markers, then marking the skin

Figure 4.6 Aliasing. The red signal sampled at the dashed vertical lines is aliased to the (smoothed) black signal, as the sampling frequency is far too low.

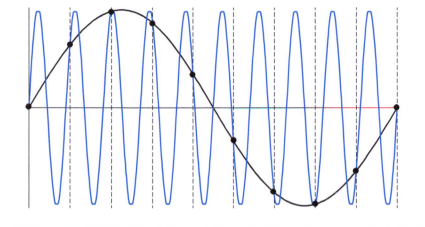

directly can be less problematic than using adhesive markers, which can fall off. A procedure sometimes used in laboratory-based research is to use markers from automatic-marker tracking systems, which are light coloured and reflective, attached to the skin with double-sided adhesive tape through small holes cut in tight-fitting clothing. This is illustrated in Figures 1.17 and 1.19 to 1.24 and, for example, in some of the video clips for quantitative analysis in the Interactive eTextbook.

- To reduce the risk of marker detachment, and to help cope with segmental movement out of the photographic plane, bands can be taped around a segment at the landmarks used to identify the 'joint centre'. This can work well, when the markers are manually digitised, for the wrist, elbow, knee and ankle joints, but is not possible for some other joints, such as the shoulder and hip.

- If axes of rotation are being estimated from anatomical landmarks, skin markers are not essential, although their use probably saves time when manually digitising; they also allow, at least in principle, automated digitising. For standard placement of markers for a two-dimensional study, see Table 5.1 and Box 6.2.

- A sufficiently high sampling frequency should be used, as discussed earlier in this chapter. The Nyquist sampling theorem requires that the sampling frequency is at least twice the maximum frequency in the signal (not twice the maximum frequency of interest) to avoid aliasing (Figure 4.6). Aliasing is a phenomenon seen in movies when wheels on cars and stage coaches, for example, appear to revolve backwards. Furthermore, the temporal resolution – the inverse of the sampling frequency – improves the precision of both the displacement data and their time derivatives. For accurate time measurements, or to reduce errors in velocities and accelerations, higher sampling frequencies may be needed (see Appendix 4.1).

- If a choice of lighting conditions is available, then natural daylight is usually preferable. If artificial lighting is used, floodlights need to be placed with care to illuminate the required area evenly and without too much shadow. Three floodlights, one mounted behind the camera (to point more or less along the optical axis of the camera) and one to each side, at 30° to the plane of movement, usually give good illumination. Careful attention must also be given to lighting when choosing the camera shutter speed.

- Whenever possible, information should be incorporated within the camera's field of view, identifying important features such as the name of the performer and date. The 'take number' is especially important when videography is used in conjunction with other data acquisition methods, such as force plates (see Chapter 5) or electromyography (see Chapter 6). When recording forces or electromyograms (EMGs) in addition to using videography, event synchronisation can be obtained by the use of an event marker, usually a light situated in the camera's field of view, triggered by the start of force or EMG data capture (a short video clip that illustrates this is available in the Interactive eTextbook).

- The recording of the movement should be as unobtrusive as possible. The performer may need to become accustomed to performing in front of a camera in an experimental context. The number of experimenters should be kept to the bare minimum in such studies.

- In controlled studies, away from competition, as little clothing as possible should be worn by the performers to minimise errors in locating body landmarks, providing that this does not affect their performance.

- In any videography study, written informed consent should be obtained from all participants; in sport, the coach may be able to provide consent for his or her athletes, but this varies from country to country and should always be checked. Furthermore, approval from an appropriate Research Ethics Committee is normally required.

The above procedures impose some unnecessary restrictions on two-dimensional videography, leading to severe practical limitations on camera placements, particularly in sports competitions, because of the requirement that the optical axis of the camera is perpendicular to the movement plane. A more flexible camera placement can be obtained, for example by the use of a two-dimensional version of the direct linear transformation (see below). This overcomes some of the camera location problems that arise in sports competitions because of spectators, officials and advertising hoardings. It requires the use of a more complex transformation from image to movement plane coordinates. Many of the above procedural steps then become redundant, but others, similar to those used in three-dimensional analysis, are introduced. This more flexible approach can also be extended to allow for camera panning. You should assess which of the steps in the above procedures could not be ensured if filming at a national-standard sports competition (see Study Task 5).

Digitising procedures

Various software packages are available for digitising and quantitative analysis of videos of sports movements. These include APAS (www.arielnet.com), Simi Motion (www.simi.com) and MaxTRAQ Educational (www.motionanalysisproducts.com). These systems have varying functionality and some idiosyncrasies. You should seek to obtain access to, and become familiar with using, such a system to undertake Study Tasks 9 and 10; APAS and MaxTRAQ Educational are fairly inexpensive for students. When digitising, attention should be paid to the following points:

- If joint centre markers are used, careful attention must be paid to their movement relative to underlying bones. If segments move in, or are seen in, a plane other than that for which the markers were placed, the marker will no longer lie along the axis through the joint as seen by the camera. To minimise errors, you need a thorough anatomical knowledge of the joints and the location of their axes of rotation with respect to superficial landmarks throughout the range of segmental orientations. It should also be noted that many joint axes of flexion–extension are not exactly perpendicular to the sagittal plane often filmed for two-dimensional analysis.
- If autotracking markers, be aware that the software will track a marker even when it moves out of alignment with the axis of rotation of the relevant joint; this obviously introduces an error.
- The alignment and scaling of the projected image must be checked; independent horizontal and vertical scalings must be performed.
- At least one recorded sequence should be digitised several times to check on operator reliability (consistency). It is also recommended that more than one person should digitise a complete sequence to check on operator objectivity. (Reliability and objectivity are considered further in Box 4.3.)
- The accuracy of digitised data can be improved by frequent checks on the accuracy of the software package used, and by careful adherence to good experimental protocols (as above), including careful calibration. The accuracy of digitised data is often assessed by the analysis of a relevant and standard criterion sequence and by carrying out checks on all calculations. Video recording of a falling object is sometimes used as a criterion sequence, as the object's acceleration is known. (Accuracy is the closeness of a measured value to the true value, which is often unknown; precision is the agreement of several measurements of the same value among themselves – somewhat similar to reliability; precision does not guarantee accuracy.)

Three-dimensional recording procedures

Some, but not all, of the procedures for two-dimensional videography also apply to three-dimensional videography. The major requirements of three-dimensional analysis are discussed in this section. It is recommended that readers should gain good experience in all aspects of two-dimensional quantitative analysis before attempting three-dimensional analysis.

- For reconstruction of the three-dimensional movement-space coordinates of a point, at least two cameras are needed. The cameras should ideally be genlocked to provide shutter (or 'time') synchronisation; as we have noted several times above, this is not possible with most inexpensive digital video cameras and camcorders.

- Furthermore, synchronisation is also needed to link the events being recorded by the two cameras (event synchronisation). Event synchronisation can be achieved by the use of synchronised character generators if the cameras can be genlocked. For cameras that cannot be genlocked, event synchronisation can be achieved simply by an event marker, such as a light switching on, placed in the fields of view of all cameras (as outlined above). Time synchronisation then needs to be performed mathematically at a later stage; obviously some error is involved in this process. It also may not be possible, again particularly in sports competitions, to include an event marker in the fields of view of the cameras. Some other event synchronisation will then need to be used, based on information available from the recorded sports movement, such as the instant of take-off in a jump.

- From two or more sets of image coordinates, some method is needed to reconstruct the three-dimensional movement-space coordinates. Several algorithms can be used for this purpose and the choice of the algorithm may have some procedural implications. Most of these algorithms involve the explicit or implicit reconstruction of the line (or ray) from each camera that is directed towards the point of interest, such as a skin marker. The location of that point is then estimated as that which is closest to the intersection of the rays from the two or more cameras.

- Flexible camera positions can be achieved with the most commonly used reconstruction algorithm, the 'direct linear transformation' (DLT). This transforms the video image coordinates to movement-space coordinates by camera calibration involving independently treated transformation parameters for each camera. The algorithm requires a minimum of six calibration (or control) points with known three-dimensional coordinates and measured image coordinates to establish the DLT (transformation) parameters, or coefficients, for each camera independently. The DLT parameters incorporate the optical parameters of the camera and linear lens distortion factors. Because of the errors in sports biomechanical data, the DLT equations also incorporate residual error terms. The equations can then be solved directly by minimisation of the sum of the squares of the residuals. Once the DLT parameters have been established for each camera, the unknown movement-space coordinates of other points, such as skin markers, can then be reconstructed using the DLT parameters and the image coordinates for all cameras. Additional DLT parameters can also be included, if necessary, to allow for symmetrical lens distortion and asymmetrical lens distortions caused by decentring of the lens elements. No improvements in accuracy are usually achieved by incorporating non-linear lens distortions. The DLT algorithms impose several experimental restrictions.

Figure 4.7 Three-dimensional DLT camera set-up. Note that the rays from the calibration spheres are unambiguous for both cameras; for clarity, only the rays from the front spheres are traced to one camera and only the rays from the rear spheres to the other camera.

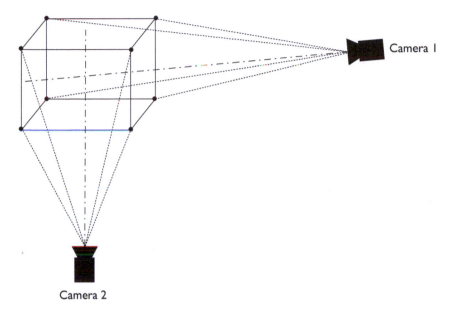

Camera 1

Camera 2

○ An array of calibration (or control) points is needed, the coordinates of which are accurately known with respect to three mutually perpendicular axes. In videography, this is usually provided by some form of calibration frame (for example, Figures 4.4(b) or 4.7) or similar structure. The accuracy of the coordinates of the calibration points is paramount, as it determines the maximum accuracy of other measurements. In filming activities such as kayaking, ski jumping, skiing or javelin flight just after release, a group of vertical calibration poles, on which markers have been carefully positioned, may be easier to use than a calibration frame. The coordinates of the markers on the poles need to be accurately measured; this often requires the use of surveying equipment. The use of calibration poles is generally more flexible and allows for a larger calibration volume than does a calibration frame. The more calibration points used, the stronger and more reliable is the reconstruction.

○ All the calibration points must be visible to each camera and their image coordinates must be clearly and unambiguously distinguishable, as in Figure 4.4(b). Calibration poles or limbs of calibration frames should not, therefore, overlap or nearly overlap, when viewed from any camera.

○ Although an angle of 90° between the optical axes of the cameras might be considered ideal, deviations from this can be tolerated if kept within a range of about

60–120°. The cameras should also be placed so as to give the best views of the performer.

○ Accurate coordinate reconstruction can only be guaranteed within the space – the calibration (or control) volume – defined by the calibration (or control) points. These should, therefore, be equally distributed within or around the volume in which the sports movement takes place. Errors depend on the distribution of the calibration points and increase if the performer moves beyond the confines of the calibration volume. This is the most serious restriction on the use of the DLT algorithm. It has led to the development of other methods which require smaller calibration objects or the 'wand' technique now used by many automatic marker-tracking systems. All of these alternatives have greater computational complexity than the relatively straightforward DLT algorithm.

○ It is often convenient to define the axes of the reference system to coincide with directions of interest for the sports movement being investigated. The International Society of Biomechanics (ISB) recommends a right-handed coordinate system, in which the x-axis corresponds to the main direction of horizontal motion, and the y-axis is vertical; this recommendation is not universally adhered to.

• If markers are used, even greater attention must be paid to their movement relative to underlying bones than in a two-dimensional study. The markers, whether points or bands (see above), must be seen only as a guide to the location of the underlying joint centres of rotation. To minimise errors, you need an even more thorough anatomical knowledge of the joints and the location of their axes of rotation with respect to superficial landmarks throughout the range of segmental orientations than for a two-dimensional study. This becomes even more essential if markers are not used.

• To circumvent the problem of a small image size, which would prevent identification of body landmarks if the calibration volume was very large, panning cameras can be used. Three-dimensional reconstruction techniques that allow two cameras to rotate freely about their vertical axis – panning – and horizontal axis – tilting – have been developed. In these techniques, the cameras must be in known positions. These approaches have also been extended to allow for variation of the focal lengths of the camera lenses during filming.

• It is obviously necessary to check the validity of these methods. This can be done by calculating the root mean squared (RMS) error between the reconstructed and known three-dimensional coordinates of points, preferably ones that have not been used to determine the DLT parameters. Furthermore, the success with which these methods reproduce three-dimensional movements can be checked, for example by filming the three-dimensional motion of a body segment of known dimensions or a rod thrown into the air. In addition, reliability and objectivity checks should be carried out on the digitised data (as, for example, in the two-dimensional study discussed in Box 4.3).

INTRODUCTION TO ON-LINE MOTION ANALYSIS SYSTEMS

Objectives and background

There are various types of on-line motion analysis system. Some, generally not favoured in sports biomechanics, use active (electrically activated) markers or magnetic sensors; they are not considered further here. The system most used in sports biomechanics uses passive reflective markers and special pulsating light sources, usually around each camera (Figure 4.8 (a); and see, for example, www.vicon.com, www.motionanalysis.com). The light is usually visible red or infra-red. The principle of operation is simple. The light sources on each camera pulse at the camera sampling frequency (usually variable and in the range 100–1000 Hz) and are synchronised with the electronic shutters of the cameras, of which there are usually between eight and 16 in a sports biomechanics laboratory set-up. The light is reflected by each marker (see Figure 4.8(b) and (c)) and these reflections are detected by the cameras to which a particular marker is visible. It should be noted that these systems only show the positions of the markers (the spots of light); unlike in the photographs in Figure 4.8(b) and (c) and in a video image, no 'person' is visible.

The resolution of the cameras used by these systems is typically better than for digital videography. The Vicon T160 camera, a high-end example, has an image resolution of 4704×3456 pixels (16 Megapixels) at up to 120 Hz, and 4704×1728 at 240 Hz; the camera can sample up to 2000 Hz, but with further loss of resolution – 240 Hz is adequate for many sports biomechanics applications.

Some of the procedures that we considered in the previous section are applicable here too, but these systems also have other procedural considerations. The procedures for on-line systems basically fall into four categories: data collection; data processing; data analysis; and data interpretation. Only the first two will concern us here (for further details of all of these procedures, see Milner, 2008, listed in Further Reading).

Data collection procedures

Hardware set-up

Some of these procedures are similar to those used for three-dimensional videography. The investigator needs to check all of the camera lens settings. The location and dimensions of the calibration volume (the term 'capture volume' is sometimes used) need to be established. This is the space in the laboratory, or elsewhere (some on-line system cameras can be used outdoors), in which the movement being analysed will take place (the movement space, if you like). For accuracy, this volume must be large enough to encompass all of the motion but not much larger, as this volume needs to be calibrated to relate the camera images to the coordinates of the movement space. The investigator then places the cameras appropriately around the calibration volume, ensuring that the amount of 'dead space' (the space seen through the camera outside of the calibration volume) is minimised in the field of view of each camera

Figure 4.8 Top: (a) Camera from a Vicon motion analysis system. Bottom: (b) left and (c) rear views of a whole-body marker set used in conjunction with the Vicon on-line motion analysis system and Visual3D. Note the use of marker clusters on the upper arm and thigh and the asymmetrical marker placements on contralateral limbs; note also the medial ankle, knee and elbow markers, used in the static trial but not in the main data collection.

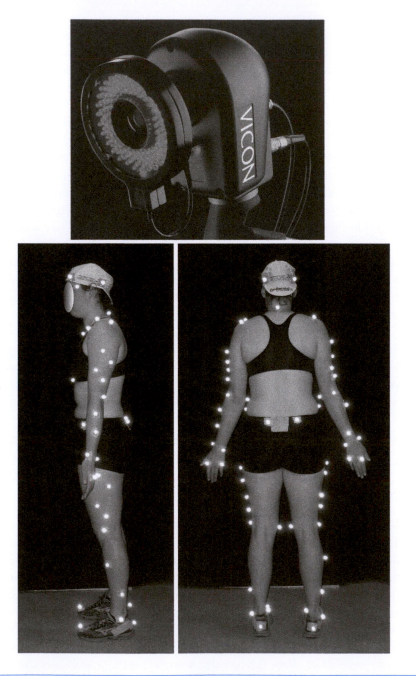

(this is done by changing the lens settings or moving the cameras). An appropriate sampling frequency for the movement being analysed is then selected. Other hardware, such as force plates (see Chapter 5) and electromyographs (see Chapter 6), can then be synchronised at an appropriate sampling frequency (which should be the same as, or an integer multiple of, the camera sampling frequency) – this synchronisation is routine in on-line systems, unlike in videography; one or more computer-controlled digital video cameras can also be properly synchronised with the system cameras.

Calibration

For a successful calibration of the movement space, the camera sensitivities should be adjusted to give good image brightness without any 'ghost' markers (ones that are not system markers); at the same time, the investigator will check for other stray reflections in each camera's field of view, and usually mask these out if no other remedy is possible. Calibration for on-line motion analysis systems is normally done in two stages: static calibration and dynamic calibration. Static calibration involves setting the origin and orientation of the fixed laboratory (or global) coordinate system, often by placing the calibration wand (Figure 4.4(c)), or a similar object, on the floor at a specific place (often, in a biomechanics laboratory, the corner of a force plate). As noted in the previous section, the ISB recommends the x-axis to be that of the main movement with the y-axis vertical; the z-axis is the third axis in the right-handed co-ordinate system. Most dynamic calibrations use the wand method, in which the wand (Figure 4.4(c)) is moved systematically by an investigator around the whole capture volume. Depending on the size of the capture volume, the wand method can give reconstruction errors (residuals) for the calibration points on the wand of less than 1 mm; an acceptable value of the residual needs to be decided for a particular set-up. It is essential to ensure that a valid calibration is maintained throughout data collection; it helps to have cameras rigidly mounted, for example on walls, rather than on tripods, although this reduces the flexibility with which the cameras can be placed.

Marker identification

Most passive on-line systems now identify markers very well. Marker identification in passive systems normally has two stages. The first stage is to ascertain which of the co-ordinate pairs (x, y) from each camera is associated with the three-dimensional coordinates of one (unspecified) marker; this involves marker tracking and is usually done in real time as data are captured. This is most commonly done by projecting the 'inverse ray' from each camera onto each marker in the movement space and finding points of near intersection of the rays from two or more cameras. Ambiguities can arise if two markers are coplanar (in the same plane) with each other and with the optical centres of the only two cameras to which the markers are visible (ghost markers can then arise). This problem can be overcome if a third camera can see the markers. Arguably, therefore, enough cameras should be used to prevent any marker ever being visible to only two cameras. Some might consider this over-restrictive, as markers and camera axes are unlikely to remain coplanar for more than a few frames with good camera placements. The second stage in marker identification is marker 'labelling', which involves deciding to which physical marker each marker 'triplet' (the three-dimensional coordinates of one marker in one image) belongs; this is by far the more troublesome of the two stages and is usually done during post-processing. It is accomplished by marker tracking and prediction of marker positions in three dimensions, to reduce ambiguities in apparent marker merging in two-dimensional camera views. The process is further supported, in some on-line systems, by having markers linked in an 'anatomical' model, which also helps correct the re-identification of temporarily obscured markers.

If markers were placed on bones, or pins attached to bones, our tasks as movement analysts would be much easier. Clearly this is rarely possible and is, generally, impossible in sports biomechanics. Instead, markers are mounted on, or above, the skin (as in Figure 4.8(b) and (c)) and are not, therefore, stationary with respect to the underlying bone; inter-marker distances change with movement. This is the main error source for data obtained from on-line motion analysis systems. Generally, the bigger the marker, the worse the problem; small markers with low inertia are better. Correct procedures can reduce errors caused by marker movements (sometime called skin movement artefacts). Marker clusters can be used to introduce redundancy, by increasing the number of markers on a segment, and to allow more flexible camera locations. Marker clusters can be deformable, when the markers are mounted on the skin, as in Figure 4.8(b) and (c), or on an elastic bandage; rigid marker clusters are mounted on a rigid plate and behave as a rigid body.

For any marker to be 'reconstructed' accurately, it needs to be visible to enough cameras; the use of at least three cameras is generally recommended (two will often, but not always, be adequate, as noted above). We need at least three markers per body segment. The movement of markers or marker clusters relative to the underlying bone must be minimised. Markers need to be in the correct places, but what are the correct places? Putting markers on bony prominences can cause errors (these have been estimated at up to 50 per cent for knee valgus–varus with markers placed on bony protuberances at the hip, knee and ankle). However, to help identify joint centres, some markers need to be placed on bony prominences near joints. On the other hand, putting markers on soft tissue also incurs movement with respect to bone and causes marker 'wobble'. Yet some mid-segment markers or marker clusters need to be placed on soft tissue. Trying to minimise errors caused by marker movement relative to underlying bones is an ongoing problem for movement analysts using on-line motion analysis systems.

To help to identify markers, to define a zero reference position for joint angles and to define joint centre locations, most passive marker-tracking systems use one or more static trials. In a static trial, the participant stands in the capture volume in a position similar to that of the person in Figure 4.8(b) and (c) but with the arms abducted towards the horizontal with the palms facing downwards. Manual identification of the markers is usually needed at this stage. Extra markers are often used in this trial to help locate joint centres; these are shown on the medial elbows, knees and ankles in Figure 4.8(b) and (c). (The static trial is, somewhat misleadingly, also called a 'static calibration trial', easily mistaken for the 'static calibration' of the movement space discussed above – the term 'static calibration trial' should, in my opinion, be avoided for this reason.)

Marker set selection and development

Many on-line motion analysis systems come with a standard (built-in) marker set, usually intended mainly for clinical gait analysis. These marker sets, normally of around three dozen or so markers (when used for the whole body), are usually derived from the New-ington–Helen Hayes marker set (see Milner, 2008, listed in Further Reading for more detail). We have measured differences between sessions (when the markers were removed then reattached by the same investigator) of more than 3° for knee flexion–extension in treadmill walking. We have also noted, with the standard marker set for the motion analysis system in our laboratory at the University of Otago, that the anterior–posterior placement of the thigh marker is crucial for correct alignment of the knee flexion–extension axis. This marker should lie in the plane containing the hip and knee joint centres and the knee flexion–extension axis, and off any muscle belly; getting this correct can be quite tricky and considerable errors arise if the marker position is wrong, particularly for knee joint movements outside the sagittal plane.

Investigators need to decide on the marker set to be used for a particular movement. You have a choice, basically, between the use of the standard marker set for a particular system, which is convenient as the system will then calculate variables such as joint angles, or the design of a customised marker set. The latter may be done in the on-line system's software or using a separate software package, such as Visual3D (www.c-motion.com/products/visual3d), a graphical package that, among other things, calculates three-dimensional joint angles from marker data. Milner (2008; see Further Reading) advises investigators to: develop and use a cluster-based marker set; introduce asymmetry into the marker set to aid tracking (as for the limbs in Figure 4.8(b) and (c)); choose a suitable marker size; use an appropriate method of marker attachment (you don't want them to fall off); and take great care with marker placement. The last of these points is absolutely crucial; poor marker placement will lead to errors (a qualification in kinanthropometry is very useful for a motion analyst working with these systems).

Data processing

Although on-line systems are designed to track and label markers automatically, and they often do this very well, investigators need to exercise considerable care to ensure this. It is essential to make sure that markers are correctly identified in each image. They will need to be identified manually during the static trials; they should then, in principle, be tracked automatically during the movement that is being analysed, but this is far from foolproof, particularly in complex sports movements. Occasionally, markers will become occluded. It is then necessary to consider how to fill any gaps in marker trajectories. Views on this vary. Milner (2008; see Further Reading) recommends automatic spline gap-filling for up to five data points; some system manuals suggest up to 15 frames at 100 Hz. It is really important not to use gap-filling automatically at peaks or changes of direction of a marker's trajectory. Some systems offer various gap-filling options, such as spline filling and pattern filling. The latter is often based on the shape of a similar trajectory, for example filling the trajectory of the left anterior superior iliac spine (ASIS) based on that of the right ASIS. Once all the trajectories have been checked and gaps dealt with appropriately, further data processing includes deleting unmarked markers (ghosts) and data filtering. Three-dimensional joint angles then need to be calculated; this is by no means a trivial task. Visual3D is an interactive graphical package that makes this task much easier, although its use does not exclude the possibility of errors, particularly those caused by inappropriate marker placements.

Some final thoughts on on-line motion analysis systems

Passive marker-tracking systems are generally preferred for sports movements. Tracking markers that are not attached to bones is a major source of error; marker clusters and well-placed markers can reduce, but not remove, these errors. Important procedures for on-line motion analysis systems include data collection (hardware set-up, calibration, marker identification, and marker set selection and development) and data processing, including inspection of all marker trajectories and gap-filling. On-line motion analysis systems, despite their sophistication and complexity, are not free from error, particularly for joint movements not in the sagittal plane; marker placements and movements are the source of most of these errors. On-line marker-tracking systems cannot be used in most, if not all, sports competitions for various reasons, many not to do with the systems themselves. (For more details on these systems, see Milner, 2008, listed in Further Reading.)

DATA PROCESSING

Noisy data

The data obtained from digitising, either before or after transformation to three-dimensional coordinates, are often referred to as 'raw' data. Many difficulties arise when processing raw kinematic data and this can lead to large errors. As noted in previous sections, some errors can be minimised by careful equipment selection and rigorous attention to experimental procedures. However, the digitised coordinates will still contain random errors (noise).

The importance of this noise removal can be seen from consideration of an extremely simplified representation of a recorded sports movement, with a coordinate (r) expressed by the equation:

$$r = 2\sin4\pi t + 0.02\sin40\pi t$$

The first term on the right-hand side of this equation ($2\sin4\pi t$) represents the motion being observed, known, in this context, as the 'signal'. The amplitude of this signal is

Figure 4.9 Simple example of noise-free data, shown by dashed black lines, and noisy data, shown by red lines. Top: (a) displacement; Middle: (b) velocity; Bottom: (c) acceleration.

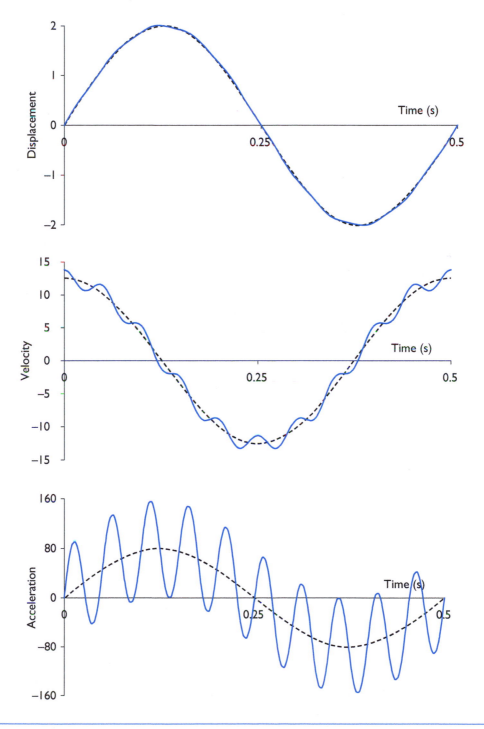

2 – in arbitrary units – and its frequency is 4π radians/s (or 2 Hz) – indicated by $\sin4\pi t$. The second term is the noise; this has an amplitude of only 1 per cent of the signal (this would be a low value for many sports biomechanics studies) and a frequency of 40π radians/s (or 20 Hz), 10 times that of the signal. The difference in frequencies is because human movement generally has a low frequency content and noise is at a higher frequency. Figure 4.9(a) shows the signal with the noise superimposed; it should be noted that the difference between the noise-free and noisy displacement curves is barely noticeable. The above equation can now be differentiated with respect to time (sorry, but this detour into the basics of differential calculus is necessary) to give velocity (v), which in turn can be differentiated with respect to time to give acceleration (a):

$$v = 8\pi\cos4\pi t + 0.8\pi\cos40\pi t$$

$$a = -32\pi^2\sin4\pi t - 32\pi^2\sin40\pi t.$$

The noise amplitude in the velocity is now 10 per cent ($0.8\pi/8\pi \times 100$) of the signal amplitude (Figure 4.9(b)). The noise in the acceleration data has the same amplitude, $32\pi^2$, as the signal, which is an intolerable error (Figure 4.9(c)). Unless the errors in the displacement data are reduced by smoothing or filtering (see Appendix 4.1), they will lead to considerable inaccuracies in velocities and accelerations and any other derived data. This will be compounded by any errors in body segment data (see below).

Body segment inertia parameters

Various body segment inertia parameters are used in movement analysis. The mass of each body segment and the segment centre of mass position are used in calculating the position of the whole-body centre of mass (see Chapter 5). These values, and segment moments of inertia, are used in calculations of net joint forces and moments using the method of inverse dynamics. The most accurate and valid values available for these inertia parameters should obviously be used. Ideally, they should be obtained from, or scaled to, the sports performer being studied. The values of body segment parameters used in sports biomechanics have been obtained from cadavers and from living persons, including measurements of the performers being filmed.

Cadaver studies have provided very accurate segmental data. However, limited sample sizes throw doubt on the extrapolation of these data to a general sports population. They are also highly questionable because of the unrepresentative samples in respect of sex, age and morphology. Problems also arise from the use of different dissection techniques by different researchers, losses in tissue and body fluid during dissection and degeneration associated with the state of health preceding death. Segment mass may be expressed as a simple fraction of total body mass or, more accurately, in the form of a linear regression equation with one or more anthropometric variables. Even the latter may cause under- or overestimation errors of total body mass as large as 4.6 per cent.

Obtaining body segment parameter data from sports performers may require sophisticated equipment and a great deal of the performer's time. Body segment data can be, or have been, obtained from living people using gamma-ray scanning or various medical imaging techniques, such as computerised tomography, magnetic resonance imaging and dual-energy X-ray absorptiometry (DXA). These may eventually supersede the cadaver data that are still too often used in sports biomechanics, but they are expensive and are not error free. Several 'mathematical' models exist which calculate body segment parameters from standard anatomical measurements, such as segment lengths and circumferences. Some of these models result in large errors even in estimates of segment volumes. Others are very time consuming, requiring up to 200 anthropometric measurements, which can take at least an hour or two to complete. Another approach, which is becoming more common, is to use a three-dimensional optical body scanner and three-dimensional computer-aided design (CAD) software. The body is scanned in height increments, for example of 2.5 mm, with hundreds of thousands of points on the body surface being scanned. All these methods require density values from other sources, usually cadavers, and most of them assume constant density throughout the segment, or throughout large parts of the segment. The greatest problems in body segment data occur for moments of inertia. Many estimations based on mathematical models, imaging or body scanning are either inaccurate or require further validation. Relative errors of 5–8 per cent in segmental moments of inertia have been reported.

Error propagation – a quick overview

Errors in the results of biomechanical data processing can be large, particularly when calculating kinetic variables from motion analysis data. This is mainly because of errors in the body segment data and linear and angular velocities and accelerations, and the combination of these errors in inverse dynamics equations (known, somewhat delightfully, as 'error propagation'). If such calculations are to be attempted, scrupulous adherence to good experimental protocols is essential. A rigorous assessment of the data processing techniques is also necessary. The topic of error analysis is a very important one and the value of sports biomechanical measurements cannot be assessed fully in the absence of a quantification of the measurement error. Error propagation in calculations can be estimated using standard formulae (see Challis, 2008, listed in Further Reading for further discussion of this somewhat advanced topic).

BOX 4.3 A CAUTIONARY TALE OF UNRELIABLE DATA

As we noted many times in Chapter 3, one of the major tasks for movement analysts is to be able to analyse coordination patterns in sport. A particular interest of some movement analysts, including me, is the variability that we find in coordination patterns, such as angle–angle diagrams (see, for example, Figure 3.12), when even a highly skilled performer repeats a movement – this variability is also observed in movement patterns seen as a function of time. Of considerable interest to applied researchers is whether we can accurately and reliably assess such movement variability in competition.

To answer this question, some of my colleagues at the University of Otago and I carried out a study to compare the reliability of estimating movement patterns in laboratory and simulated field conditions. Both conditions were recorded using a digital video camera viewing perpendicular to the sagittal plane of the runner in our laboratory. The difference between the two conditions was as follows: in the 'laboratory' condition, the participant had reflective markers attached to his skin through small holes in tight-fitting polypropylene clothing to improve identification of joint axes of rotation; in the 'simulated field' condition, no markers were used, as they cannot be used in sports competitions. Although this is not the only difference between laboratory and real field conditions, it is usually the most important one by far. The participant ran five trials in each condition at the same speed on a treadmill with equal rest periods between trials. From each trial, we selected three strides to be digitised – this means that a human operator identified each marker on each video frame, manually tracking the markers or estimating the positions of the joints in the no-marker condition. We also tracked the markers automatically using Simi Motion software (www.simi.com). Four experienced movement analysts digitised the five no-marker trials on consecutive days (these were digitised first to prevent any possible learning effects from digitising the trials with markers). Five marker trials were then auto-tracked using Simi Motion and manually tracked by the four movement analysts on consecutive days.

Several sources of variability, or variance, are present in this design. The one of interest to movement analysts is movement variability – the variance among trials. The next two sources are due to variability within and among the human operators (the four movement analysts), respectively known as intra-operator variability and inter-operator variability. The first of these, in our study, was the variance across days and the second that across the four operators. There are other sources of variance from the three two-factor and the one three-factor interactions between our three main factors – trials, days and people; these interactions will be lumped together here. We then used a statistical technique known as Analysis of Variance (ANOVA) to partition the variances between the three main effects and the several interactions. The results for the marker and the no-marker conditions are summarised in the pie charts of Figure 4.10(a) and (c) for the marker condition and Figure 4.10(b) and (d) for the no-marker condition.

Small variances across repeated attempts by the same person (across days in our study) show good intra-operator reliability; small variances across operators (across people) show good inter-operator reliability, often known as objectivity. It should be clear from Figure 4.10(a) and (c) that, when markers are used, movement variability (variance across trials) is by far the predominant source of variance. Movement variability could, therefore, be assessed both reliably and objectively in these conditions. Indeed, each human operator was not much more inconsistent than auto-tracking, which was 99.99 per cent consistent (and, therefore, reliable). Without markers, however, the picture changed dramatically: true movement variability (across trials) was then obscured by inter-operator variance (across people, Figure 4.10(d)) and intra-operator variance (across days, Figure 4.10(b) and (d)). Without markers, therefore, movement variability could not be assessed reliably or objectively; this is a dramatic finding for applied movement analysts, like me, who have focused much of their research on performance in sports competitions, in which markers cannot be attached to the performer.

Figure 4.10 Partitioning of variance (as mean squares, MS). Top left: (a) individual operator, marker condition; Top right: (b) individual operator, no-marker condition; Bottom left: (c) group of operators, marker condition; Bottom right: (d) group of operators, no-marker condition.

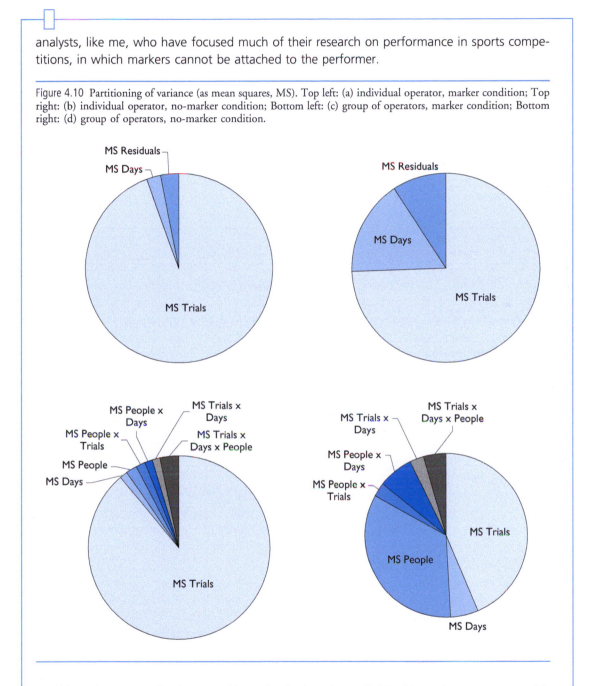

Although most studies in sports biomechanics have been digitised by only one operator, this practice ignores the importance of assessing objectivity – although, from the results of the study discussed here, this is usually justifiable if markers are used, the same is clearly not the case for no-marker conditions. The results of this study also cast a shadow on previous results from studies in sports biomechanics in which markers have not been used; this applies in particular to those – and there are far too many – in which no attempt has been made to assess reliability or objectivity. Unreliable data is clearly a big issue for the quantitative analyst wishing to focus on performance in competition; it also presents problems for qualitative analysts whose movement patterns in such conditions will be contaminated by errors.

It should be noted here (another warning!) that markers can also cause errors if they are not positioned to give good estimations of the centres of rotation of joints. Therefore, as I pointed out in the section on on-line motion analysis systems, data obtained from marker-based systems are also prone to error.

BOX 4.4 THOSE THINGS CALLED VECTORS AND SCALARS

Vector algebra has been the bane of sports biomechanics for many students who want to work in the real world of sport and exercise, providing scientific support, rather than researching. Even many quantitative movement analysts do not use vector algebra routinely in their work. In this box, I introduce only the basics – all sports biomechanics students should know these. In Appendix 4.2, I have included some further vector algebra for interested readers.

We distinguish between scalar variables, which have a magnitude but no directional quality, and vectors. Vectors have both a magnitude and a direction; their behaviour cannot be studied only by their magnitude – the direction is also important. This means that they cannot be added, subtracted or multiplied as scalars, for which we use simple algebra and arithmetic.

Mass, volume, temperature and energy are scalar quantities. Some of these are always positive – such as mass, volume and kinetic energy – whereas others depend upon arbitrary choices of datum and can be both positive and negative – temperature and potential energy come into this category. A third group often use a convention to designate a 'direction' in which the scalar 'moves'; for example, the work done by a biomechanical system on its surroundings – as in a muscle raising a weight – is, by convention, considered positive, whereas when the surroundings do work on the system, this is considered negative. Work remains, however, a scalar.

Many of the kinematic variables that are important for the biomechanical understanding and evaluation of movement in sport and exercise are vector quantities. These include linear and rotational position, displacement, velocity and acceleration. Many of the kinetic variables considered in Chapter 5, such as momentum, force and torque, are also vectors. The magnitude of a kinematic variable – the scalar part of the vector, if you like – usually has a name different from that of the vector (see Table 4.1). Interestingly, because a scalar has no implied direction, speed should always be positive: designating it as positive up or to the right and negative down or to the left converts it into a one-dimensional vector. Note that the SI system does not recognise degrees/s as a preferred unit, but I have included it in Table 4.1 as it means more to most students (and to me) than the approved unit, radians/s (π radians = 180°).

Table 4.1 Kinematic vectors and scalars.

VECTOR AND SYMBOL	SCALAR AND SYMBOL	SI UNIT
Linear		
Displacement, s or $\mathbf{s}$	Distance, s	metres, m
Velocity, v or $\mathbf{v}$	Speed, v	metres per second, m/s
Acceleration, a or $\mathbf{a}$	Acceleration, a	metres per second per second, m/s^2
Angular		
Angular displacement, θ	Angular distance, θ	radians, rad; degrees, °
Angular velocity, ω	Angular speed, ω	radians per second, rad/s; degrees per second, °/s
Angular acceleration, α	Angular acceleration, α	radians per second per second, rad/s^2; degrees per second per second, °/s^2

Scalar variables, by convention, are shown in italicised type, except for Greek symbols which are not italicised, as in Table 4.1. Vector quantities are shown in bold type, sometimes italicised, as in Table 4.1. Linear vectors can be represented graphically by a straight line arrow in the direction of the vector, with the length of the line being proportional to the magnitude of the vector. Angular vectors can also be represented graphically; in this case the direction of the arrow is found from the right-hand rule, shown diagrammatically in Figure 4.11. With the right hand orientated as in Figure 4.11, the curled fingers follow the direction of rotation and the thumb points in the direction of the angular motion vector. So, for example, the direction of the angular motion vectors (angular displacement, velocity and acceleration) for flexion–extension of the knee joint, a movement in the sagittal plane, lies along the flexion–extension axis, the transverse axis perpendicular to the sagittal plane. In the case shown here, the angular motion vector and the axis of rotation coincide. This is often, but not always, the case. See Appendix 4.2 for further information about vectors.

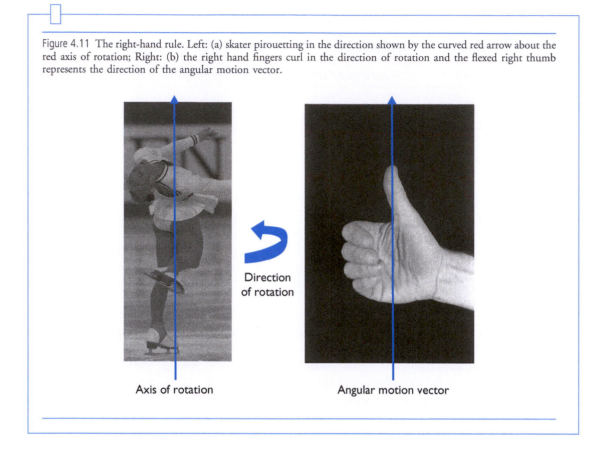

Figure 4.11 The right-hand rule. Left: (a) skater pirouetting in the direction shown by the curved red arrow about the red axis of rotation; Right: (b) the right hand fingers curl in the direction of rotation and the flexed right thumb represents the direction of the angular motion vector.

Direction of rotation

Axis of rotation

Angular motion vector

PROJECTILE MOTION

In this section, we illustrate an important example of linear (in fact, curvilinear) motion – the motion of a projectile in the air. Projectiles are bodies launched into the air that are subject only to the forces of gravity and air resistance. Projectile motion occurs frequently in sport. Often the projectile involved is an inanimate object, such as a shot or golf ball. In some activities the sports performer becomes the projectile, as in the long jump, high jump, diving and gymnastics. An understanding of the mechanical factors that govern the flight path or trajectory of a projectile is, therefore, important in sports biomechanics. The following discussion assumes that the effects of aerodynamic forces on projectile motion – both air resistance and more complex lift effects – are negligible. This is a reasonable first assumption for some, but certainly not all, projectile motions in sport; aerodynamic forces will be considered in Chapter 5. Although I introduce algebraic symbols and equations in what follows, for shorthand, I do not want to focus on the mathematical derivation of these equations, only on their importance.

Figure 4.12 Projection parameters.

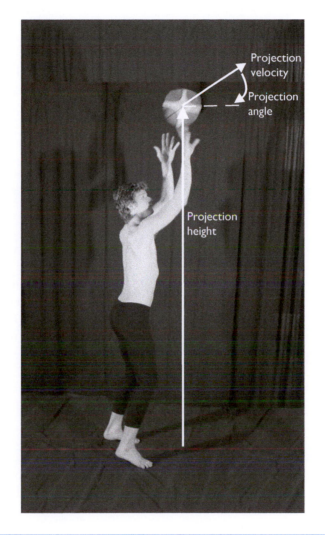

There are three parameters, in addition to gravitational acceleration, g, that determine the trajectory of a simple projectile, such as a ball, shot or hammer. These are the projection speed, angle and height (Figure 4.12). For thrown objects such as these, these three parameters are often called release speed, angle and height; for humans, the terms take-off speed, angle and height are more common. I use projection speed, angle and height to cover both types of 'projectile' – objects and humans – and consider these parameters in decreasing order of importance.

Projection speed

Projection speed (v_0) is defined as the speed of the projectile at the instant of release or take-off (Figure 4.12). When the projection angle and height are held constant, the projection speed will determine the maximum height the projectile reaches – its apex – and its range – the horizontal distance it travels. The greater the projection speed, the greater the apex and range. It is common practice to resolve a projectile's velocity vector into its horizontal and vertical components and then to analyse these independently. Horizontally a projectile is not subject to any external forces, as we are ignoring air resistance; the projectile will, therefore, have a constant horizontal velocity while in the air, as in a long jump or swimming start dive. The range (R) travelled by a projectile is the product of its horizontal projection velocity ($v_{x0} = v_0\cos\theta$) and its time of flight (t_{max}). That is:

$$R = v_{x0}t_{max}$$

To calculate a projectile's time of flight, we must consider the magnitude of the vertical component of its projection velocity (v_y). Vertically a projectile is subject to a constant acceleration due to gravity. The magnitude of the maximum vertical displacement (y_{max}), flight time (t_{max}) and range (R) achieved by a projectile can easily be determined from v_{y0} if it takes off and lands at the same level ($y_0 = 0$). This occurs, for example, in a football kick (from the ground that returns to the ground). In this case, the results are as follows:

$$y_{max} = v_{y0}^2/2g = v_0^2\sin^2\theta/2g$$

$$t_{max} = 2v_{y0}/g = 2v_0\sin\theta/g$$

$$R = 2v_0^2\sin\theta\cos\theta/g = v_0^2\sin2\theta/g$$

The range (R) equation shows that the projection speed is by far the most important of the projection parameters in determining the range achieved, because the range is proportional to the square of the release speed. Doubling the release speed increases the range fourfold.

Projection angle

The projection angle (θ) is defined as the angle between the projectile's line of travel (its velocity vector) and the horizontal at the instant of release or take-off. The value of the projection angle depends on the purpose of the activity. For example, activities requiring maximum horizontal range, such as the shot put, long jump and ski jump, tend to use smaller angles than those in which maximum height is an objective, for example the high jump or the jump of a volleyball spiker. In the absence of aerodynamic forces, all projectiles will follow a flight path that has a parabolic shape which depends upon the projection angle (Figure 4.13).

Figure 4.13 Effect of projection angle on shape of parabolic trajectory for a projection speed of 15 m/s and zero projection height. Projection angles: 30° – continuous black curve, flight time 1.53 s, range 19.86 m, maximum height 2.87 m; 45° – red curve, flight time 2.16 s, range 22.94 m, maximum height 5.73 m; 60° – dashed black curve, flight time 2.65 s, range 19.86 m, maximum height 8.60 m.

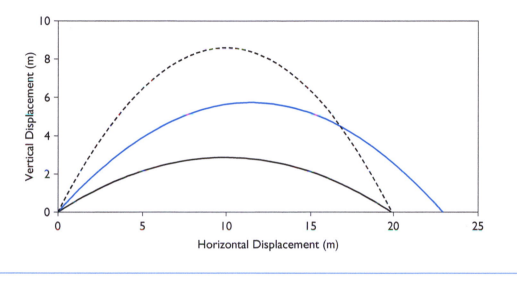

Projection height

The equations in the subsection on projection speed have to be modified if the projectile lands at a height higher or lower than that at which it was released. This is the case with most sports projectiles, for example in a shot put, a basketball shot or a long jump. At a given projection speed and angle, a greater relative projection height (y_0) will lead to a longer flight time, a greater range and a higher maximum height. The maximum height is the same as above but with the height of release added, as follows:

$$y_{max} = y_0 + v_0^2 \sin^2\theta / 2g$$

$$t_{max} = v_0 \sin\theta/g + (v_0^2\sin^2\theta + 2gy_0)^{1/2}/g$$

$$R = v_0^2\sin 2\theta/2g + v_0^2\cos\theta(\sin^2\theta + 2gy_0v_0^2)^{1/2}/g$$

The equations for the time of flight (t_{max}) and range (R) appear to be much more complicated than those for zero release height. The first of the two terms in each of these relates, respectively, to the time and horizontal distance to the apex of the trajectory. The value of these terms is exactly half of the total values in the earlier equations. The second terms relate to the time and horizontal distance covered from the apex to landing. By setting the release height (y_0) to zero, and noting that $\cos\theta\sin\theta = \sin 2\theta/2$, you will find that the second terms in the equations for the time of flight and range become equal to the first terms and that the equations are then identical to the earlier ones for which the release height was zero.

Optimum projection conditions

In many sports events, the objective is to maximise either the range or the height of the apex achieved by the projectile. As seen above, any increase in projection speed or height is always accompanied by an increase in the range and height achieved by a projectile. If the objective of the sport is to maximise height or range, it is important to ascertain the best – the optimum – angle to achieve this. Obviously maximum height is achieved when all of the available projection speed is directed vertically, when the projection angle is 90°.

As we saw above, when the projection height is zero, the range is given by $v_0^2 \sin 2\theta / g$. For a given projection speed, v_0, the range is a maximum when $\sin 2\theta$ is a maximum, that is when $\sin 2\theta = 1$ and $2\theta = 90°$; therefore, the optimum projection angle, θ, is 45°. For the more general case of a non-zero projection height, the optimum projection angle can be found from: $\cos 2\theta = g y_0 / (v_0^2 + g y \theta)$. For a good shot putter, for example, this would give a value around 42°.

Although optimum projection angles for given values of projection speed and height can easily be determined from the last equation, they do not always correspond to those recorded from the best performers in sporting events. This is even true for the shot put, for which the object's flight is the closest to a parabola of all sports objects. The reason for this is that the calculation of an optimum projection angle assumes, implicitly, that the projection speed and projection angle are independent of one another. For a shot putter, the release speed and angle are, however, not independent, because of the anatomy and mechanics of the muscles used to generate the release speed of the shot (see Chapter 6 for consideration of some of these factors). A greater release speed, and hence range, can be achieved at an angle of about 35°, which is less than the optimum projectile angle. What would be optimal for the shot – simply as a projectile – is not optimum for the shot putter. If the shot putter seeks to increase the release angle to a value closer to the optimum projectile angle, the release speed decreases and so does the range.

A similar deviation from the optimum projection angle is noticed when the activity involves the projection of an athlete's body. The angle at which the body is projected at take-off can have a large effect on the take-off speed. In the long jump, for example, take-off angles used by elite long jumpers are around 20°. To obtain the theoretically optimum take-off angle of around 42°, long jumpers would have to decrease their normal horizontal speed by around 50 per cent. This would clearly result in a drastically reduced range, as the range depends largely on the square of the take-off speed.

In many sporting events, such as the javelin and discus throws, badminton, skydiving and ski jumping, the aerodynamic characteristics of the projectile can significantly influence its trajectory. The projectile may travel a greater or lesser distance than it would have done if projected in a vacuum. Under such circumstances, the calculations of optimal projection parameters need to be modified considerably to take account of the aerodynamic forces acting on the projectile (see Chapter 5).

LINEAR VELOCITIES AND ACCELERATIONS CAUSED BY ROTATION

In this section, we show how the rotation of a body can cause linear motion. Consider the quasi-rigid body of a gymnast, shown in Figure 4.14, rotating about an axis fixed in the bar, with angular velocity ω, and angular acceleration α. The axis of rotation in the bar is fixed and we will assume that the position of the gymnast's centre of mass, C, is fixed relative to that axis. Therefore, the distance of the centre of mass from the axis of rotation (the magnitude r of the position vector r) does not change.

The linear velocity of the centre of mass of the gymnast is tangential to the circle that the centre of mass describes; its magnitude is given by $v = \omega r$. Readers who are familiar

Figure 4.14 Tangential velocity and tangential and centripetal acceleration components for a gymnast rotating about a bar. Her angular velocity vector lies along the bar, as shown by the red arrow; the position vector (dashed white arrow) runs from the bar to the gymnast's centre of mass. The tangential velocity vector (black arrow) is perpendicular to the position vector and passes posteriorly through her centre of mass. The tangential acceleration vector is also represented by the black arrow. The centripetal acceleration vector, shown by the continuous white arrow, is in the direction opposite to that of the position vector.

with basic vector algebra, or those of you who can follow Appendix 4.2, will appreciate that the tangential velocity of the centre of mass, from the cross-product rule (see Appendix 4.2), is mutually perpendicular to both the position (r) and angular velocity (ω) vectors. The angular velocity vector has a direction, perpendicularly out of the plane of the page towards you, determined by the right-hand rule, shown in Figure 4.11.

The linear acceleration of the centre of mass of the gymnast has two components, which are mutually perpendicular, as follows:

- The first component, called the tangential acceleration, has a direction identical to that of the tangential velocity and a magnitude αr.
- The second component is called the centripetal acceleration. It has a magnitude $\omega^2 r$ ($= \omega v = v^2/r$) and a direction given by the vector cross-product (see Appendix 4.2) $\omega \times v$. This direction is obtained by letting the angular velocity vector (ω) rotate towards the tangential velocity vector (v) through the right angle between them and using the vector cross-product rule of Appendix 4.2. This gives a vector ($\omega \times v$) perpendicular to both the angular velocity and tangential velocity vectors, as shown in Figure 4.14. As the velocity vector is perpendicular to the longitudinal axis of the gymnast, the direction of the centripetal acceleration vector ($\omega \times v$) is along the longitudinal axis of the gymnast towards the axis of rotation. You should note that a centripetal acceleration exists for all rotational motion. This is true even if the angular acceleration is zero, in which case the angular velocity is constant; the magnitude of the centripetal acceleration is also constant if the distance from the axis of rotation to the centre of mass is constant.

ROTATION IN THREE-DIMENSIONAL SPACE

For two-dimensional rotations of human body segments, the relative joint angle may be defined as the angle between two lines representing the proximal and distal segments; this requires only three points to define the angle. A similar procedure can be used to specify the relative angle between line representations of segments in three dimensions if the articulation is a simple hinge joint, but generally the process is more complex. There are many different ways of defining the orientation angles of two articulating rigid bodies and of specifying the orientation angles of the human performer. Most of these conventions have certain problems, one of which is to have an angle convention that is easily understood; further discussion of this topic is beyond the scope of this book.

The specification of the angular orientation of the human performer as a whole is also problematic. The representation of Figure 4.15, for example, has been used to analyse airborne movements in gymnastics, diving and trampolining. In this, rotation is specified by the somersault angle (φ) about the transverse axis through the centre of mass, the twist angle (ψ) about the longitudinal axis of the performer, and the tilt angle (θ). The last named is the angle between the longitudinal axis and the fixed plane normal to the somersault angular velocity vector.

Figure 4.15 Angular orientation showing angles of somersault (φ), tilt (θ) and twist (ψ).

SUMMARY

In this chapter, we covered the use of videography in the study of sports movements, including the equipment and methods used. The necessary features of video equipment for recording movements in sport were considered, as were the advantages and limitations of two- and three-dimensional recording of sports movements. I outlined the possible sources of error in recorded movement data and described experimental procedures that will minimise recorded errors in two- and three-dimensional movements. An introduction was provided to the use of on-line motion analysis systems. The need for smoothing or filtering of kinematic data was introduced. I also outlined briefly the requirement for accurate body segment inertia parameter data and how these can be obtained, touching briefly on some aspects of error analysis. Then, a cautionary tale of unreliable data unfolded as a warning to the analysis of data containing unacceptable measurement errors. Projectile motion was considered and equations presented to calculate the maximum vertical displacement, flight time, range and optimum projection angle of a simple projectile for specified values of the three projection parameters. Deviations of the optimal angle for the sports performer from the optimal projection angle were explained. We looked at the calculation of linear velocities and accelerations caused by rotation and concluded with a brief consideration of three-dimensional rotation.

STUDY TASKS

1 Answer all of the multiple-choice questions for Chapter 4 in the Interactive eTextbook.
   Hint: Keep repeating this until you have answered all of the questions correctly.

2 Explain why quantitative motion analysis using video (videography) is important in the study of human movement in sport.
   Hint: You may find it useful to re-read Box 1.3, 'Comparison of qualitative and quantitative movement analysis' as well as the section 'Background to quantitative motion analysis' near the start of this chapter.

3 Obtain a video of a sports activity of your choice (either by video recording, if you have a video camera, or from a website such as YouTube; www.youtube.com). Study the video carefully, frame by frame. Identify the key events that separate the various phases of the movement. Also, identify the displacements, angles, velocities and accelerations that you would need to include in a quantitative analysis of this sports activity.
   Hint: You may find it useful to re-read the subsection on 'Identifying critical features of a movement' in Chapter 2 as well as the section 'Background to quantitative motion analysis' near the start of this chapter before undertaking this task.

4 List the possible sources of error when recording human movement in sport using videography; identify which would lead to random errors and which to systematic errors.
   Hint: You should re-read the subsection on 'Sources of error in videography' before undertaking this task.

5 Briefly describe the procedures that would minimise the recorded error in a study of an essentially two-dimensional movement. Assess which of these steps could not be implemented if video recording at a national-standard sports competition. Briefly explain how these procedures would be modified for recording a three-dimensional movement.
   Hint: You should re-read the section on 'Experimental videography procedures' before undertaking this task.

6 Have your lecturer arrange, or arrange for yourself, a discussion session to consider the implications of the results of the study summarised in Box 4.3 for qualitative movement analysts.
   Hint: You should read Box 4.3 several times before undertaking this task.

7 a) A shot is released at a height of 1.89 m, with a speed of 13 m/s and at an angle of 34°. Calculate, using the equations in the section 'Projectile motion', the maximum height reached, the range and the time of flight, and the optimum

projection angle. Why do you think the release angle differs from the optimum projection angle?

b) Calculate, using the equations in the section 'Projectile motion', the maximum height reached, the range and the time of flight, and the optimum projection angle for a similar object projected with zero release height but with the same release speed and angle. Comment on the effects of changing the release height.

c) Check your answers with those in the Excel file 'Projectile motion' in the Interactive eTextbook.

d) Repeat the calculations using the Excel file 'Projectile motion' in the Interactive eTextbook for other values of the projection parameters; the file explains how to do this.

Hint: You should re-read the section on 'Projectile motion' before undertaking this study task.

8 Calculate, using the equations in the section 'Linear velocities and accelerations caused by rotation', the magnitudes of the acceleration components and the velocity of the centre of mass of a gymnast rotating about a bar and behaving as a quasi-rigid body, at a radius of 0.8 m from the axis of rotation (the bar) when the angular velocity and angular acceleration have magnitudes of 10 rad/s and -5 rad/s^2, respectively. Sketch the gymnast and draw the velocity vector and components of the acceleration vector, as well as the position and angular velocity vectors.

Hint: You should re-read the section on 'Linear velocities and accelerations caused by rotation' before undertaking this task.

9 a) In the Interactive eTextbook you will find video clips of a male athlete performing standing vertical jumps. Download the clips for the normal, model and unusual arm actions and the one with the hands kept on the hips. You will also need to download the calibration sequence for these video clips

b) If you have access to a computer with a software package for quantitative motion analysis using videography, then, after calibrating the image using the calibration sequence, digitise the normal arm condition (from frame 25 to frame 82) and unusual arm condition (from frame 25 to frame 77). You should digitise the foot, ankle, knee, hip and iliac crest. If your software package has the option, you may want to auto-track the markers wherever possible (this won't be possible when a marker is obscured). Follow carefully the instructions for the software that you are using, as these vary greatly between the various software packages that are available.

Define the knee angle as the relative angle at the knee (use the ankle, knee and hip). Define the hip angle as the relative angle at the hip (use the knee, hip and iliac crest) using our normal convention. Define the ankle angle as the relative angle at the ankle (use the foot, ankle and knee). Export the angles to the Excel file 'For Data ST9' available in the Interactive eTextbook, pasting the data for the normal arm condition into cells B2:D59 in the sheet 'Normal Arm Action' and those for the unusual arm condition into cells B2:D54 in the sheet 'Unusual Arm Action'. Angle–angle diagrams will be created automatically.

If you do not have access to a computer with a software package for quantitative motion analysis using videography, you can download an Excel file containing the appropriate angle data and angle–angle diagrams from the Interactive eTextbook.

c) Describe the changes of coordination between the relevant two joints that take place as you progress around the angle–angle diagrams with time, for all three angle couplings and both conditions.

d) Comment on the angle–angle diagrams. Does the one for the hip and the knee coupling show synchronised flexion and extension of these joints, as we postulated in Chapter 3? Are the differences in arm and leg coordination between the two jumps that you digitised reflected in the height of the two jumps? Are the heights jumped different for the two jumps you digitised compared to the one with no arm action and the one with the model arm action?

Hint: You should re-read the subsection on 'Angle–angle diagrams' in Chapter 3 as well as the subsection above on 'Digitising procedures' before undertaking this task.

10 **Case study.**

a) Answer the five multiple-choice questions for this study task in the Interactive eTextbook.

b) Plan an experimental session in which you would record several strides of an athlete running on a treadmill at three different speeds. You should carefully detail all the important procedural steps, including the use of markers (see Table 5.1 and Box 6.2). This should be written up as the methods section of the case study.

c) If you have access to a suitable digital video camera, record three complete strides at each speed; if not, download the three video clips of a young female athlete running, wearing tight-fitting black clothing and markers, from the Interactive eTextbook. You will also need to download the calibration sequence for these trials.

If you have access to a computer with a software package for quantitative motion analysis using videography, then digitise the middle stride (plus five frames before and five frames after this stride) for each of the three running speeds that you have recorded or downloaded. Define the knee angle as the relative angle at the knee (use the ankle, knee and hip). Define the hip angle as the absolute angle at the hip (use the knee and hip) to the vertical (this avoids errors if the iliac crest marker is obscured). Define the ankle angle as the relative angle at the ankle (use the foot, ankle and knee). If your software package has the option, you may want to auto-track the markers wherever possible (this won't be possible when a marker is obscured). Follow carefully the instructions for the software that you are using, as these vary greatly between the various software packages that are available. Then plot graphs of relevant kinematic variables, which you should establish by an analysis similar to that performed in Study Task 3. If you do not have access to a computer with a software package for quantitative motion analysis using videography, you can download graphs of kinematic variables for running from the Interactive eTextbook, but you will still need to justify which variables are of interest.

d) Write a report of your case study in no more than 1000 words and with no more than six graphs. Include: methods (as in (b)); results (graphs from (c)); and a brief discussion of what seem to you to be the most important results, highlighting differences between the speeds.

Hint: You should re-read the subsections on 'Two-dimensional recording procedures' and 'Digitising procedures' before undertaking this task.

SORTING AND LABELLING ACTIVITIES (INTERACTIVE ETEXTBOOK ONLY)

Sorting activity.
Labelling activity.

FURTHER READING

Bartlett, R.M. and Bussey, M. (2012) *Sports Biomechanics: Reducing Injury Risk and Improving Sports Performance*, London: Routledge. Chapter 4 provides a simple introduction to inverse dynamics without being too mathematical.

Challis, J.H. (2008) Data processing and error estimation, in C.J. Payton and R.M. Bartlett (eds) *Biomechanical Evaluation of Movement in Sport and Exercise*, London: Routledge, pp. 129–152. Chapter 8 in the book elaborates on the errors in sports biomechanical data and outlines, with clear examples, the calculation of uncertainties in derived biomechanical data.

Milner, C. (2008) Motion analysis using on-line systems, in C.J. Payton and R.M. Bartlett (eds) *Biomechanical Evaluation of Movement in Sport and Exercise*, London: Routledge, pp. 33–52. Chapter 3 in the book provides a lucid and easy-to-follow explanation of some difficult concepts. Highly recommended if you see research into sports movement as something you might wish to pursue.

Mullineaux, D.R. (2008) Research methods: sample size and variability effects on statistical power, in C.J. Payton and R.M. Bartlett (eds) *Biomechanical Evaluation of Movement in Sport and Exercise*, London: Routledge, pp. 153–175. Chapter 9 in the book, which covers pretty much what the chapter title says.

Payton, C.J. (2008) Motion analysis using video, in C.J. Payton and R.M. Bartlett (eds) *Biomechanical Evaluation of Movement in Sport and Exercise*, London: Routledge, pp. 8–32. This excellent and clearly written chapter (Chapter 2 in the book) contains much useful advice on a video study, including the reporting of such a study, which you could adapt for the case study in Study Task 10.

APPENDIX 4.1 DATA SMOOTHING, FILTERING AND DIFFERENTIATION

Introduction

Much attention has been paid to the problem of removal of noise from discretely sampled data in sports biomechanics. Solutions are not always, or entirely, satisfactory, particularly when transient signals, such as those caused by foot–ground or other impacts, are present. Noise removal is normally performed after reconstruction of the movement coordinates from the image coordinates as, for three-dimensional studies, each set of image coordinates does not contain full information about the movement coordinates. However, the noise removal should be performed before calculating other data, such as segment orientations and joint forces and moments. The reason for this is that the calculations are highly non-linear, leading to non-linear combinations of random noise, which can adversely affect the separation of signal and noise by low-pass filtering.

The two most common techniques used to remove high frequency noise from the low frequency movement coordinates use some form of digital low-pass filter or spline smoothing; the latter is normally realised through cross-validated quintic splines. Some hints to users are given in the bullet points below. Brief information on three noise-removal techniques – Butterworth digital filters, Fourier series truncation and cross-validated quintic splines – then follows for interested readers.

- Quintic splines appear to produce more accurate first and second derivatives than most other techniques that are commonly used in sports biomechanics. The two filtering techniques discussed below (Fourier series truncation and digital filters) were devised for periodic data, in which the pattern of movement is cyclical, as in Figure 4.9(a). Sporting activities that are cyclic, such as running, are obviously periodic, and some others can be considered quasi-periodic. Problems may be found in trying to filter non-periodic data, although these may be reduced by removing any linear trend in the data before filtering; this makes the first and last data values zero. The Butterworth filter often creates fewer problems in this respect than Fourier series truncation, but neither technique deals completely satisfactorily with constant acceleration motion, as for the centre of mass when a sports performer is airborne.
- The main consideration for the sports biomechanist using smoothing or filtering routines is a rational choice of filter cut-off frequency or spline smoothing parameter. A poor choice can result in some noise being retained if the filter cut-off frequency is too high, or some of the signal being rejected if the cut-off frequency is too low. As most human movement is at a low frequency, a cut-off frequency of between 4 and 8 Hz is often used; such values should not, however, be chosen arbitrarily. Lower cut-off frequencies may be preferable for slow events such as swimming, and higher ones for impacts or other rapid energy transfers. The cut-off frequency should be chosen to include the highest frequency of interest in the movement.

Figure 4.16 Residual analysis of filtered data.

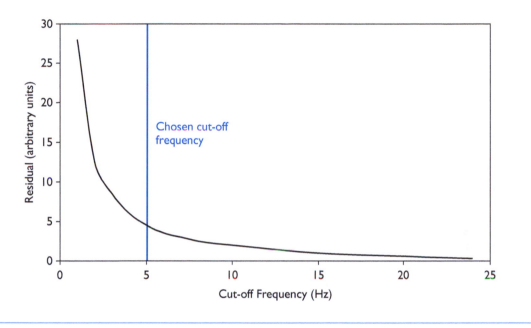

The need for data smoothness demands a minimum ratio of the sampling to cut-off frequencies of 4:1 and preferably one as high as 8:1 or 10:1 (this is much higher than the 2:1 ratio required to avoid aliasing, which was mentioned earlier in the chapter). The frame rate (or sampling frequency) used when video recording, and the digitising rate (the sampling frequency at the time of digitising the images), must allow for this.

The use of previously published filter cut-off frequencies or manual adjustment of the smoothing parameter is not recommended. Instead, a technique should be used that involves a justifiable procedure to take into account the peculiarities of each new set of data. Attempts to base the choice of cut-off frequency on some objective criterion have not always been successful. One approach is to compare the root mean square difference between the noisy data and that obtained after filtering at several different cut-off frequencies with the standard deviation obtained from repetitive digitisation of the same anatomical point. The cut-off frequency should then be chosen so that the magnitudes of the two are similar. Another approach is called residual analysis, in which the residuals between the raw and filtered data are calculated for a range of cut-off frequencies; the residuals are then plotted against the cut-off frequency, and the best value of the latter is chosen as that at which the residuals begin to approach an asymptotic value, as in Figure 4.16. Some subjective judgement is involved in assigning the cut-off frequency at which this happens.

- It is often necessary to use a different smoothing parameter or cut-off frequency for the coordinates of the different points recorded. This is particularly necessary when the frequency spectrums for the various points are different, for example, if the foot is subject to a high impact force while the arms are not.
- Finally, you should note that no automatic noise-removal algorithm will always be successful, and that the smoothness of the processed data should always be checked.

Butterworth filters

Digital low-pass filters are widely used to remove, or filter, high frequency noise from digital data. Butterworth filters (of order $2n$, where n is a positive integer) are often used in sports biomechanics, because they have a flat passband – the band of frequencies that is not affected by the filter (Figure 4.17). However, they have relatively shallow cut-offs; this can be improved by using higher-order filters. They also introduce a phase shift, which must be removed by a second, reverse filtering, which increases the order of the filter and further reduces the cut-off frequency.

Butterworth filters are recursive; that is, they use filtered values of previous data points as well as noisy data values to obtain filtered data values. This makes for faster computation but introduces problems at the ends of data sequences, at which filtered values must be estimated. This can mean that extra frames must be digitised at each end of the sequence and included in the data processing; these extra frames then have to be discarded after filtering. This can involve unwelcome extra work for the

Figure 4.17 Low-pass filter frequency characteristics.

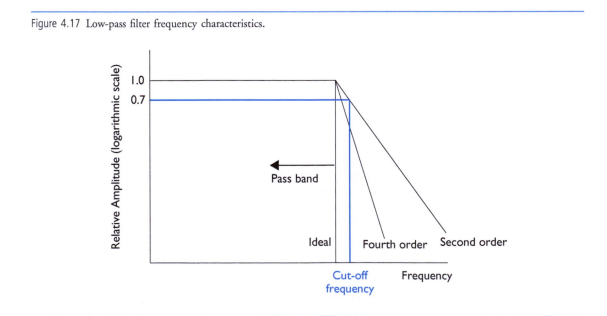

movement analyst; other solutions include various ways of padding the ends of the data sets.

The main decision for the user, as with Fourier series truncation, is the choice of cut-off frequency (discussed briefly above). The filtered data are not obtained in analytic form, so a separate numerical differentiation process must be used. Although Butterworth filtering appears to be very different from spline fitting (see below), the two are, in fact, closely linked.

Fourier series truncation

The first step in Fourier series truncation is the transformation of the noisy data into the frequency domain by means of a Fourier transformation. This, in essence, replaces the familiar representation of displacement as a function of time (the time domain), as in Figure 4.18(a), by a series of sinusoidal waves of different frequencies. This 'frequency domain' representation of the data is then presented as amplitudes of the sinusoidal components at each frequency – the harmonic frequencies – as in Figure 4.18(b), or as a continuous curve. Figure 4.19(a) shows the frequency domain representation of the simplified data of Figure 4.18(a). The data are then filtered to remove high-frequency noise. This is done by reconstituting the data up to the chosen cut-off frequency and truncating the number of terms in the series from which it is made up. For the simplified data of Figure 4.19(a), if the cut-off frequency was, say, 4 Hz, then the second frequency term would be rejected as noise.

In this simplified case, the noise would have been removed perfectly, as the time domain signal of Figure 4.19(b) demonstrates. There would be no resulting errors in the velocities and accelerations. The major decision here concerns the choice of cut-off frequency, and similar principles to those described above can be applied. Unlike digital filters, the cut-off can be infinitely steep, as in Figure 4.17, but this is not necessarily the case. The filtered data can be represented as an equation and can be differentiated analytically. This technique requires the raw data points to be sampled at equal time intervals, as do digital low-pass filters (see above).

Quintic spline curve fitting

Many techniques used for the smoothing and differentiation of data in sports biomechanics involve the use of spline functions. These are a series of polynomial curves joined – or pieced – together at points called knots. This smoothing technique, which is performed in the time domain, can be considered to be the numerical equivalent of drawing a smooth curve through the data points. Indeed, the name 'spline' is derived from the flexible strip of rubber or wood used by draftsmen for drawing curves. Splines are claimed to represent the smoothness of human movement while rejecting

Figure 4.18 Displacement data represented in: Top: (a) the time domain; Bottom: (b) the frequency domain.

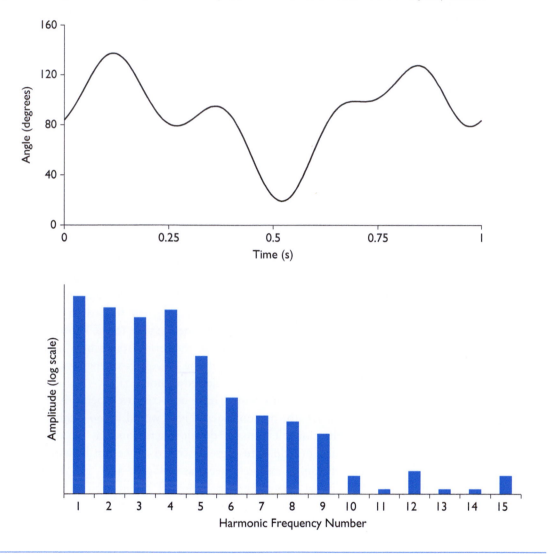

the normally distributed random noise in the digitised coordinates. Many spline techniques have a knot at each data point, obviating the need for the user to choose optimal knot positions. The user has simply to specify a weighting factor for each data point and select the value of the smoothing parameter, which controls the extent of the smoothing; generally the weighting factor should be the inverse of the estimate of the variance of the data point. This is easily established in sports biomechanics by repeated digitisation of a video sequence. The use of different weighting factors for different points can be useful, particularly if points are obscured from the camera and therefore have a greater

Figure 4.19 Simplified examples of: Top (a) noisy data in the frequency domain; Bottom (b) same data in the time domain after removal of noise by filtering by Fourier series truncation.

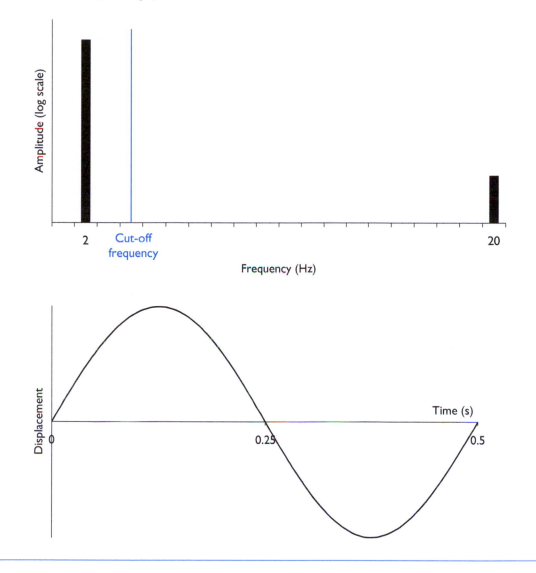

variance than ones that can be seen clearly. Inappropriate choices of the smoothing parameter can cause problems of over-smoothing (Figure 4.20(a) and (b)) or under-smoothing (Figure 4.20(c) and (d)).

Generalised cross-validated quintic splines do not require the user to specify the error in the data to be smoothed, but instead automatically select an optimum smoothing parameter. Computer programs for spline smoothing are available in various software packages, such as MATLAB, and on the Internet (see for example,

Figure 4.20 Top: over-smoothing. Left: (a) velocity; Right: (b) acceleration. Middle: under-smoothing. Left: (c) velocity; Right: (d) acceleration. Bottom: optimum smoothing. Left: (e) velocity; Right: (f) acceleration.

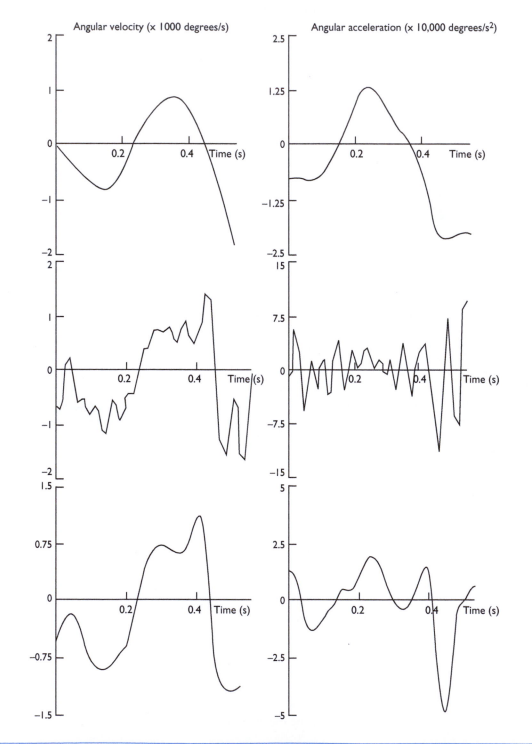

http://isbweb.org/software/sigproc.html), and allow a choice of automatic or user-defined smoothing parameters. Generalised cross-validation can accommodate data points sampled at unequal time intervals. Splines can be differentiated analytically. Quintic splines are continuous up to the fourth derivative, which is a series of interconnected straight lines; this allows accurate generation of the second derivative, acceleration.

APPENDIX 4.2 BASIC VECTOR ALGEBRA

The vector in Figure 4.21(a) can be designated F (magnitude F) or OP (magnitude OP). Vectors can often be moved in space parallel to their original position, although some caution is necessary for force vectors (see Chapter 5). This allows easy graphical addition and subtraction as in Figure 4.22(a) to (f). Note that the vector F in Figure 4.21(a) is equal in magnitude but opposite in direction to the vector G in Figure 4.21(b); if the direction of a vector is changed by 180°, the sign of the vector changes, hence $G = -F$.

Vector addition and subtraction

When two or more vector quantities are added together the process is called 'vector composition'. Most vector quantities, including force, can be treated in this way. The single vector resulting from vector composition is known as the resultant vector or simply the resultant. In Figure 4.22 the vectors added are shown in black, the resultants in red, and the graphical solutions for vector addition are shown between dashed vertical lines.

Figure 4.21 Vector representation. Left: (a) vector F; Right (b) vector $G = -F$.

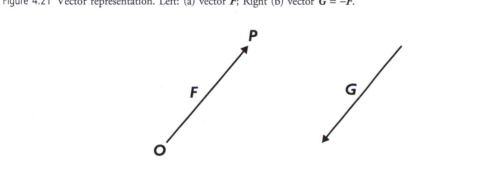

Figure 4.22 Vector addition. Top: (a) with same direction; Second line: (b) in opposite directions; Third line: (c) using vector triangle; Fourth line: (d) using vector parallelogram; Fifth line: (e) using vector polygon; Bottom lines: (f) vector subtraction.

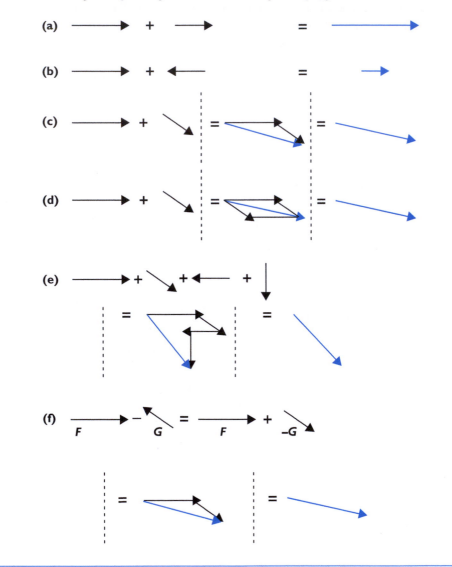

The addition of two or more vectors having the same direction results in a vector that has the same direction as the original vectors and a magnitude equal to the sum of the magnitudes of the vectors being added, as shown in Figure 4.22(a). If vectors directed in exactly opposite directions are added, the resultant has the direction of the longer vector and a magnitude that is equal to the difference in the magnitudes of the two original vectors, as in Figure 4.22(b).

When the vectors to be added lie in the same plane but not in the same or opposite directions, the resultant can be found using the vector triangle approach. The tail of the second vector is placed on the tip of the first vector. The resultant is then drawn from the tail of the first vector to the tip of the second, as in Figure 4.22(c). An alternative approach is to use a vector parallelogram, as in Figure 4.22(d). The vector triangle is more useful as it easily generalises to the vector polygon of Figure 4.22(e).

Although graphical addition of vectors is very easy for two-dimensional problems, the same is not true for three-dimensional ones. Component addition of vectors using trigonometry can be more easily generalised to the three-dimensional case. This technique is introduced for a two-dimensional example in the next but one sub-section.

The subtraction of one vector from another can be tackled graphically simply by treating the problem as one of addition, as in Figure 4.22(f); that is $J = F - G$ is the same as $J = F + (-G)$. Vector subtraction is also often used to find the relative motion between two objects.

Vector resolution and components

Determining the perpendicular components of a vector is often useful in sports biomechanics. Examples include the normal and frictional components of ground reaction force, and the horizontal and vertical components of a projectile's velocity vector. It is, therefore, sometimes necessary to resolve a single vector into two or three perpendicular components – a process known as vector resolution. This is essentially the reverse of vector composition and can be achieved using a vector parallelogram or vector triangle. This is illustrated by the examples in Figure 4.23, where the red arrows are the original vector and the black ones are its components. The vector parallelogram approach is more usual as the components then have a common origin, as in Figure 4.23(a).

Most angular motion vectors obey the rules of resolution and composition, but this is not true for angular displacements.

Figure 4.23 Vector resolution. Left: (a) using vector parallelogram; Right: (b) using vector triangle.

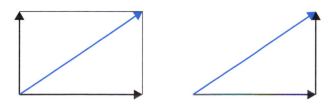

Vector addition and subtraction using vector components

Vector addition and subtraction can also be performed on the components of the vector using the rules of simple trigonometry. For example, consider the addition of the three vectors represented in Figure 4.24(a). Vector *A* is a horizontal vector with a magnitude (proportional to its length) of 1 unit. Vector *B* is a vertical vector of magnitude −2 units (it points vertically downwards, hence it is negative). Vector *C* has a magnitude of 3 units and is at 120° measured anticlockwise from a right-facing horizontal line.

Figure 4.24 Vector addition using components. Top: (a) vectors to be added; Second line: (b) their components; Third line: (c) components of resultant; Bottom: (d) resultant.

Figure 4.25 Vector cross-product.

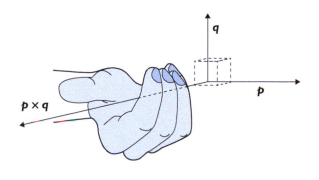

The components of the three vectors are summarised below (see also Figure 4.24(b)). The components (R_x, R_y) of the resultant vector $R = A + B + C$ are shown in Figure 4.24(c). The magnitude of the resultant is then obtained from the magnitudes of its two components, using Pythagoras' theorem ($R^2 = R_x^2 + R_y^2$), as $R = (0.25 + 0.36)^{1/2} = 0.78$. Its direction to the right horizontal is given by the angle, θ, whose tangent is R_y/R_x. That is, $\tan\theta = -1.2$, giving $\theta = 130°$. The resultant R is rotated anticlockwise 130° from the right horizontal, as shown in Figure 4.24(d). (A second solution for $\tan\theta = -1.2$ is $\theta = -50°$, which would have been the answer if R_x had been +0.5 and R_y had been −0.6.)

Vector	Horizontal component (x)	Vertical component (y)
A	1	0
B	0	−2
C	$3\cos120° = -3\cos60° = -1.5$	$3\sin120° = 3\sin60° = 2.6$
A + B + C	−0.5	0.6

Vector multiplication

The rules for vector multiplication do not follow the simple algebraic rules for multiplying scalars.

Vector (cross) product

The product of two vectors (or vector cross-product) is useful in rotational motion, as, for example, it enables angular motion vectors to be related to translational motion vectors (see below). It will be stated here in its simplest case for two vectors at right angles, as in Figure 4.25. The vector product of two vectors p and q inclined to one another at right angles is defined as a vector $p \times q$ of magnitude equal to the product (pq) of the magnitudes of the two given vectors. Its direction is perpendicular to both vectors p and q in the direction in which the thumb points if the curled fingers of the right hand point from p to q through the right angle between them.

Scalar (dot) product

The scalar (dot) product of two vectors can be used, for example, to calculate power (a scalar, P) from force (F) and velocity (v), which are both vectors, using $P = F.v$. The dot product is a scalar so has no directional property. It is calculated as the product of the magnitudes of the two vectors and the cosine of the angle between them. It can also be calculated from the components of the vectors. For example, if $F = F_x + F_y$ and $v = v_x + v_y$ then $P = (F_x + F_y).(v_x + v_y)$. Now, the angle between the force and velocity along the same axis is 0°, so the cosine of that angle is 1; however, the angle between the force and velocity along different axes is 90°, so the cosine of that angle is 0. Hence, $P = F_x v_x + F_y v_y$. Please note that power does NOT have x and y components, as it is a scalar.

5 What causes sports movements? Forces and moments of force

Knowledge assumed
The importance of movement patterns for qualitative analysis (Chapters 1 to 3)
The body's cardinal planes and axes of movement (Chapter 1)
Simple algebraic manipulation (Chapter 4)
Quantitative analysis of sports movements (Chapter 4)
Basic vector algebra (Chapter 4)

INTRODUCTION

In Chapter 4, we covered quantitative motion analysis in sports biomechanics, particularly videography. In the final two chapters of this book, we will explore how sports movements are generated. In this chapter, we will consider the forces that affect the movement of the sports performer. This branch of knowledge is often called 'kinetics', and is subdivided into linear and angular (rotational) kinetics; it deals with the action of forces and moments of force in producing or changing motion. We will also look at how we measure the forces and pressures acting on the sports performer.

BOX 5.1 LEARNING OUTCOMES

After reading this chapter you should be able to:

- appreciate how and why the variation with time of the forces acting on a sports performer can be viewed as another movement pattern that can be evaluated both qualitatively and quantitatively
- define force and identify the external forces acting in sport and how they affect movement
- understand the laws of linear kinetics and related concepts such as linear momentum
- calculate, from segmental and kinematic data, the position of the centre of mass of the human performer
- identify the ways in which rotation is acquired and controlled in sports movements
- understand the laws of angular kinetics and related concepts such as angular momentum
- appreciate why the measurement of the external forces acting on the sports performer is important in analysing sports movements
- outline the procedures to be used when measuring force and pressure
- evaluate the information that can be obtained from force and pressure measurements.

FORCES IN SPORT

A force can be considered as the pushing or pulling action that one object exerts on another. Forces are vectors; they possess both a magnitude and a directional quality. The latter is specified by the direction in which the force acts and by the point on an object at which the force acts – its point of application. Alternatively, the total directional quality of the force can be given by its line of action, as in Figure 5.1.

The effects of a force are not altered by moving it along its line of action. Its effects on rotation – though not on linear motion – are changed if the force is moved parallel

Figure 5.1 Directional quality of force.

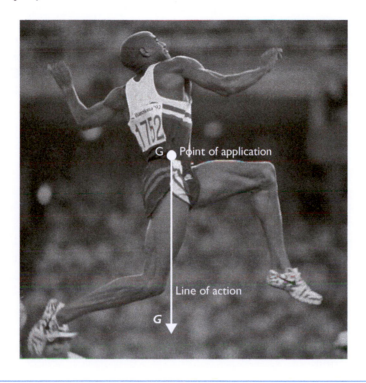

to the original direction and away from its line of action. A moment of force, also known as a torque (a turning effect), is then introduced; this is an effect tending to rotate the object (see below).

The SI unit of force is the newton (N) and the symbol for a force vector is *F*. One newton is the force that, when applied to a mass of one kilogram (1 kg), causes that mass to accelerate at 1 m/s^2 in the direction of the force application. A sports performer experiences forces both internal to and external to the body. Internal forces are generated by the muscles and transmitted by tendons, bones, ligaments and cartilage; these will be considered in Chapter 6. The main external forces, the combined effect of which determines the overall motion of the body, are as follows.

Weight

Weight is a familiar force (Figure 5.1) attributable to the gravitational pull of the earth. It acts vertically downwards through the centre of gravity of an object towards the centre of the earth. The centre of gravity (G in Figure 5.1) is an imaginary point at which the weight of an object can be considered to act. For the human performer, there is little difference between the positions of the centre of mass (see later) and the centre of gravity. The former is the term preferred in most modern sports biomechanics literature and will be used in the rest of this book. One reason for this preference is that the centre of gravity is a meaningless concept in weightless environments, such as space shuttles. An athlete with a mass of 50 kg has a weight (G) of about 490 N at sea level, at which the standard value of gravitational acceleration, g, is assumed to be 9.81 m/s^2.

Reaction forces

Reaction forces are the forces that the ground or other external surface exerts on the sports performer as a reaction to the force that the performer exerts on the ground or surface. This principle is known as Newton's third law of linear motion or the law of action–reaction. The vertical component of force acting on a person performing a standing vertical jump – with no arm action – is shown as a function of time in Figure 5.2. This movement pattern shows the period during which the jumper is on the ground (A), then in the air (B) and, finally, during landing (C). The component of the reaction force tangential to the surface, known as friction or traction, is crucially important in sport and is considered in the next subsection.

Friction

The ground, or other, contact force acting on an athlete (Figure 5.3(a)) can be resolved into two components (see Appendix 4.2), one (F_n) normal (perpendicular) and one (F_t) tangential to the contact surface (Figure 5.3(b)). The former component is the normal force and the latter is the friction, or traction, force. 'Traction' is the term used when the force is generated by interlocking of the contacting objects, such as spikes penetrating a Tartan track; this interaction between objects is known as 'form locking'. In friction, the force is generated by 'force locking', in which no surface penetration occurs. Without friction or traction, movement in sport would be very difficult.

If an object, such as a training shoe (Figure 5.4(a)), is placed on a sports surface material, such as Tartan, it is possible to investigate how the friction force changes. The forces acting on the plane are shown in the 'free-body diagram' of the shoe removed from its surroundings, but showing the forces that the surroundings exert on it (Figure 5.4(b)). Because the shoe is not moving, these forces are in equilibrium. Resolving the weight of the shoe (G) along (F_t) and normal (F_n) to the plane, the magnitudes of the components are, respectively: $F_t = G\sin\theta$; $F_n = G\cos\theta$. Dividing F_t by F_n, we get $F_t/F_n = \tan\theta$. If the angle of inclination of the plane (θ) is increased, the friction force will eventually be unable to resist the component of the shoe's weight down the slope and the shoe will begin to slide. The ratio of F_t/F_n (= $\tan\theta$) at which this occurs is called the coefficient of (limiting) static friction (μ_s). The maximum sliding friction force that can be transmitted between two bodies is: $F_{t\ max} = \mu_s\ F_n$. This is known as Newton's law of friction and refers to static friction, just before there is any relative movement between the two surfaces. It also relates to conditions in which only the friction force prevents relative movement. For such conditions, the maximum friction force depends only on the magnitude of the normal force pressing the surfaces together and the coefficient of static friction (μ_s). This coefficient depends only on the materials and nature (such as roughness) of the contacting surfaces and is, to a large extent, independent of the area of contact. The coefficient of friction should exceed 0.4 for safe walking on normal floors, 1.1 for running and 1.2 for all track and field events.

In certain sports in which spikes or studs penetrate or substantially deform a surface, the tangential (usually horizontal) force is transmitted by interlocking surfaces – traction – rather than by friction. Form locking then generates the tangential force, which is usually

Figure 5.2 Vertical component of ground reaction force in a standing vertical jump with no arm action: (A) on the ground before take-off for the jump; (B) in the air; (C) landing.

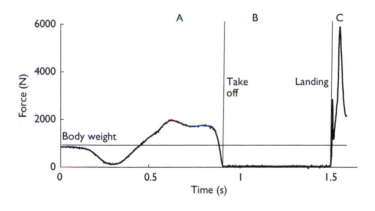

Figure 5.3 Left: (a) sagittal plane ground reaction force; Right: (b) its tangential (F_t) and normal (F_n) components.

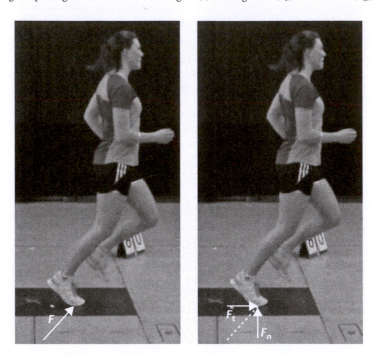

Figure 5.4 Left: (a) training shoe on an inclined plane; Right: (b) its free-body diagram.

greater than that obtainable from static friction. For such force generation, a traction coefficient can be defined similarly to the friction coefficient above.

Once the two surfaces are moving relative to one another, as when skis slide over snow, the friction force between them decreases and a coefficient of kinetic friction is defined such that: $F_t = \mu_k F_n$, noting $\mu_k < \mu_s$. This coefficient is relatively constant up to a speed of about 10 m/s. Kinetic friction always opposes relative sliding motion between two surfaces.

Friction not only affects translational motion, it also influences rotation, such as when swinging around a high bar or pivoting on the spot. At present there is no agreed definition of, nor agreed method of measuring, rotational friction coefficients in sport. Frictional resistance also occurs when one object tends to rotate or roll along another, as for a hockey ball rolling across an Astroturf pitch. In such cases it is possible to define a coefficient of rolling friction. The resistance to rolling is considerably less than the resistance to sliding and can be established by allowing a ball to roll down a slope from a fixed height (1 m is often used) and then measuring the horizontal distance that it rolls on the surface of interest. In general, for sports balls rolling on sports surfaces, the coefficient of rolling friction is around 0.1.

Reducing friction

To reduce friction or traction between two surfaces it is necessary to reduce the normal force or the coefficient of friction. In sport, the latter can be done by changing the materials of contact, and the former by movement technique. Such a technique is known as unweighting, in which the performer imparts a downward acceleration to his or her centre of mass (Figure 5.5(a)), thereby reducing the normal ground contact force to below body weight (Figure 5.5(b)). This technique is used, for example, in some turning skills in skiing and is often used to facilitate rotational movements.

Large coefficients of friction are detrimental when speed is wanted and friction opposes this. In skiing straight runs, kinetic friction is minimised by treating the base of the skis with wax. This can reduce the coefficient of friction to below 0.1. At the high speeds associated with skiing, frictional melting occurs, which further reduces the coefficient of friction to as low as 0.02 at speeds above 5 m/s. The friction coefficient is also affected by the condition of the snow–ice surface. In ice hockey and in figure and speed skating, the sharpened blades minimise the friction coefficient in the direction

Figure 5.5 Unweighting. Left: (a) forces acting on jumper; Right: (b) force platform record.

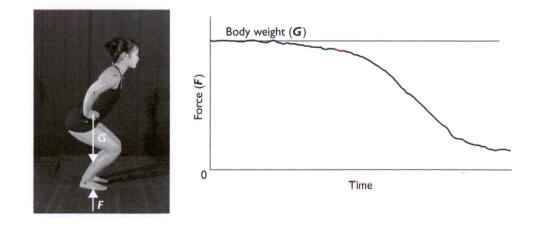

parallel to the blade length. The high pressures involved cause localised melting of the ice, which, along with the smooth blade surface, reduces friction. Within the human body, where friction causes wear, synovial membranes of one form or another excrete synovial fluid to lubricate the structures involved, resulting in frictional coefficients as low as 0.001. This occurs in synovial joints, synovial sheaths (such as that of the long head of the biceps brachii), and synovial sacs and bursae that protect tendons, for example at the tendon of quadriceps femoris near the patella.

Increasing friction

A large coefficient of friction or traction is often needed to permit quick changes of velocity or large accelerations. To increase friction, it is necessary to increase either the normal force or the friction coefficient. The normal force can be increased by weighting, the opposite process from unweighting. Other examples of increasing the normal force include the use of inverted aerofoils on racing cars and the technique used by skilled rock and mountain climbers of leaning away from the rock face. To increase the coefficient of friction, a change of materials, conditions or locking mechanism is necessary. The last of these can lead to a larger traction coefficient through the use of spikes in, for instance, javelin throwing and running, in which large velocity changes occur. Studs and cleats on sports boots and shoes have a similar, though lesser, effect.

Starting, stopping and turning

As noted above, form locking is very effective when large accelerations are needed. However, the use of spikes or studs makes rotation more difficult. This requires a compromise in general games, in which stopping and starting and rapid direction changes are combined with turning manoeuvres necessitating sliding of the shoe on the ground. When starting, the coefficient of friction or traction limits a runner's performance. A larger value on synthetic tracks compared with cinders, about 0.85 compared with 0.65, allows the runner a greater forward inclination of the trunk and a more horizontally directed leg drive and horizontal impulse. The use of starting blocks has similar benefits, with form locking replacing force locking. With lower values of the coefficient of friction, the runner must accommodate by using shorter strides. Although spikes can increase traction, energy is necessary to pull them out of the surface and it is questionable whether they confer any benefit when running on dry, dust-free synthetic tracks. When stopping, a sliding phase can be beneficial, unless a firm anchoring of the foot is required, as in the delivery stride of javelin throwing. Sliding is possible on cinder tracks and on grass and other natural surfaces; this potential is used by the grass and clay court tennis player. On synthetic surfaces, larger friction coefficients limit sliding; an athlete has to accommodate by unweighting, by hip and knee flexion. When turning, a large coefficient of friction requires substantial unweighting to permit a reduction in the moment of force needed to generate the turn. Without this unweighting, the energy demands of turning increase with rotational friction. In turning and stopping techniques in skiing, force locking is replaced by form locking using the edges of the skis; this substantially increases the force on the skis.

Effects of contact materials

The largest friction coefficients occur between two absolutely smooth, dry surfaces, owing to microscopic force locking at an atomic or molecular level. Many dry, clean, smooth metal surfaces in a vacuum adhere when they meet; in most cases, attempts to slide one past the other produce complete seizure. This perfect smoothness is made use of with certain rubbers in rock climbing shoes and racing tyres for dry surfaces. In the former case, the soft, smooth rubber adheres to the surface of the rock; in the latter, localised melting of the rubber occurs at the road surface. However in wet or very dusty conditions the loss of friction is substantial, as adhesion between the rubber and surface is prevented. The coefficient of friction reduces for a smooth tyre from around 5.0 on a dry surface to around 0.1 on a wet one. A compromise is afforded by treaded tyres with dry and wet surface friction coefficients of around 1.0 and 0.4 respectively. The treads allow water to be removed from the contact area between the tyre and road surface. Likewise, most sports shoes have treaded or cleated soles, and club and racket grips are rarely perfectly smooth. In some cases, the cleats on the sole of a sports shoe will also provide some form locking with certain surfaces.

Pulley friction

Passing a rope around the surface of a pulley makes it easier to resist a force of large magnitude at one end by a much smaller force at the other end because of the friction between the rope and the pulley. This principle is used, for example, in abseiling techniques in rock climbing and mountaineering. It also explains the need for synovial membranes to prevent large friction forces when tendons pass over bony prominences.

Buoyancy

Buoyancy is the force experienced by an object immersed, or partly immersed, in a fluid. It always acts vertically upwards at the centre of buoyancy (CB in Figure 5.6). The magnitude of the buoyancy force (B) is expressed by Archimedes' principle 'the upthrust is equal to the weight of fluid displaced', and is given by $B = V\rho g$, where V is the volume of fluid displaced, ρ is the density of the fluid and g is gravitational acceleration. The buoyancy force is large in water – pure fresh water has a density of 1000 kg/m^3 – and much smaller, but not entirely negligible, in air, which has a density of around 1.23 kg/m^3. For a person or an object to float and not sink, the magnitudes of the buoyancy force and the weight of the object must be equal, so that $B = G$.

Figure 5.6 Buoyancy force. Left: (a) forces acting – **B** is buoyancy force, **G** is swimmer's weight; Right: (b) forces in equilibrium with same line of action.

The swimmer in Figure 5.6 will only float if her average body density is less than or equal to the density of water. How much of her body is submersed will depend on the ratio of the two densities. If the density of the swimmer is greater than that of the water, she will sink. It is easier to float in sea water, for which the density is around 1020 kg/m^3, than in fresh water. For the human body, the relative proportions of tissues will determine whether sinking or floating occurs. Typical densities for body tissues are: fat 960 kg/m^3; muscle 1040–1090 kg/m^3; bone 1100 kg/m^3 (cancellous) to 1800 kg/m^3 (compact). The amount of air in the lungs is also very important. Most Caucasians can float with full inhalation whereas most people with a negroid body type cannot float even with full inhalation because of their different body composition, which is surely a factor contributing to the shortage of world-class black swimmers. Most people cannot float with full exhalation. Women float better than men because of an inherently higher proportion of body fat and champion swimmers have, not surprisingly, higher proportions of body fat than other elite athletes.

Fluid dynamic forces

Basic fluid mechanics

All sports take place within a fluid environment; the fluid is air (a gas) in running, water (a liquid) in underwater turns in swimming, or both, for example in sailing. Unlike solids, fluids flow freely and their shape is only retained if enclosed in a container; particles of the fluid alter their relative positions whenever a force acts. Liquids have a volume that stays the same while the shape changes. Gases expand to fill the whole volume available by changing density. This ability of fluids to distort continuously is vital to sports motions as it permits movement. Although fluids flow freely, there is a resistance to this flow, known as the 'viscosity' of the fluid. Viscosity is a property causing shear stresses between adjacent layers of moving fluid, leading to a resistance to motion through the fluid.

In general, the instantaneous velocity of a small element of fluid will depend both on time and its spatial position. A small element of fluid will generally follow a complex path, known as the 'path line' of the element of fluid. An imaginary line that lies tangential to the direction of flow of the fluid particles at any instant is called a 'streamline'; streamlines have no fluid flow across them.

An important principle for understanding fluid dynamics in sport is Bernoulli's principle, which, in essence, states that reducing the flow area, as for fluid flow past a runner, results in an increase in fluid speed and a decrease in fluid pressure. There are two very important ratios of fluid forces in sport. The Reynolds number is important in all fluid flow in sport; it is the ratio of the inertial force in the fluid to the viscous force. The 'Reynolds number' is calculated as $v\,l/\upsilon$ where v is a 'characteristic speed', usually the relative velocity between the fluid and an object, l is some 'characteristic length' of the object and υ is the 'kinematic viscosity' of the fluid. The 'Froude number' is the square root of the ratio of inertial to gravity forces; it is important whenever an interface between two fluids occurs and waves are generated, as happens in almost all water sports. The Froude number is calculated as $v/\sqrt{(l\,g)}$ where v and l are the characteristic speed and length, as above, and g is gravitational acceleration.

Laminar and turbulent flow

In laminar flow, the fluid particles move only in the direction of the flow. The fluid can be considered to consist of discrete plates (or laminae) flowing past one another. Laminar flow occurs at moderate speeds past objects of small diameter, such as a table tennis ball. In laminar flow energy is exchanged only between adjacent layers of the flowing fluid. Turbulent flow is predominant in sport. The particles of fluid have fluctuating velocity components in both the main flow direction and perpendicular to it. Turbulent flow is best thought of as a random collection of rotating eddies or vortices; energy is exchanged by these turbulent eddies on a greater scale than in laminar flow.

The type of flow that exists under given conditions depends on the Reynolds number. For low Reynolds numbers the fluid flow is laminar. At the 'critical' Reynolds number, the flow passes through a transition region and then becomes turbulent at a slightly higher Reynolds number. The Reynolds number at which flow changes from laminar to turbulent depends very much on the object past which the fluid flows. Consider a fairly flat boat hull moving through stationary water. Let us use the distance along the hull from the bow as the 'characteristic length' for the 'local' Reynolds number of the water flow past that point on the hull. Furthermore, we will define the characteristic speed as that of the boat moving through the water. For this example, the critical Reynolds number is in the range 100,000–3,000,000, depending on the nature of the flow in the water away from the boat and the surface roughness of the hull. The fluid flow close to the hull (in the 'boundary layer' discussed below) will change from laminar to turbulent at the point along the hull where the 'local' Reynolds number equals the critical value. If this does not happen, the flow will remain laminar along the whole length of the hull. For flow past a ball, the ball diameter is used as the characteristic length and the characteristic speed is the speed of the ball relative to the air. The critical Reynolds number, depending on ball roughness and flow conditions outside the boundary layer, is in the range 100,000–300,000.

The boundary layer

When relative motion occurs between a fluid and an object, as for flow of air or water past the sports performer, the fluid nearest the object is slowed down because of its viscosity. The region of fluid affected in this way is known as the boundary layer. Within this layer, the relative velocity of the fluid and object changes from zero at the surface of the object to the 'free stream' velocity, which is the difference between the velocity of the object and the velocity of the fluid outside the boundary layer.

Figure 5.7 Separation points (S) on a smooth ball for boundary layer flow that is: Top: (a) laminar; Bottom: (b) turbulent – T indicates transition from laminar to turbulent boundary flow.

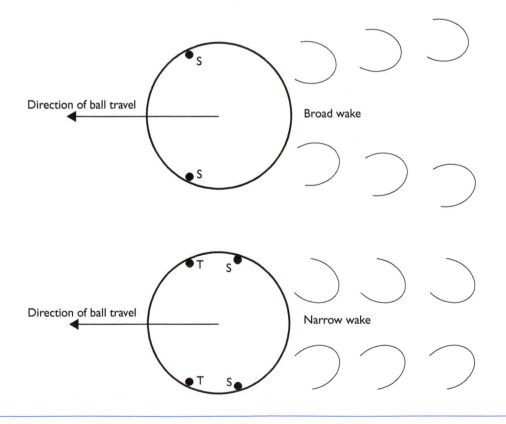

The slowing down of the fluid is accentuated if the flow of the fluid is from a wider to a narrower cross-section of the object, as the fluid is then trying to flow from a low-pressure region to a high-pressure region. Some of the fluid in the boundary layer may lose all of its kinetic energy. The boundary layer then separates from the body at the separation points (S in Figure 5.7), leaving a low-pressure area, known as the wake, behind the object.

An object moving from a region of low pressure to one of high pressure experiences a drag force, which will be discussed below. The boundary layer separation, which leads to the formation of the wake, occurs far more readily if the fluid flow in the boundary layer is laminar (Figure 5.7(a)) than if the flow is turbulent (Figure 5.7(b)). This is because kinetic energy is more evenly distributed across a turbulent boundary layer, enabling the fluid particles near the boundary to resist the increasing pressure better. Figure 5.7 shows the difference in the separation point (S) positions and the size of the wake between laminar and turbulent boundary layers on a ball. The change from laminar to turbulent boundary layer flow will occur, for a given object and conditions, at a speed related to the critical Reynolds number. The change occurs at the transition point (T, Figure 5.7(b)), and the relationship between the transition and separation points is very important. If separation occurs before its transition to turbulent flow, a large wake is formed (Figure 5.7(a)), whereas transition to turbulent flow upstream of the separation point results in a smaller wake (Figure 5.7(b)).

Drag forces

For an object symmetrical with respect to the fluid flow, such as a non-spinning table tennis ball, the fluid dynamic force acts in the direction opposite to the motion of the object and is termed a 'drag' force. Drag forces resist motion and, therefore, generally restrict sports performance. They can, however, have beneficial propulsive effects, as in swimming and rowing. To maintain a runner in motion at a constant speed against a drag force requires an expenditure of energy equal to the product of the drag force and the speed. If no such energy is present, as for a projectile, the object will decelerate at a rate proportional to the area presented by the object to the fluid flow (the so-called 'frontal' area, A) and inversely proportional to the mass of the body, m. The ratio of mass to frontal area (m/A) is crucial in determining the effect that air resistance has on projectile motion. A shot, with a very high ratio of mass to frontal area, is hardly affected by air resistance, whereas a cricket ball, with only one-sixteenth the ratio of mass to frontal area of the shot, is far more affected. A table tennis ball (one-two hundred and fiftieth the ratio of mass to frontal area of the shot) has a greatly altered trajectory.

Pressure drag

Pressure drag, or wake drag, contributes to the fluid resistance experienced by, for example, projectiles and runners. This is the major drag force in most sports and is caused by boundary layer separation leaving a low-pressure wake behind the object. The object, tending to move from a low-pressure to a high-pressure region, experiences a drag force. The pressure drag can be reduced by minimising the disturbance that the object causes to the fluid flow, a process known as streamlining. An oval shape, similar to a rugby ball, has only two-thirds of the pressure drag of a spherical ball with the same frontal area. The pressure drag is very small on a streamlined aerofoil shape, such as the cross-section of a glider wing. Streamlining is very important in motor car and motor cycle racing, and in discus and javelin throwing. Swimmers and skiers can reduce the pressure drag forces acting on them by adopting streamlined shapes. The adoption of a streamlined shape is of considerable advantage to downhill skiers.

If we increase the speed of an object through a fluid – such as a ball through the air – we find a dramatic change in the drag as the boundary layer flow changes from laminar to turbulent. As this transition occurs, at the critical Reynolds number, the drag decreases by about 65 per cent. Promoting a turbulent boundary layer is an important mechanism in reducing pressure drag if the speed is close to the value necessary to achieve the critical Reynolds number. At such speeds, which are common in ball sports, roughening the surface promotes turbulence in the boundary layer, encouraging this decrease in drag. The nap of tennis balls and the dimples on golf balls are examples of roughness helping to induce boundary layer transition, thereby reducing drag. Within the Reynolds number range 110,000–175,000, which corresponds to ball speeds off the tee of 45–70 m/s, the dimples on a golf ball cause the drag coefficient to decrease proportionally to speed. The drag force then increases only proportionally to speed, rather than speed squared, benefiting the hard-hitting player.

Many sports balls are not uniformly rough. Then, within a speed range somewhat below the critical Reynolds number, it is possible for roughness elements on one part of the ball to stimulate transition of the boundary layer to turbulent flow, while the boundary layer flow on the smoother portion of the ball remains laminar. This is very important, for example, in cricket, in which the asymmetrical disposition of the ball's seam accounts for the lateral movement of the ball known as swing. The seam promotes turbulence in the boundary layer on the 'rough' side of the ball, on which the seam is upstream of the separation point, as in Figure 5.7(b), while separation occurs on the other ('smooth') side of the ball, as in Figure 5.7(a). The asymmetrical wake causes the ball to swing towards the side to which the seam points. For reverse swing to occur, the ball must be released above the critical speed for the smooth side of the ball, which can only be done by bowlers who can achieve such speeds. The boundary layer becomes turbulent on both hemispheres before separation. On the rough side, the turbulent boundary layer thickens more rapidly and separates earlier than on the smooth side. The result is the reversal of the direction of wake displacement and, therefore, of swing.

Skin friction drag

Skin friction drag is the force caused by friction between the molecules of fluid and a solid boundary. It is only important for streamlined bodies for which separation – and pressure drag – has been minimised. Unlike pressure drag, skin friction drag is reduced by having a laminar as opposed to a turbulent boundary layer. This occurs because the rate of shear at the solid boundary is greater for turbulent flow. Reduction of skin friction drag is important for racing cars, racing motor cycles, gliders, hulls of boats, skiers and ski-jumpers, and swimmers. It is minimised by reducing the roughness of the surfaces in contact with the fluid.

Wave drag

Wave drag occurs only in sports in which an object moves through both water and air. As the object moves through the water, the pressure differences at its boundary cause the water level to rise and fall and waves are generated. The energy of the waves is provided by the object, which experiences a resistance to its motion. The greater the speed of the body, the larger the wave drag, which is important in most aquatic sports. Wave drag also depends on the wave patterns generated and the dimensions of the object. The drag is often expressed as a function of the Froude number. Speedboats and racing yachts are designed to plane – to ride high in the water – at their highest speeds so that wave drag – and pressure drag – are then very small. In swimming the wave drag is small compared with the pressure drag, unless the swimmer's speed is above about 1.6 m/s, when a bow wave is formed.

Other forms of drag

Spray-making drag occurs in some water sports because of the energy involved in generating spray. It is usually negligible, except perhaps during high-speed turns in surfing and windsurfing. Induced drag arises from a three-dimensional object that is generating lift. It can be minimised by having a large aspect ratio – the ratio of the dimension of the object perpendicular to the flow direction to the dimension along the flow direction. Long, thin wings on gliders minimise the induced drag, whereas a javelin has entirely the wrong shape for this purpose.

Lift forces

If an asymmetry exists in the fluid flow around a body, the fluid dynamic force will act at some angle to the direction of motion and can be resolved into two component forces. These are a drag force opposite to the flow direction and a lift force perpendicular to the flow direction. Such asymmetry may be caused in three ways. For a discus or javelin, for example, it arises from an inclination of an axis of symmetry of the body to the direction of flow (Figure 5.8(a)). Another cause is asymmetry of the body (Figure 5.8(b)); this is the case for sails, which act similarly to the aerofoil-shaped wings of an aircraft, and the hands of a swimmer, which function as hydrofoils. The Magnus effect (Figure 5.8(c)) occurs when rotation of a symmetrical body, such as a ball, produces asymmetry in the fluid flow.

Figure 5.8 Generation of lift. Top: (a) inclination of an axis of symmetry; Middle: (b) body asymmetry; Bottom: (c) Magnus effect.

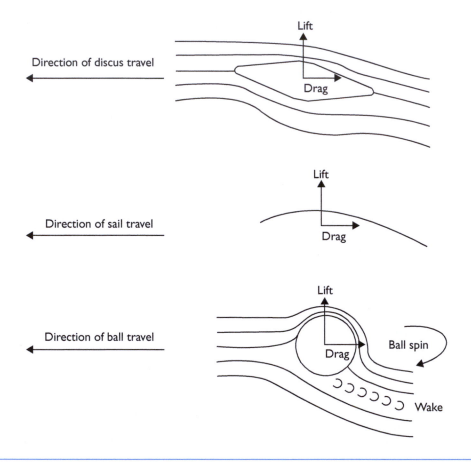

Swimmers use a mixture of lift and drag forces for propulsion, with their hands acting as rudimentary hydrofoils. A side view of a typical path of a front crawl swimmer's hand relative to the water is shown in Figure 5.9(a). In the initial and final portions of the pull phase of this stroke (marked 'i' and 'f' in Figure 5.9(a)) only the lift force (L) can make a significant contribution to propulsion. In the middle region of the pull phase (marked 'm'), the side view would suggest that drag (D) is the dominant contributor. However, a view from in front of the swimmer (Figure 5.9(b)) or below (Figure 5.9(c)) shows an S-shaped pull pattern in the sideways plane. These sideways movements of the hands generate significant propulsion through lift forces perpendicular to the path of travel of the hand (Figure 5.9(c)). Swimmers need to develop a 'feel' of the water flow over their hands, and to vary the hand 'pitch' angle with respect to the flow of water to optimise the propulsive forces throughout the stroke. The shape of both oars and paddles suggests that they can also behave as hydrofoils. In rowing, for

Figure 5.9 Typical path of a swimmer's hand relative to the water. Top and left: (a) side view; Bottom: (b) view from in front of the swimmer; Right: (c) view from below the swimmer.

example, the propulsive forces generated are a combination of both lift and drag components and not just drag. The velocity of the oar or paddle relative to the water is the crucial factor. If this is forwards at any time when the oar is submerged, the drag is in the wrong direction to provide propulsion. Only a lift force can fulfil this function (see Figure 5.9). The wing paddle in kayaking was developed to exploit this propulsive lift effect.

Many ball sports involve a spinning ball. Consider, for example, a ball moving through a fluid, and having backspin as in Figure 5.8(c). The top of the ball is moving in the same direction as the air relative to the ball, while the bottom of the ball is moving against the air stream. The rotational motion of the ball is transferred to the thin boundary layer adjacent to the surface of the ball. On the upper surface of the ball this 'circulation' imparted to the boundary layer reduces the difference in velocity across the boundary layer and delays separation. On the lower surface of the ball, the boundary layer is moving against the rest of the fluid flow, known as the free stream. This increases the velocity difference across the boundary layer and separation still occurs. The resulting wake has, therefore, been deflected downwards, as can be seen in Figure 5.8(c). Newton's laws of motion imply that the wake deflection is due to a force provided by the ball acting downwards on the air and that a reaction moves the ball away from the wake. This phenomenon is known as the Magnus effect. For a ball with backspin, the force acts perpendicular to the motion of the ball – it is a lift force.

Golf clubs are lofted so that the ball is undercut, producing backspin. This varies from approximately 50 Hz for a wood to 160 Hz for a nine-iron. The lift force generated can even be sufficient to cause the initial ball trajectory to be curved slightly upwards. The lift force increases with the spin and substantially increases the length of drive compared to that with no spin. The main function of golf ball dimples is to assist the transfer of the rotational motion of the ball to the boundary layer of air to increase the Magnus force and give optimum lift. Backspin and topspin are used in games such as tennis and table tennis, both to vary the flight of the ball and to alter its bounce. In cricket, a spin bowler usually spins the ball so that it is rotating about the axis along which it is moving (its velocity vector), and the ball only deviates when it contacts the ground. However, if the ball's spin axis does not coincide with its velocity vector, the ball will also move laterally through the air. A baseball pitcher also uses the Magnus effect to 'curve' the ball; at a pitching speed of 30 m/s the spin imparted can be as high as 30 Hz, which gives a lateral deflection of 0.45 m in 18 m. A soccer ball can be made to swerve, or 'bend', in flight by moving the foot across the ball as it is kicked. This causes rotation of the ball about the vertical axis. If the foot is moved from right to left as the ball is kicked, the ball will swerve to the right. Slicing and hooking of a golf ball are caused, inadvertently, by sidespin imparted at impact. In crosswinds, the relative direction of motion between the air and the ball is changed; a small amount of sidespin, imparted by 'drawing' the ball with a slightly open club face or 'fading' the ball with a slightly closed club face depending on the wind direction, can then increase the length of the drive.

A negative Magnus effect can also occur for a ball travelling below the critical Reynolds number. This happens when the boundary layer flow remains laminar on the side of the ball moving in the direction of the relative air flow, as the Reynolds number here remains below the critical value. On the other side of the ball, the rotation increases the relative speed between the air and the ball so that the boundary layer becomes turbulent. If this happens on a back-spinning ball, laminar boundary layer flow will occur on the top surface and turbulent on the bottom surface (the opposite case to Figure 5.8(c)). The wake will be deflected upwards, the opposite from the normal Magnus effect discussed above, and the ball will plummet to the ground under the action of the negative lift force. Reynolds numbers in many ball sports are close to the critical value, and the negative Magnus effect may, therefore, be important. It has occasionally been proposed as an explanation for certain unusual ball behaviour in, for example, the 'floating' serve in volleyball.

Impact forces

Impact forces occur whenever two or more objects collide. They are usually very large and of short duration compared to other forces acting. The most important impact force for the sport and exercise participant is that between that person and some external object, for example a runner's foot striking a hard surface. These forces can be positive biologically as they can promote bone growth, providing that they are not too large; large impact forces are one factor that can increase the injury risk to an athlete.

An example of an impact force is shown by the force peak just after the start of the landing phase (C) in Figure 5.2.

Impacts involving sports objects, such as a ball and the ground, can affect the technique of a sports performer. For example, the spin imparted by the server to a tennis ball will affect how it rebounds, which will influence the stroke played by the receiver. Impacts of this type are termed oblique impacts and involve, for example, a ball hitting the ground at an angle other than 90°, as in a tennis serve, and a bat or racket hitting a moving ball. If the objects at impact are moving along the line joining their centres of mass, the impact is 'direct', as when a ball is dropped vertically onto the ground. Direct impacts are unusual in sport, in which oblique impacts predominate.

COMBINATIONS OF FORCES ON THE SPORTS PERFORMER

In sport, more than one external force usually acts on the performer and the effect produced by the combination of these forces will depend on their magnitudes and relative directions. Figure 5.10(a) shows a biomechanical system, here a runner, isolated (conceptually) from the surrounding world. The effects of those surroundings, which for the runner are weight and ground reaction force, are represented on the diagram as force vectors. As I mentioned above, such a diagram is known as a 'free-body diagram', which should be used whenever carrying out a biomechanical analysis of 'force systems'. The effects of different types of force system can be considered as follows.

Statics is a very useful, and mathematically simple and powerful branch of mechanics. It is used to study force systems in which the forces are in equilibrium, such that they have no resultant effect on the object on which they act, as in Figure 5.6(b). In that figure, the buoyancy force, B, and the weight of the swimmer, G, share the same line of action and are equal in magnitude but have opposite directions, so that $B = G$. This approach may seem to be somewhat limited in sport, in which the net, or resultant, effect of the forces acting is usually to cause the performer or object to accelerate, as in Figure 5.10(a). In this figure, the resultant force can be obtained by moving the ground reaction force, F, along its line of action, which passes through the centre of mass in this case, giving Figure 5.10(b). As the resultant force passes through the runner's centre of mass, the runner can be represented as a point, the centre of mass, at which the entire runner's mass is considered to be concentrated; only changes in linear motion will occur for such a force system. The resultant of F and G will be the net force acting on the runner. This net force equals the mass of the runner, m, multiplied by the acceleration, a, of the centre of mass. Symbolically, this is written as $m\,a = F + G$. This is one form of Newton's second law of motion (see Box 5.2).

More generally, as in Figure 5.10(c), the resultant force will not act through the centre of mass; a moment of force – also called a torque – will then tend to cause the runner to rotate about his or her centre of mass. The magnitude of this moment of force about a point – here the centre of mass – is the product of the force and its

Figure 5.10 Forces on a runner. Left: (a) free-body diagram of dynamic force system with ground reaction force through centre of mass; Middle: (b) resultant force (note that the vectors have, for clarity, been magnified fourfold from (a); Right: (c) free-body diagram with ground reaction force not through centre of mass.

moment arm, which is the perpendicular distance of the line of action of the force from that point. Rotation will be considered in detail later in this chapter.

It is possible to treat dynamic systems of forces, such as those represented in Figure 5.10, using the equations of static equilibrium. To do this, however, we need to introduce an 'imaginary' force into the dynamic system, which is equal in magnitude to the resultant force but opposite in direction, to produce a quasi-static force system. This imaginary force is known as an 'inertia' force. Its introduction allows the use of the general and very simple equations of static equilibrium for forces (F) and moments of force (M): $\sum F = 0$; $\sum M = 0$; that is, the vector sum ($\sum$) of all the forces, including the imaginary 'inertia' forces, is zero and the vector sum of all the moments of force, including the imaginary 'inertia' moments, is also zero (see Appendix 4.2 for a simple graphical method of calculating vector sums). These vector equations of static equilibrium can be applied to all force systems that are static or have been made quasi-static through the use of inertia forces. How the vector equations simplify to the scalar equations used to calculate the magnitudes of forces and moments of force will depend on how the forces combine to form the system of forces. Two-dimensional systems of forces are known as 'planar' force systems and have forces acting in one plane only; three-dimensional force systems are known as 'spatial' force systems. Force systems can be classified as follows.

Figure 5.11 Levers as examples of parallel force systems. Left: (a) first-class lever; Right: (b) third-class lever. Note: F_m is the muscle force, F_j the joint force and F_r the resistance; r_m is the muscle moment arm (the force arm) and r_r the resistance arm.

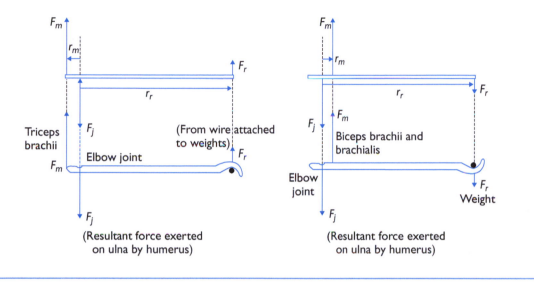

- Linear (also called collinear) force systems consist of forces with the same line of action, such as the forces in a tug-of-war rope or the swimmer in Figure 5.6(b). No moment equilibrium equation is relevant for such systems as all forces act along the same line.
- Concurrent force systems have the lines of action of the forces passing through a common point, such as the centre of mass. The collinear system in the previous paragraph is a special case. The runner in Figure 5.10(a) is an example of a planar concurrent force system and many spatial ones can also be found in sports movements. As all forces pass through the centre of mass, no moment equilibrium equation is relevant.
- Parallel force systems have the lines of action of the forces all parallel; they can be planar, as in Figure 5.6(a), or spatial. The tendency of the forces to rotate the object about some point means that the equation of moment equilibrium must be considered. The simple cases of first-class and third-class levers in the human musculoskeletal system are examples of planar parallel force systems and are shown in Figure 5.11(a) and (b). The moment equilibrium equation in these examples reduces to the 'principle of levers'. This states that the product of the magnitudes of the muscle force and its moment arm, sometimes called the force arm, equals the product of the resistance and its moment arm, called the resistance arm. Symbolically, using the notation of Figure 5.11: $F_m\, r_m = F_r\, r_r$. The force equilibrium equation leads to $F_j = F_m + F_r$ and $F_j = F_m - F_r$ for the joint force (F_j) in the first-class and third-class levers of Figure 5.11(a) and (b), respectively. It is worth mentioning here that the example of a second-class lever sometimes used in sports

biomechanics textbooks – a person rising onto the toes, treating the floor as the fulcrum – is contrived. Few, if any, such levers exist in the human musculoskeletal system. This is not surprising as they represent a class of mechanical lever intended to enable a large force to be moved by a small one, as in a wheelbarrow. The human musculoskeletal system, by contrast, achieves speed and range of movement but requires relatively large muscle forces to accomplish this against resistance.

• Finally, general force systems may be planar or spatial, have none of the above simplifications and are the ones normally found in sports biomechanics, such as when analysing the various soft tissue forces acting on a body segment. These force systems will not be covered further in this book.

The vector equations of statics and the use of inertia forces can aid the analysis of the complex force systems that are commonplace in sport. However, many sports biomechanists feel that the use of the equations of static equilibrium obscures the dynamic nature of force in sport, and that it is more revealing to deal with the dynamic equations of motion, an approach that I prefer. In sport, force systems almost always change with time, as in Figure 5.2, which shows the vertical component of ground reaction force recorded from a force platform during a standing vertical jump. The effect of the force at any instant is reflected in an instantaneous acceleration of the performer's centre of mass. The change of the force with time determines how the velocity and displacement of the centre of mass change, and it is important to remember this.

MOMENTUM AND THE LAWS OF LINEAR MOTION

Inertia and mass

The inertia of an object is its reluctance to change its state of motion. Inertia is directly measured or expressed by the mass of the object, which is the quantity of matter of which the object is composed. It is more difficult to accelerate an object of large mass, such as a shot, than one of small mass, such as a dart. Mass is a scalar, having no directional quality; the SI unit of mass is the kilogram (kg).

Momentum

Linear momentum (more usually just called momentum) is the quantity of motion possessed by a particle or rigid body, measured by the product of its mass and the velocity of its centre of mass. It is a very important quantity in sports biomechanics. As it is the product of a scalar and a vector, it is itself a vector whose direction is identical to that of the velocity vector. The unit of linear momentum is kg·m/s.

BOX 5.2 NEWTON'S LAWS OF LINEAR MOTION

These laws completely determine the motion of a point, such as the centre of mass of a sports performer, and are named after the great British scientist of the seventeenth century, Sir Isaac Newton. They have to be modified to deal with the rotational motion of the body as a whole or a single body segment, as below. They have limited use when analysing complex motions of systems of rigid bodies, but these are beyond the scope of this book.

First law (law of inertia)

An object will continue in a state of rest or of uniform motion in a straight line (constant velocity) unless acted upon by external forces that are not in equilibrium. Straight-line skating is a close approximation to this state; a skater can glide across the ice at almost constant velocity as the coefficient of friction is so small. To change velocity, the blades of the skates need to be turned away from the direction of motion to increase the force acting on them. In the flight phase of a long jump the horizontal velocity of the jumper remains almost constant, as air resistance is small. However, the vertical velocity of the jumper changes continuously because of the jumper's weight – an external force caused by the gravitational pull of the earth.

Second law (law of momentum)

The rate of change of momentum of an object is proportional to the force causing it and takes place in the direction in which the force acts. For an object of constant mass, such as the human performer, this law simplifies to: the mass multiplied by the acceleration of that mass is equal to the force acting. When a ball is kicked, in soccer for example, the acceleration of the ball will be proportional to the force applied to the ball by the kicker's foot and inversely proportional to the mass of the ball.

Third law (law of interaction)

For every action, or force, exerted by one object on a second, there is an equal and opposite force, or reaction, exerted by the second object on the first. The ground reaction force experienced by the runner of Figure 5.3 is equal and opposite to the force exerted by the runner on the ground (F); this latter force would be shown on a free-body diagram of the ground (we don't often draw these!).

Impulse of a force

Newton's second law of linear motion (the law of momentum) can be expressed symbolically at any time, t, as $F = \mathrm{d}p/\mathrm{d}t = \mathrm{d}(m\,v)/\mathrm{d}t$. That is, F, the net external force acting on the body, equals the rate of change with time ($\mathrm{d}/\mathrm{d}t$) of momentum ($p = m\,v$). For an object of constant mass (m), this equation becomes: $F = \mathrm{d}p/\mathrm{d}t = m\,\mathrm{d}v/\mathrm{d}t = m\,a$, where v

is velocity and a is acceleration. If we now sum these symbolic equations over a time interval we can write: $\int\mathbf{F}\,dt = \int d(m\,\mathbf{v})$; this equals $m\int d\mathbf{v}$, if m is constant. The symbol $\int$ is called an integral, which is basically the summing of instantaneous forces. The left side, $\int\mathbf{F}\,dt$, of this equation is the impulse of the force, for which the SI unit is newton-seconds, N·s. This impulse equals the change of momentum of the object ($\int d(m\,\mathbf{v})$ or $m\int d\mathbf{v}$ if m is constant). This equation is known as the impulse–momentum equation and, with its equivalent form for rotation, is an important foundation of the study of human movement in sport (see also Appendix 2.1). The impulse is the area under the force–time curve over the time interval of interest and can be calculated graphically or, usually, numerically. The impulse of force can be found from a force–time pattern, such as Figure 5.2 or Figure 5.12, which is easily obtained from a force plate.

The impulse–momentum equation can be rewritten for an object of constant mass (m) as $F\Delta t = m\Delta v$, where F is the mean value of the force acting during a time interval Δt during which the velocity of the object changes by Δv (the Greek symbol delta, Δ, simply designates a change). The change in the horizontal velocity of a sprinter from the gun firing to leaving the blocks depends on the horizontal impulse of the force exerted by the sprinter on the blocks (from the second law of linear motion) and is inversely proportional to the mass of the sprinter. In turn, the impulse of the force exerted by the blocks on the sprinter is equal in magnitude but opposite in direction to that exerted, by muscular action, by the sprinter on the blocks (from the third law of linear motion). Obviously, a large horizontal velocity off the blocks is desirable. However, a compromise is needed as the time (Δt) spent in achieving the required impulse adds to the time spent running after leaving the blocks to give the recorded race time. The production of a large impulse of force is also important in many sports techniques of hitting, kicking and throwing for maximising the speed of the object involved. In javelin throwing, for example, the release speed of the javelin depends on the impulse applied to the javelin by the thrower during the delivery stride and the impulse applied by ground reaction and gravity forces to the combined thrower–javelin system throughout the preceding phases of the throw. In catching a ball, the impulse required to stop the ball is determined by the mass (m) and change in velocity (Δv) of the ball. The catcher can reduce the mean force (F) acting on his or her hands by increasing the duration of the contact time (Δt) by 'giving' with the ball.

FORCE–TIME GRAPHS AS MOVEMENT PATTERNS

Consider an international volleyball coach who wishes to assess the vertical jumping capabilities of his or her squad members. Assume that this coach has access to a force plate, a device that records the variation with time of the contact force between a person and the surroundings (see below). The coach uses the force plate to record the force–time graph exerted by the players performing standing vertical jumps (see, for

Figure 5.12 Standing vertical jump time series. Top: (a) acceleration; Middle: (b) velocity; Bottom: (c) displacement.

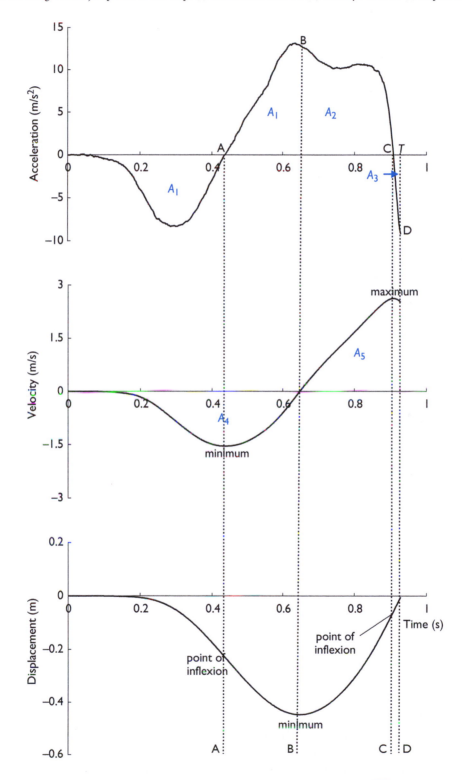

example, Figure 5.2). These graphs provide another movement pattern for both the qualitative and the quantitative movement analyst; our world is exceedingly rich in such patterns. Each player's force–time graph, after subtracting his or her weight, is easily converted to an acceleration–time graph (Figure 5.12(a)) as acceleration equals force divided by the player's mass, where the acceleration is that of the jumper's centre of mass.

Qualitative evaluation of a force–time or acceleration–time pattern

In Chapter 3, we saw how important it is for a qualitative analyst to be able to interpret angle–time and displacement–time patterns qualitatively. Force–time or acceleration–time patterns are far less likely to be encountered by the qualitative movement analyst and are not so revealing about other kinematic patterns – velocity and displacement – as are graphs of displacement or angle against time. However, if you are prepared to accept that the velocity equals the area between the horizontal zero-acceleration line – the time (t) axis of the graph – and the acceleration curve from the start of the movement at time 0 up to any particular time, and that areas below the time axis are negative and those above positive, then several key points on the velocity–time graph follow.

- At time A in Figure 5.12(a), the area (A_1) under the time axis and above the acceleration–time curve from O to A reaches its greatest negative value, so the vertical velocity of the jumper's centre of mass also reaches its greatest negative value there, corresponding to a zero acceleration. We can then sketch the velocity graph in Figure 5.12(b) up to time A, noting that it must be a smooth curve.
- At time B in Figure 5.12(a), the area under the acceleration–time curve from A to B and above the time axis is $+ A_1$ – the same magnitude as before but now positive. So the net area between the acceleration–time curve and the time axis from O to B is $-A_1 + A_1 = 0$. The vertical velocity of the jumper's centre of mass at B is, therefore, zero; we can now sketch the vertical velocity curve from A to B in Figure 5.12(b).
- From B to C the area between the acceleration–time curve and the time axis is positive, so the area (A_2) reaches its greatest positive value at C. Now we can sketch the vertical velocity curve from B to C in Figure 5.12(b).
- Finally, from C to take-off at D (time T), we have a small negative area, A_3, and the vertical velocity decreases from its largest positive value by this small amount before take-off, as in Figure 5.12(b).

By similar reasoning, if you are prepared to accept that displacement of the jumper's centre of mass equals the area between the horizontal zero-velocity line – the time axis of the graph – and the velocity curve from the start of the movement at 0 up to any particular time, and, again, that areas below the time axis are negative and those above positive, then several key points on the displacement–time graph follow.

- At time B in Figure 5.12(b), the area ($-A_4$) under the time axis and above the vertical velocity–time curve from O to B reaches its greatest negative value, so the vertical displacement of the jumper's centre of mass also reaches its greatest negative value there, corresponding to a zero velocity. We can then sketch the displacement graph in Figure 5.12(c) up to B. Please note that this is the lowest point reached by the jumper's centre of mass, at full hip and knee flexion, before the jumper starts to rise.
- At time T in Figure 5.12.b, the area (A_5) under the velocity–time curve from B to D and above the time axis is positive so the vertical displacement reaches its greatest positive value while the jumper is still on the force plate at take-off, T. Now we can sketch the vertical displacement curve from B to D in Figure 5.12(c).

Note again, as in Chapter 2, the trend of peaks or, more obviously in this case, troughs is acceleration then velocity then displacement.

Quantitative evaluation of a force–time or acceleration–time pattern

Our volleyball coach may wish to obtain, from this acceleration–time curve, values for the magnitude of the vertical velocity at take-off and the maximum height reached by the player's centre of mass. The process of obtaining velocities and displacements from accelerations qualitatively was outlined above. The quantitative process for doing the same thing is referred to, mathematically, as integration; it can be performed graphically or, usually, numerically. If quantitative acceleration data are available – the numbers from which Figure 5.12(a) was plotted, if you like – we can integrate the acceleration data to obtain the velocity–time graph, as in Figure 5.12(b), which can, in turn, be integrated to give the displacement–time graph of Figure 5.12(c). Most quantitative ways of doing these integrations basically involve determining areas as above, but for increasing small time intervals from left to right. The resulting graphs, with numbered axes as in Figure 5.12, would be more accurate than the 'sketched' qualitative ones but the shapes should be very similar if the qualitative analyst understood well the process of obtaining the velocity and displacement patterns. Our volleyball coach could now simply read the vertical take-off velocity (v_T) for each player from graphs such as Figure 5.12(b) at take-off, T (see Study Task 3). We can calculate the maximum height (h) reached by a player's centre of mass by equating his or her take-off kinetic energy, $\frac{1}{2}mv_T^2$, to the potential energy at the peak of the jump, mgh, where m is the player's mass and g is gravitational acceleration, so $h = v_T^2/(2g)$.

It can be very useful when interpreting force–time patterns, both qualitatively and quantitatively, to view the force–time pattern and a video recording (or images from an on-line motion analysis system) simultaneously. Two ways of doing this, for the vertical force from a squat standing vertical jump synchronised with digital video footage using Simi Motion, are shown in the Interactive eTextbook.

DETERMINATION OF THE CENTRE OF MASS OF THE HUMAN BODY

We have seen in the previous sections that the most important application of the laws of linear motion in sports biomechanics is in expressing, completely, the motion of a sports performer's centre of mass, which is the unique point about which the mass of the performer is evenly distributed. The effects of external forces upon the sports performer can, therefore, be studied by the linear motion of the centre of mass and by rotations about the centre of mass. It is often found that the movement patterns of the centre of mass vary between highly skilled and less skilful performers, providing a simple tool for evaluating technique. Furthermore, the path of the centre of mass is important, for example, in studying whether a high jumper's centre of mass can pass below the bar while the jumper's body segments all pass over the bar, and how high above the hurdle a hurdler's centre of mass needs to be to just clear the hurdle.

The position of the centre of mass is a function of age, sex and body build, and changes with breathing, ingestion of food and disposition of body fluids. It is doubtful whether it can be pinpointed to better than 3 mm. In the fundamental or anatomical reference position (see Chapter 1), the centre of mass lies about 56–57 per cent of a male's height from the soles of the feet, the figure for females being 55 per cent. In this position, the centre of mass is located about 40 mm inferior to the navel, roughly midway between the anterior and posterior skin surfaces. The position of the centre of mass is highly dependent on the orientation of a person's body segments. For example, in a piked body position the centre of mass of a gymnast may lie outside the body.

The segmentation method is generally used in sports biomechanics to determine the position of the whole-body centre of mass. In this method, the following information is required:

- The masses of the individual body segments, usually as proportions of the total body mass.
- The locations of the centres of mass of those segments in the position to be analysed. This requirement is usually met by a combination of the pre-established location of each segment's centre of mass with respect to the end points of the segment, and the positions of those end points on a video image, for example the ankle joint in Figure 5.13(a). The end points can be joint centres or terminal points and are estimated in the analysed body position from the camera viewing direction (Figure 5.13). The anatomical landmarks used to estimate joint centre positions are shown in Table 5.1 and Box 6.2. It is worth noting that even for the apparently sagittal plane movement in Figure 5.13(b), in which the markers were carefully placed according to Table 5.1 and Box 6.2 with the lifter in the fundamental reference posture but with the palms facing backwards when holding the bar, some markers no longer exactly overlay joint axes of rotation.

Figure 5.13 Determination of whole-body centre of mass. Top: (a) simplified example for Study Task 4 – red circles represent appropriate joint centres (for clarity, H = hip and W = wrist) or terminal points (see also Table 5.1); Bottom: (b) normal example with markers placed on the body in the reference position and with some markers obscured.

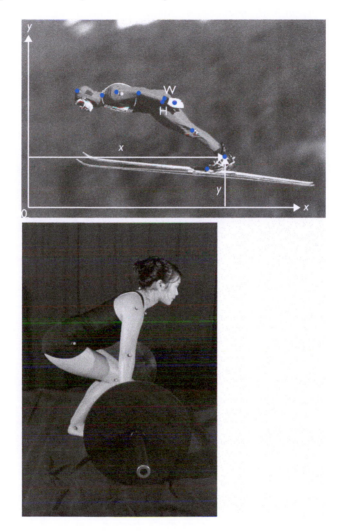

The ways of obtaining body segment data, including masses and locations of centres of mass, were briefly outlined in Chapter 4. The positions of the segmental end points are obtained from some visual record, usually a video recording of the movement. For the centre of mass to represent the system of segmental masses, the moment of mass (similar to the moment of force) of the centre of mass must be identical to the sum of the moments of body segment masses about any given axis. The calculation can

Table 5.1 Calculation of the two-dimensional position of the whole-body centre of mass; cadaver data adjusted to correct for fluid loss.

SEGMENT	MASS FRACTION $m' = m_i / m$	LENGTH RATIO[1,2] lr	x-COORDINATE PROXIMAL x_p	DISTAL x_d	MASS CENTRE[3] x_m	MOMENT $= m'x_m$	y-COORDINATE PROXIMAL y_p	DISTAL y_d	MASS CENTRE[3] y_m	MOMENT $= m'y_m$
Head and neck	0.081	0.500								
Trunk	0.497	0.450								
Right upper arm	0.028	0.436								
Right forearm	0.016	0.430								
Right hand	0.006	0.506								
Right thigh	0.101	0.433								
Right calf	0.046	0.433								
Right foot	0.014	0.449								
Left upper arm	0.028	0.436								
Left forearm	0.016	0.430								
Left hand	0.006	0.506								
Left thigh	0.101	0.433								
Left calf	0.046	0.433								
Left foot	0.014	0.449								
Whole body	1.000	—	—	—	—	$=\Sigma m'x_m$	—	—	—	$=\Sigma m'y_m$

Notes:
1. Using simple ratios, although many biomechanists use regression equations.
2. Defined as the distance of the centre of mass from the proximal point divided by the distance from the proximal to the distal point. Joint centre locations are given in Box 6.2. The proximal point is the proximal joint and the distal point is the distal joint except for the following; for the head and neck, the 'proximal' point is the top (vertex) of the head and the distal point is the midpoint of a line joining the tip of the spinous process of the seventh cervical vertebra (C7) and the suprasternal notch (or of the line joining the two shoulder joint centres; for the trunk, the proximal point is the same as the distal point for the head and neck and the distal point is the midpoint of the line joining the hips; for the hand, the distal point is the third metacarpophalangeal joint (the third knuckle); for the foot, the proximal point is the most posterior point on the heel (calcaneus), and the distal point is the end of the second toe.
3. $x_m = x_p + lr(x_d - x_p)$; $y_m = y_p + lr(y_d - y_p)$

be expressed symbolically as: $m\,\boldsymbol{r} = \sum m_i\,\boldsymbol{r}_i$, or $\boldsymbol{r} = \sum (m_i\,/\,m)\,\boldsymbol{r}_i$, where m_i is the mass of segment number i, m is the mass of the whole body (the sum of all of the individual segment masses $\sum m_i$); $m_i\,/m$ is the fractional mass ratio of segment number i; and $\boldsymbol{r}$ and $\boldsymbol{r}_i$ are the position vectors, respectively, of the centre of mass of the whole body and the mass of segment number i. In practice, the position vectors are specified by their two-dimensional $(x,\,y)$ or three-dimensional $(x,\,y,\,z)$ coordinates. Table 5.1 on page 226 shows the calculation process for a two-dimensional case with given segmental mass fractions and position of centre of mass data (see also Study Task 4).

FUNDAMENTALS OF ANGULAR KINETICS

Almost all human motion in sport and exercise involves rotation (angular motion), for example the movement of a body segment about its proximal joint. In Chapter 4, we considered the kinematics of angular motion. In this section, our focus will be on the kinetics of such motions.

Moments of inertia

In linear motion, the reluctance of an object to move (its inertia) is expressed by its mass. In angular motion, the reluctance of the object to rotate depends also on the distribution of that mass about the axis of rotation, and is expressed by the moment of inertia. The SI unit for moment of inertia is kilogram-square metres ($kg{\cdot}m^2$); moment of inertia is a scalar quantity. An extended (straight) gymnast has a greater moment of inertia than a piked or tucked gymnast and is, therefore, more 'reluctant' to rotate. This makes it more difficult to somersault in an extended, or layout, position than in a piked or tucked position. Formally stated, the moment of inertia is the measure of an object's resistance to accelerated angular motion about an axis. It is equal to the sum of the products of the masses of the object's elements and the squares of the distances of those elements from the axis of rotation. Moments of inertia can be expressed in terms of the radius of gyration, k, such that the moment of inertia, I, is the product of the mass, m, and the square of the radius of gyration: $I = m\,k^2$.

The moments of inertia for rotation about any point on a three-dimensional rigid body are normally expressed about three mutually perpendicular axes of symmetry; the moments of inertia about these axes are called the principal moments of inertia. For the sports performer in the anatomical reference position, the three principal axes of inertia through the centre of mass correspond with the three cardinal axes. The moment of inertia about the longitudinal axis is much smaller – about one-tenth – of the moment of inertia about the other two axes, and that about the medio-lateral axis is slightly less than that about the anteroposterior axis. It is worth noting that rotations about the intermediate principal axis, here the mediolateral axis, are unstable, whereas those about the principal axes with the greatest and smallest moments of inertia are stable. This is another factor making layout somersaults difficult, unless the body is realigned to make the moment of inertia about the mediolateral, or somersault, axis greater than that about the anteroposterior axis.

For the sports performer, movements of the limbs other than in symmetry away from the anatomical reference position result in a misalignment between the body's cardinal axes and the principal axes of inertia. This has important consequences for the generation of aerial twist in a twisting somersault.

BOX 5.3 LAWS OF ANGULAR MOTION

The laws of angular motion are analogous to Newton's three laws of linear motion.

Principle of conservation of angular momentum (law of inertia)

A rotating body will continue to turn about its axis of rotation with constant angular momentum unless an external moment of force acts on it. The magnitude of the moment of force about an axis of rotation is the product of the force and its moment arm, which is the perpendicular distance from the axis of rotation to the line of action of the force.

Law of momentum

The rate of change with time (d/dt) of angular momentum (L) of a body is proportional to the moment of force (M) causing it and has the same direction as the moment of force. This is expressed symbolically by the following equation, which holds true for rotation about any axis fixed in space: $M = dL/dt$. If we now rearrange this equation by multiplying by dt, and integrate it, we obtain: $\int M \, dt = \int dL = \Delta L$; that is, the impulse of the moment of force equals the change of angular momentum (ΔL). If the impulse of the moment of force is zero, this equation reduces to $\Delta L = 0$ or L = constant, which is a mathematical statement of the first law of angular motion.

The last equation in the previous paragraph can be modified by writing $L = I \omega$ where I is the moment of inertia and ⬚ is the angular velocity of the body if, and only if, the axis of rotation is fixed in space or is a principal axis of inertia of a rigid body or quasi-rigid body. Then, and only then, $M = d(I \omega)/dt$. Furthermore, if, and only if, I is constant (for example for an individual rigid or quasi-rigid body segment), $M = I \alpha$, where α is the angular acceleration. The restrictions on the use of the equations in this paragraph compared with the universality of the equations in the previous paragraph should be carefully noted.

The angular motion equations for three-dimensional rotations are far more complex than the ones above and will not be considered in this book.

Third law (law of interaction of law of reaction)

For every moment of force that is exerted by one object on another, an equal and opposite moment of force is exerted by the second object on the first. In Figure 5.14(a), the forward and upward swing of the long jumper's legs (thigh flexion) evokes a reaction causing the forward and downward motion of the trunk (trunk flexion). As the two moments of force are both within the jumper's body, there is no change in her angular momentum; the two moments involved produce equal but opposite impulses. In Figure 5.14(b), the ground provides the reaction to the action moment of force generated in the racket arm and upper body, although this is not apparent because of the extremely high moment of inertia of the earth. If the tennis player played the same shot with his feet off the ground, there would be a moment of force on his lower body causing it to rotate counter to the movement of the upper body, lessening the angular momentum in the arm–racket system.

Figure 5.14 Action and reaction. Top: (a) airborne; Bottom: (b) with ground contact.

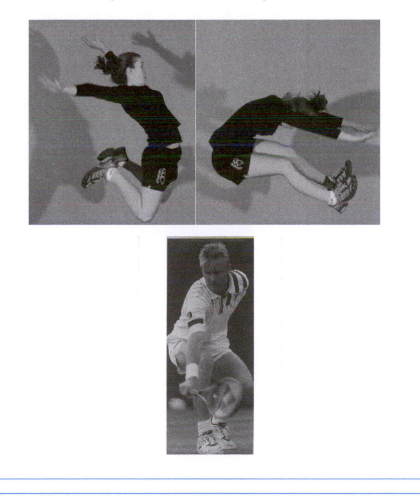

Minimising inertia

The law of momentum (Box 5.3) allows the derivation of the principle of minimising inertia. The increase in angular velocity and, therefore, the reduction in the time taken to move through a specified angle will be greater if the moment of inertia of the whole chain of body segments about the axis of rotation is minimised. Hence, for example, in running – and particularly in sprinting – the knee of the recovery leg is flexed to minimise the duration of the leg recovery phase.

Angular momentum of a rigid body

For a rigid body rotating about either an axis fixed in space, as in Figure 5.15(a), or a principal axis of inertia, it can be shown that, for planar motion, the angular momentum (L) is the product of the body's moment of inertia about the axis (I) and its angular velocity (ω); that is, $L = I\,\omega$. The direction of the angular momentum vector L, which is the same as that of ω, is given by allowing the position vector r to rotate towards the velocity vector v through the right angle indicated in Figure 5.15(a). By the right-hand rule, the angular momentum vector is into the plane of the page. The SI unit of angular momentum is kg·m^2/s.

Figure 5.15 Angular momentum. Left: (a) single rigid body; Right: (b) part of a system of rigid bodies.

Angular momentum of a system of rigid bodies

For planar rotations of systems of rigid bodies, for example the sports performer, each rigid body can be considered to rotate about its centre of mass (G), with an angular velocity ω_2. This centre of mass rotates about the centre of mass of the whole system (O), with an angular velocity ω_1, as for the bat of Figure 5.15(b). The derivation will not be provided here, but the result is that the magnitude of the angular momentum of the bat is: $L = m\,r^2\,\omega_1 + I_g\,\omega_2$. The first term, owing to the motion of that rigid body's centre of mass about the system's centre of mass, is known as the 'remote' angular momentum. The latter, owing to the rigid body's rotation about its own centre of mass, is the 'local' angular momentum. For an interconnected system of rigid body segments, representing the sports performer, the total angular momentum is the sum of the angular momentums of each of the segments calculated as in the above equation. The ways in which angular momentum is transferred between body segments can then be studied for sports activities such as running, airborne manoeuvres in gymnastics or the flight phase of the long jump.

GENERATION AND CONTROL OF ANGULAR MOMENTUM

A net external moment of force is needed to alter the angular momentum of a sports performer. Traditionally in sports biomechanics, three mechanisms of inducing rotation, or generating angular momentum, have been identified, although they are, in fact, related.

Force couple

A force couple consists of a parallel force system of two equal and opposite forces (F) which are a certain distance apart (Figure 5.16(a)). The net translational effect of these two forces is zero and they cause only rotation. The net torque (note the use of this word here rather than 'moment of force') of the force couple is: $M = 2r \times F$. The $\times$ sign in this equation tells us that the position vector, r, and the force vector, F, are

Figure 5.16 Generation of rotation. Left: (a) force couple; Right: (b) the torque (or moment) of the couple.

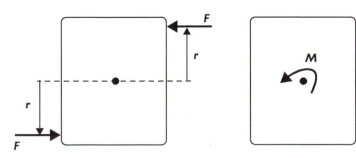

Figure 5.17 Generation of rotation. Top left: (a) an eccentric force; Top right: (b) addition of two equal and opposite collinear forces acting through the centre of mass, G; Bottom left: (c) equivalence to a 'pure' force and a torque; Bottom right: (d) checking of linear motion.

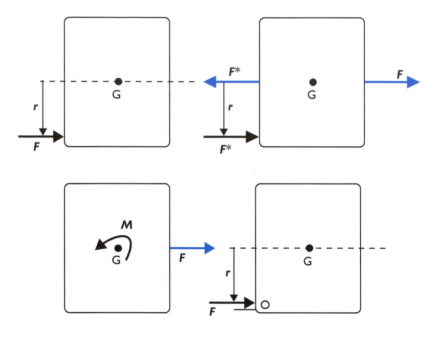

multiplied vectorially (see Appendix 4.2). The resulting torque vector has a direction perpendicular to, and into, the plane of this page. Its magnitude ($2rF$) is the magnitude of one of the forces (F) multiplied by the perpendicular distance between them ($2r$).

The torque (or moment of force) can be represented as in Figure 5.16(b) and has the same effect about a particular axis of rotation wherever it is applied along the body. In the absence of an external axis of rotation, the body will rotate about an axis through its centre of mass. The swimmer in Figure 5.6(a) is acted upon by a force couple of her weight and the equal, but opposite, buoyancy force.

Eccentric force

An eccentric force ('eccentric' means 'off-centre') is effectively any force, or resultant of a force system, that is not zero and that does not act through the centre of mass of an object. This constitutes the commonest way of generating rotational motion, as in Figure 5.17(a).

The eccentric force here can be transformed by adding two equal and opposite forces at the centre of mass, as shown by the red arrows in Figure 5.17(b), which will have no net effect on the object. The two forces indicated in Figure 5.17(b) with an asterisk can then be considered together and constitute an anticlockwise force couple, which can be replaced by a torque M as in Figure 5.17(c). This leaves a 'pure' force (F) acting through the centre of mass, which causes only linear motion, $F = \mathrm{d}(mv)/\mathrm{d}t$; the torque M causes only rotation, $M = \mathrm{d}L/\mathrm{d}t$. The magnitude of the torque (or moment of force), M, is Fr.

This example could be held to justify the use of the term 'torque' for the turning effect of an eccentric force in general, although, strictly, 'torque' is defined as the moment of a force couple (as above, where the torque replaced a force couple). The two terms, torque and moment of force, are often used interchangeably. Although there is a strong case for abandoning the use of the term 'moment of force' or 'force couple' entirely in favour of 'torque', given the various other uses of the term 'moment' in biomechanics, 'torque' is not a term that most students feel comfortable with.

Checking of linear motion

Checking of linear motion occurs when an already moving body is suddenly stopped at one point. An example is the foot plant of a javelin thrower in the delivery stride, although the representation of such a system as a quasi-rigid body is of limited use. This, as shown in Figure 5.17(d), is merely a special case of an eccentric force. It is best considered in that way to avoid misunderstandings that exist in the literature, such as the misconception that O is the instantaneous centre of rotation. This last sentence begs the question of where the instantaneous centre of rotation does lie in such cases.

Consider a rigid body that is simultaneously rotating with angular velocity, ω, about its centre of mass while moving linearly, as in Figure 5.18(a). The whole body has the same linear velocity (v), as in Figure 5.18(b), but the tangential velocity owing to rotation (v_t) depends on the displacement (r) from the centre of mass, G, such that $v_t = \omega \times r$, as in Figure 5.18(c). Adding v and v_t gives the net linear velocity (Figure 5.18(d)) that at some point P (which need not lie within the body) is zero; this point is called the instantaneous centre of rotation and its position usually changes with time.

Consider now a similar rigid body acted upon by an impact force, as in Figure 5.18(e), which is similar to Figure 5.17(d). There will, in general, be a point R that will experience no net acceleration. By Newton's second law of linear motion, the magnitude of the acceleration of the centre of mass of the rigid body, mass m, is $a_g = F/m$. From the second law of rotation (see Box 5.3), the magnitude ($F\,c$) of the moment of the force F is equal to the product of the moment of inertia of the body about its centre of mass (I_g) and its angular acceleration (α). That is $F\,c = I_g\,\alpha$. This gives a tangential acceleration ($\alpha\,r$) that increases linearly with distance (r) from G. The net acceleration profile then appears as in Figure 5.18(f). At point R ($r = b$), the two accelerations are equal and opposite and, therefore, cancel to give a zero net acceleration. The position of R is given by equating F/m ($= a_g$) to $F\,b\,c/I_g$, the tangential acceleration at R. That is, $b\,c = I_g/m$. If R is a fixed centre of rotation then Q is known as the centre of percussion, defined as that point at which a force may be applied without causing an acceleration at another specific point, the centre of rotation. The above equation

Figure 5.18 Instantaneous centre of rotation and centre of percussion. Top: (a) rigid body undergoing linear and angular motion; (b) linear velocity profile; (c) tangential velocity profile; (d) net velocity profile and instantaneous centre of rotation (P); Bottom: (e) impact force on a rigid body at the centre of percussion; (f) net acceleration profile and centre of percussion (Q).

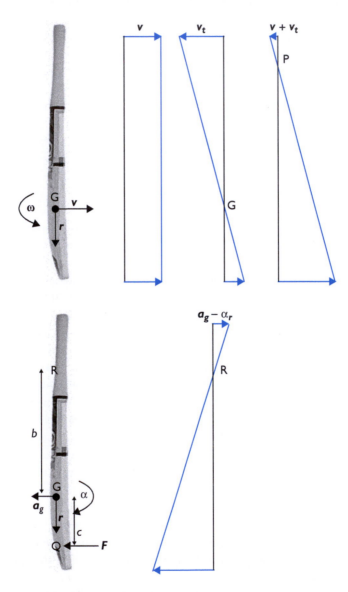

shows that Q and R can be reversed. The centre of percussion is important in sports where objects, such as balls, are struck with other objects, such as bats and rackets. If the impact occurs at the centre of percussion, no force is transmitted to the hands. For an object such as a cricket bat, the centre of percussion will lie some way below the centre of mass, whereas for a golf club, with the mass concentrated in the club head, the centres of percussion and mass more nearly coincide. Variation in grip position will alter the position of the centre of percussion. If the grip position is a long way from the centre of mass and the centre of percussion is close to the centre of mass, then the position of the centre of percussion will be less sensitive to changes in grip position. This is achieved by moving the centre of mass towards the centre of percussion, as for golf clubs with light shafts and heavy club heads, and cricket bats for which the mass of the bat is built up around the centre of percussion. Much tennis racket design has evolved towards positioning the centre of percussion nearer to the likely impact spot. The benefits of such a design feature include less fatigue and a reduction in injury.

The application of the centre of percussion concept to a generally non-rigid body, such as the human performer, is problematic. However, some insight can be gained into certain sports movement techniques. Consider a reversal of Figure 5.18(e) such that Q is high in the body and R is at the ground (similar to Figure 5.17(d)). Let F be the reaction force experienced by a thrower who is applying force to an external object. If F is directed through the centre of percussion, there will be no resultant acceleration at R (the foot–ground interface). A second example relates Figure 5.18(e) to the braking effect when the foot lands in front of the body's centre of mass. The horizontal component of the impact force will oppose relative motion and cause an acceleration distribution, as in Figure 5.18(f), with all body parts below R decelerated and only those above R accelerated. This is important in, for example, javelin throwing, where it is desirable not to slow the speed of the object to be thrown during the final foot contacts of the thrower.

Transfer of angular momentum

The principle of transfer of angular momentum from segment to segment is sometimes considered to be a basic principle of coordinated movement. Consider, for example, the skater in Figure 4.11(a); if she moved her arms fully away from her, to a 90° abducted position, she would decrease her speed of rotation; if she moved them into her body, she would rotate faster. This is sometimes interpreted in terms only of the two 'quasi-static' end positions – fully abducted arms, and arms drawn into the body. The former position has a large moment of inertia, and hence low speed of rotation; the latter position has a low moment of inertia and high speed of rotation. However, from the abducted-arms to the tucked-arms position, the arms lose angular momentum as they move towards the body, 'transferring' some of their angular momentum to the rest of the body, which, therefore, turns faster. A more complex example is the hitch kick technique in the flight phase of the long jump, in which the arm and leg motions transfer angular momentum from the trunk to the limbs to prevent the jumper from rotating forwards too early in the flight phase.

Figure 5.19 Trading of angular momentum between axes of rotation. Left: (a) at take-off; Right: (b) after asymmetrical arm movement in a backward somersault (with twist).

(a)   (b)

Trading of angular momentum

The term 'trading of angular momentum' is often used to refer to the transfer of angular momentum from one axis of rotation to another. For example, the model diver – or gymnast – in Figure 5.19 takes off with angular momentum ($L = L_{som}$) about the somersault axis. The diver then adducts her left arm, or performs some other asymmetrical movement, by a muscular moment of force that evokes an equal but opposite counter-rotation of the rest of the body to produce an angle of tilt. No external moment of force has been applied so the angular momentum (L) is still constant about a horizontal axis (sometimes called the axis of momentum) but now has a component (L_{twist}) about the twisting axis. The diver has 'traded' some somersaulting angular momentum for twisting, or longitudinal, angular momentum and will now both somersault and twist. It is often argued that this method of generating twisting angular momentum is preferable to 'contact twist' (twist generated when in contact with an external surface), as it can be more easily removed by re-establishing the original body position before landing. This can avoid problems in gymnastics, trampolining and diving caused by landing or entering the water with residual twisting angular momentum. The crucial factor in generating airborne twist is to establish a tilt angle and, approximately, the twist rate is proportional to the angle of tilt. In practice, many sports performers use both the contact and the airborne mechanisms to acquire twist.

Three-dimensional rotation

Rotational movements in airborne activities in diving, gymnastics and trampolining, for example, usually involve three-dimensional, multi-segmental movements. The mathematical analysis of the dynamics of such movements is beyond the scope of this book. The three-dimensional dynamics of even a rigid or quasi-rigid body are far from simple. For example, in two-dimensional rotation of such bodies, the angular momentum and angular velocity vectors coincide in direction. If a body with principal moments of inertia that are not identical – as is the case for the sports performer – rotates about an axis that does not coincide with one of the principal axes, then the angular velocity vector and the angular momentum vectors do not coincide. A movement known as 'nutation' can result. Nutation also occurs, for example, when performing an airborne pirouette with asymmetrical arm positions. The body's longitudinal axis is displaced away from its original position of coincidence with the angular momentum vector and describes a cone around that vector. Furthermore, the equation of conservation of angular momentum applies to an inertial frame of reference, such as one moving with the centre of mass of the performer but always parallel to a fixed, stationary frame of reference. The conservation of angular momentum does not generally apply to a frame of reference fixed in the performer's body and rotating with it.

MEASUREMENT OF FORCE

BOX 5.4 WHY MEASURE FORCE OR PRESSURE?

- To provide further movement patterns for the use of the qualitative analyst.
- To highlight potential risk factors, particularly in high-impact activities.
- To evaluate, for example, the foot-strike patterns of runners or the balance of archers.
- To provide the external inputs for internal joint moment and force calculations (inverse dynamics, see Bartlett and Bussey, 2012, listed in 'Further reading').
- The forces and moments of force can be further processed to provide other movement information (see below).

Most force measurements in sport use a force plate, which measures the contact force components (see Figure 5.20) between the ground, called the ground contact force, or another surface, and the sports performer. The measured force acting on the force plate has the same magnitude as, but opposite direction from, the reaction force exerted on the performer by the force plate, by the law of interaction (action–reaction).

Figure 5.20 Ground contact force (F_x, F_y, F_z) and moment (or torque) (M_x, M_y, M_z) components that act on the sports performer.

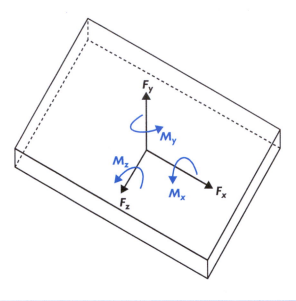

Force plates are widely used in research into the loading on the various joints of the body. In such research, movement data from videography, or an on-line motion analysis system (Chapter 4), are used with force, moment of force and centre of pressure data to calculate the resultant forces and moments at body joints. The two recording systems need to be synchronised for such investigations, as I outlined in the previous chapter.

Force plates can be obtained in a variety of sizes. The most commonly used ones have a relatively small contact area, for example 600 mm × 400 mm for the Kistler type 9281B11 (www.kistler.com) or 508 mm × 643 mm for the AMTI model OR6-5-1 (www.amtiweb.com). Solid force plates generally weigh between 310 and 410 N; honeycombed force plates are much lighter and reasonably portable. When in use, force plates are normally bolted to a base plate which is set in concrete.

Forces of interaction between the sports performer and items of sports equipment can also be measured using other force transducers, often purpose built or adapted for a particular application. Such transducers have been used, for example, to measure the forces exerted by a rower on an oar, by a cyclist on his or her bike's pedals, or by a skier (Figure 5.21). Such examples are now quite commonplace. Many of the principles discussed in this chapter for force plates also apply to force transducers in general. Further consideration of operation of these devices will not be undertaken in this book.

One limitation of force plates is that they do not show how the applied force is distributed over the contact surface, for example the shoe or the foot. This information can be obtained from pressure plates, pads and insoles, which will be considered in the next section.

Figure 5.21 Force transducers used to measure forces on a ski. Courtesy of Dr Stefan Lindinger, University of Salzburg, Austria.

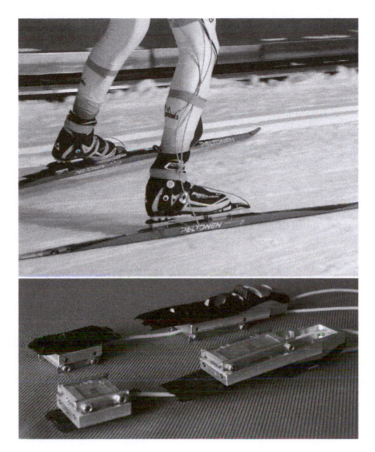

Force plates used for the evaluation of sports performance are sophisticated electronic devices and are generally very accurate. Essentially, they can be considered as weighing systems that are responsive to changes in the displacement of a sensor or detecting element. They incorporate force transducers, which convert the force into an electrical signal. The transducers are mounted on the supports of the rigid surface of the force plate, usually one support at each of the four corners of a rectangle. One transducer is used, at each support, to measure each of the three force components, one of which is perpendicular to the plate and two tangential to it; for ground contact forces, there are usually one vertical and two horizontal force components, and we will use this example in what follows. The transducers are normally strain gauges, as in AMTI plates, or piezoelectric, as in Kistler plates. The signals from the transducers are amplified and may undergo other electrical modification. The amplified and modified signals are converted to digital signals for computer processing. The signal is then sampled at discrete time intervals, expressed as the sampling frequency. The Nyquist sampling theorem (see Chapter 4) requires a sampling frequency at least twice that of the highest signal frequency. It should be remembered that, although the frequency content of much human movement is low, many force plate applications involve impacts, which have a higher frequency content. A sampling frequency as high as 500 Hz or 1 kHz may, therefore, be appropriate.

Accurate (valid) and reliable force plate measurements depend on adequate system sensitivity, a low force detection threshold, high linearity, low hysteresis, low crosstalk and the elimination of cable interference, electrical inductance, and temperature and humidity variations. The plate must be sufficiently large to accommodate the movement under investigation. Extraneous vibrations must be excluded. Mounting instructions for force plates are specified by the manufacturers. The plate is normally sited on the bottom floor of a building in a large concrete block. If mounted outdoors, a large concrete block sited on pebbles or gravel is usually a suitable base and attention must be given to problems of drainage. The main measurement characteristics of a force plate are considered in Appendix 5.1. Most commercial force plates that are mounted according to their manufacturers' specifications will meet the required measurement characteristics exemplified in Box 5.5. In addition, a good temperature range (−20–70°C) and a relatively light weight may be important. Also, any variation in the recorded force with the position on the plate surface at which it is applied should be less than 2–3 per cent in the worst case.

BOX 5.5 GUIDELINE VALUES FOR FORCE PLATE CHARACTERISTICS

Linearity	≤ 0.5 per cent of full scale deflection
Hysteresis	≤ 0.5 per cent of full scale deflection
Crosstalk	≤ 3 per cent
Natural frequency	≥ 800 Hz
Maximum frequency ratio	≤ 0.2
(of signal frequency to natural frequency)	
Damping ratio	0.5 to 0.8 (0.707 optimum)

Experimental procedures

General

A force plate, if correctly installed and mounted and used with appropriate auxiliary equipment, is generally simple to use. When used with an analog-to-digital (A–D) converter and computer, the timing of data collection is important. This can be achieved, for example, by computer control of the collection time, by the use of photoelectric triggers or by sampling only when the force exceeds a certain threshold. When using a force plate with video recording, synchronisation of the two will be required. This can be done in several ways, such as causing the triggering of the force plate data collection to illuminate a light in the field of view of the cameras (see Chapter 4 and Study Task 8).

The sensitivity of the overall system will need to be adjusted to prevent saturation while ensuring the largest possible use of the equipment's range. This can often be done by trial-and-error adjustments of amplifier gains; this should obviously be done before the main data collection. If the manufacturers have recommended warm-up times for the system amplifiers, then these must be carefully observed.

Care must be taken in the experimental protocol, if the performer moves onto the plate, to ensure that foot contact occurs with little (preferably no) targeting of the plate by the performer. This may, for example, require the plate to be concealed by covering the surface with a material similar to that of the surroundings of the plate. Obviously the external (or ecological) validity of an investigation will be compromised if changes in movement patterns occur to ensure foot contact on the plate. Also important for ecological validity, particularly when recording impacts, is matching the plate surface to that which normally exists in the sport being studied. The aluminium surfaces normally used for force plates are unrepresentative of most sports surfaces.

Calibration

It is essential that the force plate system should be able to be calibrated to minimise systematic errors. The overall system will require regular calibration checks, even if this is not necessary for the force plate itself. Calibration of the amplifier output as a function of force input will usually be set by the manufacturers and may require periodic checking. The vertical channel is easily calibrated under static loading conditions by use of known weights. If these are applied at different points across the plate surface, the variability of the recorded force with its point of application can also be checked. The horizontal channels can also be statically calibrated, although not so easily. One method of doing this involves attaching a cable to the plate surface, passing the cable over a frictionless air pulley at the level of the plate surface, and adding weights to the free end of the cable. Obviously this cannot be done while the plate is installed in the ground flush with the surrounding surface. There appears to be little guidance provided to users on the need for, or regularity of, dynamic calibration checks on force plates. The tendency of piezoelectric transducers to drift may mean that zero corrections are required and strain gauge plates may need more frequent calibration checks than do piezoelectric ones.

Crosstalk can be checked by recording the outputs from the two horizontal channels when only a vertical force, such as a weight, is applied to the plate. A similar procedure can be used for assessing crosstalk on the vertical channel if horizontal forces can be applied. Positions of the point of force application can be checked by placing weights on the plate at various positions and comparing these with centre of pressure positions calculated from the outputs from the individual vertical force transducers. As errors in these calculations are problematic when small forces are being recorded, small as well as large weights should be included in such checks. Finally, the natural frequency (see Appendix 5.1) can be checked by lightly striking the plate with a metal object and using an oscilloscope to show the ringing of the plate at its natural frequency. This should be carried out, of course, in the location in which the plate is to be used.

Data processing

Processing of force plate signals is relatively simple and accurate, compared with most data in sports biomechanics. The example data of Figure 5.22 were obtained from a standing long jump. The three mutually perpendicular (orthogonal) components of the ground contact force (Figures 5.20 and 5.22(a)) are easily obtained by summing the outputs of individual transducers. As the plate provides whole-body measurements, these forces (F) can be easily converted to the three components of centre of mass acceleration (a) simply by dividing by the mass of the performer ($F = ma$, Figure 5.22(b)), after subtracting the performer's weight from the vertical force component. The coordinates of the point of application of the force, the centre of pressure (Figure 5.22(c)), on the plate working surface can also be calculated. The accuracy of the centre of pressure calculations in particular depends on careful calibration of the force plate; this accuracy deteriorates at the beginning and end of any contact phase, when the calculation of centre of pressure involves the division of small forces by other small forces.

The moment of the ground contact force about the vertical axis perpendicular to the plane of the plate – the frictional moment of force, sometimes called the free moment – (Figure 5.22(d)) can be easily calculated. With appropriate knowledge of the position of the performer's centre of mass, in principle at one instant only, the component moments of the ground contact force (Figure 5.22(d)) can also be calculated about the two horizontal and mutually perpendicular axes passing through the performer's centre of mass and parallel to the plate.

From the force–time and moment–time data, integration can be performed to find overall or instant-by-instant changes in centre of mass velocity and whole-body angular momentum. Absolute magnitudes of these variables at all instants (Figures 5.22(e) and (f)) can be calculated only if their values are known at least at one instant. These values could be obtained from videography or another motion analysis system. They are easily obtained if the performer is at rest on the plate at some instant, when both linear and angular momentum are zero. If absolute velocities are known, then the changes in position – displacement – can be found by integration. In this case, absolute values of the position of the centre of mass with respect to the plate coordinate system (Figure 5.22(g)) can be obtained if that position is known for at least one instant. Again, that value could be obtained from videography or an on-line motion analysis system. Alternatively, the horizontal coordinates can be obtained from the centre of pressure position with the person stationary on the plate, and the vertical coordinate as a fraction of the person's height.

Figure 5.22 Force plate variables (as anteroposterior (x, red), longitudinal (y, black) and mediolateral (z, dashed red) components, except for power) as functions of time for a standing long jump. Top: (a) force; (b) centre of mass acceleration; Second line: (c) point of force application (x, z only); (d) moment of force (torque); Third line: (e) centre of mass velocity; (f) whole-body angular momentum; Fourth line: (g) centre of mass displacement; (h) load rate; Bottom: (i) whole-body power.

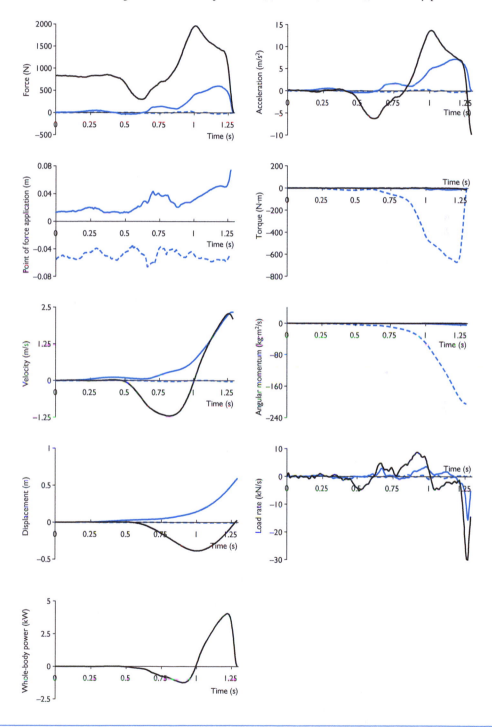

Figure 5.23 Left: (a) Side view of force vectors for a standing long jump; Right: (b) centre of pressure path from above (S shows the start of the movement and T take-off). Note: (a) and (b) are not to the same scale.

The load rate (Figure 5.22(h)) can be calculated as the rate of change with time (d/dt) of the contact force (dF/dt). The load rate has often been linked to injury. Other calculations that can be performed include whole-body power ($P = \boldsymbol{F}.\boldsymbol{v}$) (Figure 5.22(i)), which, you should note, does not have x, y and z components, as power is a scalar (see also Appendix 4.2).

All the above variables can be presented graphically as functions of time, as in Figure 5.22, providing the qualitative analyst with a rich new set of movement patterns and the quantitative analyst with further useful data. In addition, the forces acting on the performer can be represented as instantaneous force vectors, arising from the instantaneous centres of pressure (a side view is shown in Figure 5.23(a)). Front, top and three-dimensional views of the force vectors are also possible. The centre of pressure path can also be shown superimposed on the plate surface (Figure 5.23(b)).

MEASUREMENT OF PRESSURE

As we noted in the previous section, force plates provide the position of the point of application of the force, also called the centre of pressure, on the plate. This is the point at which the force can be considered to act, although the pressure is distributed over the plate and foot. Indeed, there may be no pressure acting at the centre of pressure when, for example, it is below the arch of the foot or between the feet during double stance. Information about the distribution of pressure over the contacting surface is required, for example, to examine the areas of the foot on which forces are concentrated during the stance phase in running to improve running shoe design. In such cases, a pressure platform or pressure pad must be used. These devices consist of a set of force transducers with a small contact area over which the mean pressure for that area of contact (pressure = force ÷ area) is calculated. For just a few selected regions of the contact surface, pressures can be measured using individual sensors; problems with this approach include choosing the appropriate locations and movement of the sensors during the activity being studied.

Various types of pressure plate are commercially available, and have been mostly used for the measurement of pressure distributions between the foot or shoe and the ground. They have been used only to a limited extent in sport, partly because their usually small size causes targeting problems for the performer. Also, the distribution of pressure is altered if the platform is covered with a sports surface. Pressure pads have been developed for the measurement of contact pressures between parts of the body and the surroundings. Specialist applications have included pads for the study of the dorsal pressures on the foot

Figure 5.24 A plantar pressure insole system – pedar® (www.novel.de). Courtesy of Dr Stefan Lindinger, University of Salzburg, Austria.

within a shoe. Plantar pressure insoles are commercially available (for example, Figure 5.24) and can be used to measure the plantar pressure distribution between the foot and the shoe. This is generally more important, for the sports performer, than the pressure between the shoe and the ground measured by pressure plates. These insoles allow data collection for several foot strikes and do not cause problems of targeting.

All pressure insoles have certain drawbacks for use in sport. First, they require cabling and a battery pack to be worn by the performer. Secondly, the insole may alter the pressure distribution because of its thickness. Thirdly, all commercially available devices currently only record the normal component of stress (pressure), not the tangential (shear) components. Furthermore they are susceptible to mechanical damage and crosstalk between the individual sensors. The durability of the sensors is a function of thickness – the thicker they are, the more durable – but mechanical crosstalk also increases with sensor thickness. Although very thin sensors may be suitable for static and slowly changing pressure measurements, durability is important in sports applications involving rapid pressure changes, such as foot strike. Pressure plates, pads and insoles suitable for use in sports biomechanics are based on capacitive, conductive or piezoelectric transducers (for further details, see Lees and Lake, 2008, listed in Further Reading).

Data processing

Many data processing and data presentation options are available to help analyse the results from pressure measuring devices. In principle, all of the data processing options available for force plates also apply to pressure plates. In addition, displays of whole-foot pressure distributions are available, similar to those shown in Figure 5.25 for pressure insoles. The centre of pressure path – the gait line – measured from pressure insoles and plates is far less sensitive to error than for force plates. Pressure insole software usually provides for many displays of the pressure–time information. The software also allows the user to define areas of the foot of special interest (up to eight, normally) and then to study those areas individually as well as the foot as a whole. The information available includes the following:

- Three-dimensional colour-coded wireframe displays of the summary maximum pressure distributions at each sensor (the maximum pressure picture) and the pressure distribution at each sample time (see the Interactive eTextbook for these and other graphics examples and video clips). Monochrome versions of these are shown in Figure 5.25(a) and (b), displayed as if viewing the right foot from below or the left from above; these can usually be animated in the system software so that the user can see how the pressure patterns evolve over time. These are fascinating patterns of movement that, to date, have been little used by qualitative analysts.
- Force (sum of all sensor readings), maximum pressure and contact area as functions of time for the whole foot and any specified region of the foot.

Figure 5.25 Pedar® insole data displays. Left: (a) and (b) pressure distributions as three-dimensional displays of (a) summary maximum pressures (maximum pressure picture) and (b) pressure distribution at one sample time, both for running at medium speed; Right: (c) centre of pressure paths (shown by the curved lines from heel to toe). Colour coding is explained in the Interactive eTextbook. Courtesy of Dr Stefan Lindinger, University of Salzburg, Austria.

- Bar charts of the peak pressure, force, contact area and the pressure–time integral for all regions of the foot.
- The centre of pressure path, or gait line (Figure 5.25(c)).

SUMMARY

In this chapter, we considered linear kinetics, which is important for an understanding of human movement in sport and exercise. This included the definition of force, the identification of the various external forces acting in sport and how they combine, and the laws of linear kinetics and related concepts, such as linear momentum. We addressed how friction and traction influence movements in sport and exercise, including reducing and increasing friction and traction. Fluid dynamic forces were also considered; the importance of lift and drag forces both on the sports performer and on objects for which the fluid dynamics can impact on a player's movements were outlined. We emphasised both qualitative and quantitative aspects of force–time graphs. The segmentation method for calculating the position of the whole-body centre of mass of the sports performer was explained. The vitally important topic of rotational kinetics was covered, including the laws of rotational kinetics and related concepts such as angular momentum and the ways in which rotation is acquired and controlled in sports movements. The use of force plates in sports biomechanics was covered, including the equipment and methods used, and the processing of force plate data. The procedures for calibrating a force plate were outlined, along with those used to record forces in practice. The different ways in which force plate data can be processed to obtain other movement variables were covered. The value of contact pressure measurements in the study of sports movements was covered. Some examples were provided of the ways in which pressure transducer data can be presented to aid analysis of sports movements.

STUDY TASKS

1   Answer all of the multiple-choice questions for Chapter 5 in the Interactive eTextbook.
    Hint: Keep repeating this until you have answered all the questions correctly.

2   a) List the external forces that act on the sports performer and, for each force, give an example of a sport in which that force will be very important.
    b) Define and explain the three laws of linear kinetics and give at least two examples from sport, other than the examples in this chapter, of the application of each law.
    Hint: You may wish to re-read the sections on 'Combinations of forces on the sports performer' and 'Momentum and the laws of linear motion' before undertaking this task.

3   Download the Excel spreadsheet 'Vertical Jump Force Plate Data' for a standing vertical jump from the Interactive eTextbook. The sample times (t) and magnitudes of the vertical ground reaction force (F) are shown in the first two columns of the spreadsheet. The force–time graph is shown in the worksheet 'Force Time Series'.
    a) Obtain the vertical accelerations (a) in the third column (C) by noting the jumper's weight (G) when standing still at the start of the sequence and using $a = gF/G$, where $g = 9.81$ m/s^2. This calculation has been done for you for cells C2–4 (with the jumper's weight as 843 N); you simply need to apply ('cut and paste') the formula to the remaining cells in column C.
    b) Use a simplified numerical integration formula for the change in the magnitude of the vertical velocity from one time interval, i, to the next, $i+1$, over sampling time Δt: $\Delta v = (a_i + a_{i+1})\Delta t/2$, noting $v = 0$ at $t = 0$ (this has been entered for you in cell D2). The velocities are calculated in column D of the spreadsheet. This calculation has been done for you for cells D3–4; you simply need to apply the formula to the remaining cells in column D.
    c) Use a similar numerical integration formula for the change in magnitude of the centre of mass vertical displacement (y) from one time interval, i, to the

next, $i+1$, over sampling time Δt: $\Delta y = (v_i + v_{i+1})\Delta t/2$, defining $y = 0$ at $t = 0$ (this has been entered for you in cell E2). The displacements are calculated in column E of the spreadsheet. This calculation has been done for you for cells E3–4; you simply need to apply the formula to the remaining cells in column E.

d) Time-series graphs of the vertical acceleration, velocity and displacement of the centre of mass will now appear in the worksheets 'Acceleration Time Series', 'Velocity Time Series' and 'Displacement Time Series', respectively. Compare your graphs with Figure 5.12; they should be identical. If they are not, check very carefully your cutting and pasting of formulas into Excel cells (you need to paste formulas not values).

e) What was the jumper's take-off velocity (see cell E467)? Calculate, by equating the kinetic energy at take-off to the potential energy at the peak of the jump, the maximum height reached by the centre of mass.

Hint: You should re-read the section on 'Force–time graphs as movement patterns' before undertaking this task. If you are unfamiliar with performing simple calculations in Microsoft Excel, simply follow the procedures above to paste the calculations in rows 3 and 4 into the remaining cells in the appropriate row; for further help, go to the online Excel help site, or see your tutor.

4   a) Photocopy or scan Figure 5.13(a), or download Figure 5.13 from the Interactive eTextbook. Measure the x- and y-coordinates of each of the segment end points marked on the ski jumper (these should all be obvious from Figure 5.13(a) and Table 5.1; the hip and wrist markers are labelled H and W respectively, for clarity). Then use a photocopy or scan of Table 5.1, or download it from the Interactive eTextbook, to calculate the position of the ski jumper's whole-body centre of mass in the units of the image. Assume that the joints on the right side of the body have identical coordinates to those on the left side. If you are having problems with the calculations, then download the Excel file 'Whole Body Centre of Mass Table' from the Interactive eTextbook. You will then only need to type the x- and y-coordinates of the red circles on Figure 5.13(a) into the appropriate columns of the Excel worksheet. Finally, as a check on your calculation, whichever way you did it, mark the resulting centre of mass position on your figure. If it looks silly, check your calculations and repeat until the centre of mass position appears reasonable.

b) Repeat for Figure 5.13(b). You will need to estimate the positions of the obscured markers on the wrist, knuckle and toe, and to measure the midpoint of the line joining the markers on the seventh cervical vertebra and the suprasternal notch. Assume that the joints on the left side of the body have identical coordinates to those on the right side. Again, you can use the 'Whole Body Centre of Mass Table', but please try to do one row of the calculations – say for the trunk – by hand so that you understand the process better.

Hint: You may wish to re-read the section on 'Determination of the centre of mass of the human body' before undertaking this task.

5   Carry out the inclined plane experiment, mentioned in the section on friction, to calculate the coefficient of friction between the material of a sports surface and a training shoe and other sports objects. You only need a board covered with the relevant material, a shoe and a protractor.

Hint: You may wish to re-read the subsection on 'Friction' before undertaking this task.

6   Obtain a video recording of top class diving, trampolining or gymnastics, for example from YouTube. Carefully analyse some airborne movements that do not involve twisting, including the transfer of angular momentum between body segments. Repeat for movements involving twisting; consider in particular the ways in which performers generate twist in somersaulting movements.

Hint: You should re-read the section on 'Generation and control of angular momentum' before undertaking this task.

7   Outline how you would statically calibrate a force plate, how you would check for variability of the recorded force with its point of application on the plate surface, how you would check for crosstalk, and how you would check the accuracy of centre of pressure calculations.

Hint: You may wish to re-read the subsection on 'Experimental procedures' in 'Measurement of force' before undertaking this task.

8   Describe two ways in which you might be able to synchronise the recording of forces from a force plate with a video recording of the movement. This may require some careful thought.

Hint: You may wish to re-read the subsection on 'Experimental procedures' in 'Measurement of force' before undertaking this task.

9   Visit the Interactive eTextbook and look at the various graphical examples and video clips available there – from pressure plates and insoles – of the movement patterns available to a qualitative movement analyst. Assess which of these you think could be of routine use to a qualitative analyst and which are best thought of as back-up information that might occasionally be useful.

Hint: You might wish to re-read relevant sections on movement patterns in Chapter 3 before undertaking this task.

10 **Case study**.

a) Answer the five multiple-choice questions for this study task in the Interactive eTextbook.

b) Download the Excel spreadsheet 'Long Jump Force Plate Data' from the Interactive eTextbook.

c) From the data for 'Long Jump 1' in the Excel spreadsheet, plot all relevant graphs of variables against time (see Figure 5.22).

d) If you have access to a force plate, perform an experiment involving a standing long jump from the plate, with a countermovement and normal arm action; collect force and moment of force data for all three components. Make notes of the procedures involved for the methods section for your case study report. (If you do not have access to a force plate, you will find a dataset of forces and moments of force for a standing long jump with a countermovement and normal arm action in the worksheet 'Long Jump 2' in the Excel spreadsheet 'Long Jump Force Plate Data'. In this case, you will need to base the methods section of your case study report on information in the section 'Measurement of force' in this chapter.)

e) From your recorded force and moment of force components (or those in the Excel worksheet 'Long Jump 2'), calculate all of the other variables that appear in the worksheet 'Long Jump 1' and plot graphs of them all against time, as in part (c).

f) Compare the results you obtain with those from part (c) (Figure 5.22).

g) Write a report of your case study in no more than 1000 words, including no more than ten graphs. This should include: methods; results (comparing the two long jumps); and discussion, focusing on the differences between the two long jumps.

Hint: You should re-read the subsection on 'Data processing' in 'Measurement of force' and revisit Study Task 3 before undertaking this study task.

SORTING AND LABELLING ACTIVITIES (INTERACTIVE ETEXTBOOK ONLY)

Sorting activity.
Labelling activity.

FURTHER READING

Bartlett, R.M. and Bussey, M. (2012) *Sports Biomechanics: Reducing Injury and Improving Sports Performance*, London: Routledge. Chapter 4 provides a simple introduction to inverse dynamics without being too mathematical.

Lees, A. and Lake, M. (2008) Force and pressure measurement, in C.J. Payton and R.M. Bartlett (eds) *Biomechanical Evaluation of Movement in Sport and Exercise*, London: Routledge. Good coverage of force and pressure measurement in sport.

APPENDIX 5.1 FORCE PLATE CHARACTERISTICS

Linearity

Linearity is expressed as the maximum deviation from linearity as a percentage of full scale deflection. For example, in Figure 5.26(a), linearity would be expressed as $y/Y \times 100$ per cent. Although good linearity is not essential for accurate measurements, as a non-linear system can be calibrated, it is useful and does make calibration easier. A suitable figure for a force plate for use in sports biomechanics would be 0.5 per cent of full scale deflection or better.

Hysteresis

Hysteresis exists when the input–output relationship depends on whether the input force is increasing or decreasing, as in Figure 5.26(b). Hysteresis can be caused, for example, by the presence of deforming mechanical elements in the force transducers. It is expressed as the maximum difference between the output voltage for the same force, increasing and decreasing, divided by the full scale output voltage. It should be 0.5 per cent of full scale deflection or less.

Range

The range of forces that can be measured must be adequate for the application and the range should be adjustable. If the range is too small for the forces being measured, the output voltage will saturate (reach a constant value), as shown in Figure 5.26(c). Suitable maximum ranges for many sports biomechanics applications would be −10 kN to +10 kN for the two horizontal axes and −10 kN to +20 kN for the vertical axis.

Sensitivity

Sensitivity is the change in the recorded signal for a unit change in the force input, or the slope of the idealised linear voltage–force relationships of Figure 5.26. The sensitivity decreases with increasing range. Good sensitivity is essential as it is a limiting factor in the accuracy of the measurement. In most modern force plate systems, an analog-to-digital (A–D) converter is used and is usually the main limitation on the overall system resolution. An 8-bit A–D converter divides the input into an output that can take one of 256 (2^8) discrete values. The resolution is then 100/255 per cent, approximately 0.4 per cent. A 12-bit A–D converter will improve the resolution to about 0.025 per cent. In a force plate system with adjustable range, it is essential to choose the range that just avoids saturation, so as to achieve optimum sensitivity. For example, consider that the maximum vertical force to be recorded is 4,300 N, an 8-bit A–D converter is used, and a choice of ranges of 10,000 N, 5,000 N and 2,500 N is available. The best available range is 5,000 N, and the force would be recorded to approximately the nearest 20 N (5,000/255). The percentage error in the maximum force is then only about 0.5 per cent (20 × 100/4,300). A range of 10,000 N would double this error to about 1 per cent. A range of 2,500 N would cause saturation, and the maximum force recorded would be 2,500 N, an underestimate of over 40 per cent (compare with Figure 5.26(c)).

Figure 5.26 Force plate characteristics. Top: (a) linearity; Middle: (b) hysteresis (simplified); Bottom: (c) output saturation and effect of range on sensitivity.

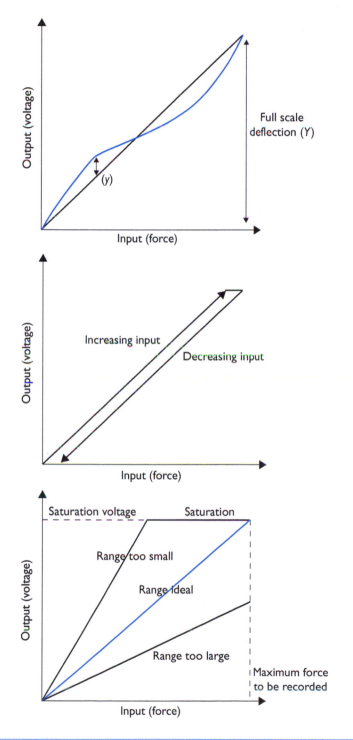

Crosstalk

Force plates are normally used to measure force components in more than one direction. The possibility then exists of forces in one component direction affecting the forces recorded by the transducers used for the other components. The term 'crosstalk' is used to express this interference between the recording channels for the various force components. Crosstalk must be small, preferably less than 3 per cent.

Dynamic response

Forces in sport almost always change rapidly as a function of time. The way in which the measuring system responds to such rapidly changing forces is crucial to the accuracy of the measurements and is called the 'dynamic response' of the system. The considerations here relate mostly to the mechanical components of the system. A representation of simple sinusoidally varying input and output signals of a single frequency (ω) as a function of time is presented in Figure 5.27.

The ratio of the amplitudes (maximum values) of the output to the input signal is called the amplitude ratio (A). The time by which the output signal lags the input signal is called the phase lag. This is often expressed as the phase angle (ϕ), which is the time lag multiplied by the signal frequency.

In practice, the force signal will contain a range of frequency components, each of which could have different phase lags and amplitude ratios. The more different these are across the range of frequencies present in the signal, the greater will be the distortion of the output signal. This will reduce the accuracy of the measurement. We therefore require the following:

Figure 5.27 Representation of force input and recorded output signals as a function of time.

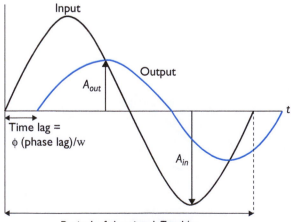

Figure 5.28 Steady-state frequency response characteristics of a typical second-order force plate system. Top: (a) amplitude plot; Bottom: (b) phase plot for damping ratios of: 2 (overdamped case shown by the dashed red curve), 0.707 (critically damped case shown by the continuous black curve), and 0.2 (underdamped case shown by the continuous red curve).

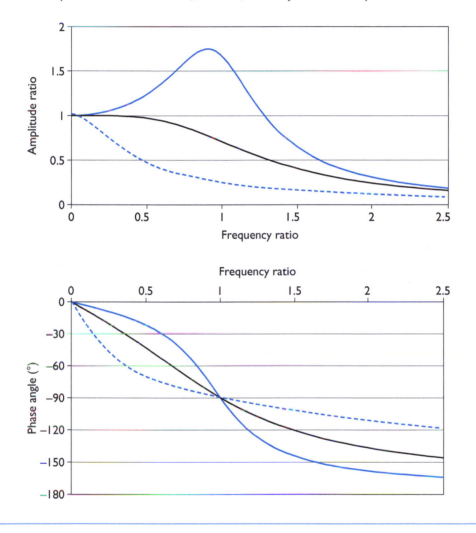

- All the frequencies present in the force signal should be equally amplified; this means that there should be a constant value of the amplitude ratio A (system calibration can allow A to be considered as 1, as in Figure 5.28).
- The phase lag (or phase angle, ϕ) should be small.

A force plate is a measuring system consisting, essentially, of a mass m, a spring of stiffness k and a damping element c, rather like a racing car's suspension system; some simple models of the human lower extremity also use such a mass–spring–damper model. The 'steady-state' frequency response characteristics of such a system

Figure 5.29 Transient response characteristics of a second-order force plate system for damping ratios of: 2 (overdamped case shown by the dashed red curve), 0.707 (critically damped case shown by the continuous black curve), and 0.2 (underdamped case shown by the continuous red curve). The output signal 'settles' to the input signal (the dashed black horizontal line) far quicker for the critically damped case than for the other two.

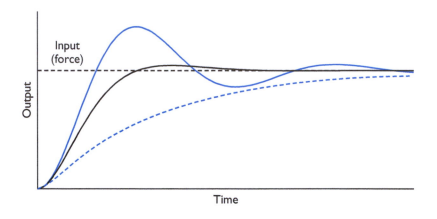

are usually represented by the unique series of non-dimensional curves of Figure 5.28. The response of such a system to an instantaneous change of the input force is known as its 'transient' response and can be represented as in Figure 5.29.

In these two figures:

- ζ is the 'damping ratio' of the system, $c/\sqrt{(4km)}$
- ω_n is the 'natural frequency', $\sqrt{(k/m)}$ – the frequency at which the plate will vibrate if struck and then allowed to vibrate freely
- ω is the signal frequency (as in Figure 5.27).

To obtain a suitable transient response, the damping ratio needs to be around 0.5–0.8 to avoid under- or overdamping. A value of 0.707 is considered ideal, as in Figure 5.29, as this ensures that the output follows the input signal – reaches steady state – in the shortest possible time.

Careful inspection of Figure 5.28 allows the suitable frequency range to be established for steady-state response to achieve a nearly constant amplitude ratio (Figure 5.28(a)) and a small phase lag (Figure 5.28(b)), with $\zeta = 0.707$. The frequency ratio ω'/ω_n, where ω' is the largest frequency of interest in the signal, must be small, ideally less than 0.2. Above this value, the amplitude ratio (Figure 5.28(a)) starts to deviate from a constant value and the phase lag increases and becomes very dependent on the frequency, causing errors in the output signal. For impact forces, the natural frequency should be 10 times the equivalent frequency of the impact, which can exceed 100 Hz in sports activities. The natural frequency must, therefore, be as large as possible to record the frequencies of interest. The structure must be relatively light but stiff, to give a high natural frequency; this consideration relates not only to the plate but also to its mounting. A high natural frequency, of around 1000 Hz, would be desirable for most applications in sports biomechanics. Among the highest natural frequencies specified for commercial plates are: for one piezoelectric plate, 850 Hz, all three channels; for two strain gauge plates, (a) 1000 Hz for the vertical channel, 550 Hz for the two horizontal channels, and (b) 1500 Hz (vertical) and 320 Hz (horizontal). However, the value specified for a particular plate may not always be found in practical applications, particularly if not mounted according to the manufacturer's instructions.

6   The anatomy of human movement

Knowledge assumed
Axes and planes of movement
(Chapter 1)
Analysis of sports movements
(Chapters 1 to 4)
Relationship between force
and movement (Chapter 5)
Basic muscle physiology
(see Further Reading)

INTRODUCTION

In this chapter we will consider the anatomical principles that apply to movement in sport and how the movements of the sports performer are generated. Anatomy is an old branch of science, in which the use of Latin names is still common in the English-speaking world. As most sports biomechanics students do not, understandably, speak Latin, the use of Latin words will be avoided, unless necessary, in this chapter; so, for example, Latin names for the various types of joint are not used. Where this avoidance is not possible, and this includes the naming of most muscles, some brief guidance on the grammar of this antique language is given. We shall also look at how electromyography can be used in the study of muscle activation patterns in sports movements and the use of isokinetic dynamometry in recording muscle torques.

BOX 6.1 LEARNING OUTCOMES

After reading this chapter you should be able to:

- identify the functions of the skeleton and give examples of each type of bone
- describe typical surface features of bone and how these can be recognised superficially
- understand the tissue structures involved in the joints of the body and the factors contributing to joint stability and mobility
- identify the features of synovial joints and give examples of each class of these joints
- understand the features and structure of skeletal muscles
- classify muscles both structurally and functionally
- describe the types and mechanics of muscle contraction and appreciate how tension is produced in muscle
- understand how the total force exerted by a muscle can be resolved into components depending on the angle of pull
- appreciate the applications of electromyography to the study of sports skills
- understand why the recorded EMG differs from the physiological signal and how to use EMG measuring equipment in sports movements
- describe the main methods of quantifying the EMG signal in the time and frequency domains
- appreciate how and why isokinetic dynamometry is used to record the net muscle torque at a joint.

THE SKELETON AND ITS BONES

In this section, the functions of the human skeleton and the form, nature and composition of its bones will be considered. There are 206 bones in the human skeleton, of which 177 engage in voluntary movement. The functions of the skeleton are: to

Figure 6.1 The human skeleton.

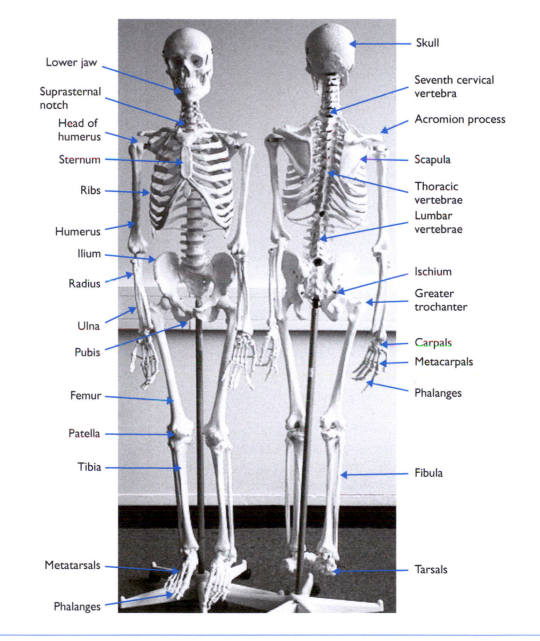

- Skull
- Lower jaw
- Seventh cervical vertebra
- Suprasternal notch
- Acromion process
- Head of humerus
- Sternum
- Scapula
- Ribs
- Thoracic vertebrae
- Humerus
- Lumbar vertebrae
- Ilium
- Radius
- Ischium
- Ulna
- Greater trochanter
- Pubis
- Carpals
- Metacarpals
- Phalanges
- Femur
- Patella
- Tibia
- Fibula
- Metatarsals
- Tarsals
- Phalanges

protect vital organs such as the brain, heart and lungs; to provide rigidity for the body; to provide muscle attachments whereby the bones function as levers, allowing the muscles to move them about the joints; to enable the manufacture of blood cells; and to provide a storehouse for mineral metabolism.

The skeleton, shown in Figure 6.1, is often divided into the axial skeleton, comprising the skull, lower jaw, vertebrae, ribs, sternum, sacrum and coccyx, which is mainly protective, and the appendicular skeleton, consisting of the shoulder girdle (clavicles and scapulae) and upper limbs, and the pelvic girdle and lower limbs, which functions in movement.

Bone structure

Macroscopically, there are two types of bone tissue: cortical, or compact, bone and trabecular, or cancellous, bone. The first forms the outer shell, or cortex, of a bone and has a dense structure. The second has a loose latticework structure of trabeculae or cancelli; the spaces – or interstices – between the trabeculae are filled with red marrow in which red blood cells form. Cancellous bone tissue is arranged in concentric layers, or lamellae, and its cells, called osteocytes, are supplied with nutrients from blood vessels passing through the red marrow. The lamellar pattern and material composition of the two bone types are similar. Different porosity is the principal distinguishing feature, and the distinction between the two types might be considered somewhat arbitrary. Biomechanically, the two types of bone should be considered as one material with a wide range of densities and porosities. It can be classified as a composite material in which the strong but brittle mineral element is embedded in a weaker but more ductile one consisting of collagen and ground substance. Like many similar but inorganic composites, such as carbon-reinforced fibres, which are important in sports equipment, this structure gives a material whose strength-to-weight ratio exceeds that of either of its constituents.

With the exception of the articular surfaces, bones are wholly covered with a membrane known as the periosteum. This has a strong outer layer of fibres of a protein, collagen, and a deep layer that produces cells called osteoblasts, which participate in the growth and repair of the bone. The periosteum also contains capillaries, which nourish the bone, and it has a nerve supply. It is sensitive to injury and is the source of much of the pain from fracture, bone bruises and shin splints. Muscles generally attach to the periosteum, not directly to the bone, and the periosteum attaches to the bone by a series of root-like processes.

Classification of bones

Bones can be classified according to their geometrical characteristics and functional requirements, as follows:

• Long bones occur mostly in the appendicular skeleton and function for weight-bearing and movement. They consist of a long, central shaft, known as the body or diaphysis, the central cavity of which consists of the medullary canal, which is filled with fatty yellow marrow. At the expanded ends of the bone, the compact shell is very thin and the trabeculae are arranged along the lines of force transmission. In the same region, the periosteum is replaced by smooth, hyaline articular cartilage. This has no blood supply and is the residue of the cartilage from which the bone formed. Examples of long bones are the humerus, radius and ulna of the upper limb, the femur, tibia and fibula of the lower limb, and the phalanges of the fingers and toes (see Figure 6.1).

- Short bones are composed of cancellous tissue and are irregular in shape, small, chunky and roughly cubical; examples are the carpal bones of the hand and the tarsal bones of the foot.
- Flat bones are basically a sandwich of richly veined cancellous bone within two layers of compact bone. They serve as extensive flat areas for muscle attachment and, except for the scapulae, enclose body cavities. Examples are the sternum, ribs and ilium.
- Irregular bones are adapted to special purposes and include the vertebrae, sacrum, coccyx, ischium and pubis.
- Sesamoid bones form in certain tendons; the most important example is the patella (the kneecap).

The surface of a bone

The surface of a bone is rich in markings that show its history; some examples are shown in Figure 6.2. Some of these markings can be seen at the skin surface and many others can be easily felt (palpated) – some of these are the anatomical landmarks used to estimate the axes of rotation of the body's joints (see Box 6.2), which are crucially important for quantitative biomechanical analysis of human movement in sport.

- Lumps on bones known as tuberosities or tubercles – the latter are smaller than the former – and projections, known as processes, show attachments of strong fibrous cords, such as tendons. The styloid processes on the radius and ulna (Figure 6.2(a)) are used to locate the wrist axis of rotation in the sagittal plane. The acromion process on the scapula (see Figure 6.1) is often used to estimate the shoulder joint axis of rotation in the sagittal plane (see Box 6.2).
- Ridges and lines indicate attachments of broad sheets of fibrous tissue known as aponeuroses or intermuscular septa.
- Grooves (known as furrows or sulci), holes (foramina), notches and depressions (fossae) often suggest important structures, for example grooves for tendons. The suprasternal notch (see Figure 6.1) is often used to establish the trunk–neck boundary for centre of mass calculations (see Table 5.1).
- A projection from a bone was defined above as a process, while a rounded prominence at the end of a bone is termed a condyle, the projecting part of which is sometimes known as an epicondyle. The humeral epicondyles (Figure 6.2(b)) and the femoral condyles (Figure 6.2(c)) are used, respectively, to locate the elbow and knee axes of rotation in the sagittal plane.

Figure 6.2 Surface features of bones. From top: (a) at the wrist; (b) at the elbow; (c) at the knee; (d) at the ankle.

• Special names are given to other bony prominences. The greater trochanter on the lateral aspect of the femur, shown in Figure 6.1, is often used to estimate the position of the hip joint centre. The medial and lateral malleoli, at the distal ends of the tibia and fibula, respectively (Figure 6.2(d)), are used to locate the ankle axis of rotation in the sagittal plane.

BOX 6.2 LOCATION OF MAIN JOINT SAGITTAL AXES OF ROTATION AND JOINT CENTRES OF ROTATION (SEE ALSO TABLE 5.1)

Joint	Sagittal axis	Joint centre
Shoulder	About 10 per cent of the distance between the most lateral point on the lateral border of the acromion process and the elbow joint axis, below the acromion process (see Figure 6.1).	At the centre of the head of the humerus (cannot be palpated).
Elbow	Along line joining the medial and lateral epicondyles of the humerus (see Figure 6.2(b)).	Midway along that line.
Wrist	Along line joining styloid processes on radius and ulna (see Figure 6.2(a)).	Midway along that line.
Hip	Approximately along line joining the most proximal palpable point on the greater trochanter on the femur to the equivalent point on the contralateral femur (perhaps 1 per cent of the distance from this point to the knee axis of rotation, superior to the greater trochanter; see Figure 6.1).	At the centre of the head of the femur (cannot be palpated).
Knee	Along line joining medial and lateral condyles on femur (see Figure 6.2(c)).	Midway along that line.
Ankle	Along line joining most palpable point of tibial (medial) malleolus and most lateral point on fibular (lateral) malleolus (see Figure 6.2(d)).	Midway along that line.

Bone fracture

The factors affecting bone fracture, such as the mechanical properties of bone and the forces to which bones in the skeleton are subjected during sport, will not be discussed in detail here (for further information, see Bartlett and Bussey, 2012, listed in Further Reading).

The loading of living bone is complex because of the combined nature of the forces, or loads, applied and because of the irregular geometric structure of bones. For example, during the activities of walking and jogging, the tensile and compressive stresses along the tibia are combined with transverse shear stresses, caused by torsional loading associated with lateral and medial rotation of the tibia. Although the tensile stresses are, as would be expected, much larger for jogging than walking, the shear stresses are greater for the latter activity. Most fractures are produced by such a combination of several loading modes.

After fracture, bone repair is effected by two types of cell, known as osteoblasts and osteoclasts. Osteoblasts deposit strands of fibrous tissue, between which ground substance is later laid down, and osteoclasts dissolve or break up damaged or dead bone. Initially, when the broken ends of the bone are brought into contact, they are surrounded by a mass of blood. This is partly absorbed and partly converted, first into fibrous tissue then into bone. The mass around the fractured ends is called the callus. This forms a thickening, for a period of months, which will gradually be smoothed away, unless the ends of the bone have not been correctly aligned. In that case, the callus will persist and form an area where large mechanical stresses may occur, rendering the region susceptible to further fracture.

THE JOINTS OF THE BODY

Joints, also known as articulations, occur between the bones or cartilage of the skeleton. They allow free movement of the various parts of the body or more restricted movements, for example during growth or childbirth. Other tissues that may be present in the joints of the body are dense, fibrous connective tissue, which includes ligaments, and synovial membrane. The nature and biomechanical functions of these and other structures associated with joints will not be considered here.

Joint classification

Overall, joints are classified according to the movement they allow. In fibrous joints, the edges of the bone are joined by thin layers of the fibrous periosteum, as in the suture joints of the skull, where movement is undesirable. With age these joints disappear as the bones fuse. These are immovable joints. Ligamentous joints occur between two bones. The bones can be close together, as in the interosseus talofibular ligament, which allows only a little movement, or further apart, as in the broad and flexible interosseus membrane of fibrous tissue between the ulna and radius, which permits free movement. These are not true joints and are classed as slightly movable. Cartilaginous joints either consist of hyaline cartilage, as in the joint between the sternum and first rib, or fibrocartilage, as in the intervertebral discs. Cartilaginous joints are classed as slightly movable.

The third classification of joint has a joint cavity surrounded by a sleeve of fibrous tissue, the ligamentous joint capsule, which unites the bones. Friction between the bones is minimised by smooth hyaline cartilage. Although cartilage has been traditionally regarded as a shock absorber, this role is now considered unlikely. The functions of the cartilage in such joints are mainly to help to reduce stresses between the contacting surfaces, by widely distributing the joint loads, and to allow movement with minimal friction. The inner surface of the capsule is lined with the delicate synovial membrane, the cells of which exude the synovial fluid that lubricates the joint. This fluid converts potentially compressive solid stresses into equally distributed hydrostatic ones, and nourishes the bloodless hyaline cartilage. These freely moveable or synovial joints (Figure 6.3) are the most important in human movement. The changing relationship of the bones to each other during movement creates spaces filled by synovial folds and fringes attached to the synovial membrane. When filled with fat cells these are called fat pads. In certain synovial joints, such as the sternoclavicular and distal radio-ulnar joints, fibrocartilaginous discs occur that wholly or partially divide the joint. Synovial joints can be classified as follows, based mainly on how many degrees of rotational freedom the joint allows (Figure 6.3):

Figure 6.3 Classification of synovial joints: (a) plane joint; (b) hinge joint; (c) pivot joint; (d) condyloid joint; (e) saddle joint; (f) ball and socket joint.

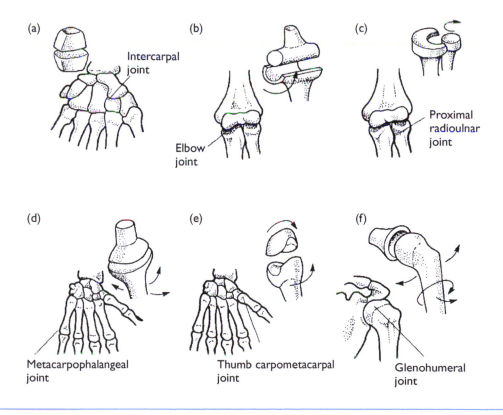

- Plane joints (also known as gliding or irregular joints) are joints in which only slight gliding movements occur. These joints have an irregular shape. Examples are the intercarpal joints of the hand (Figure 6.3(a)), the intertarsal joints of the foot, the acromioclavicular joint and the heads and tubercles of the ribs. The joints are classed in the literature both as non-axial, because they glide more or less on a plane surface, and multiaxial. The latter term is presumably used because the surfaces are not plane but have a large radius of curvature and, therefore, an effective centre of rotation some considerable distance from the bone. The former description seems more useful. Although individual joint movements are small, combinations of several of these joints, as in the carpal region of the hand, can result in significant motion.

- Hinge joints are joints in which the concave surface of one bone glides partially around the convex surface of the other. Examples are the elbow (Figure 6.3(b)) and ankle joints and the interphalangeal joints of the fingers and toes. The knee is not a simple hinge joint, although it appears that way when bearing weight. Hinge joints are uniaxial, permitting only the movements of flexion and extension.

- Pivot joints are joints in which one bone rotates about another. This may involve the bones fitting together at one end, with one rotating about a peg-like pivot in the other, as in the atlanto-axial joint between the first and second cervical vertebrae. The class is also used to cover two long bones lying side by side, as in the proximal radioulnar joint of Figure 6.3(c). These joints are uniaxial, permitting rotation about the longitudinal axis in the transverse plane.

- Condyloid joints are classified as biaxial joints, permitting flexion–extension and abduction–adduction (and, therefore, circumduction). The class is normally used to cover two slightly different types of joint. One of these has a spheroidal surface that articulates with a spheroidal depression, as in the metacarpophalangeal or 'knuckle' joints (Figure 6.3(d)) – 'condyloid' means 'knuckle-like'. These joints are potentially triaxial but lack the musculature to perform rotation about the longitudinal axis. The other type, which is sometimes classified separately as ellipsoidal joints, is similar in most respects except that the articulating surfaces are ellipsoidal rather than spheroidal, as in the wrist joint.

- Saddle joints consist of two articulating saddle-shaped surfaces, as in the thumb carpometacarpal joint, shown in Figure 6.3(e). These are biaxial joints, with the same movements as other biaxial joints but with a greater range of movement.

- Ball and socket joints, also known as spheroidal joints, have the spheroidal head of one bone fitting into the cup-like cavity of the other, as in the hip joint and the shoulder (or glenohumeral) joint. The latter is shown in Figure 6.3(f). These are triaxial joints, permitting movements in all three planes.

Joint stability and mobility

The stability, or immobility, of a joint is the joint's resistance to displacement. It depends on the following factors:

- The shape of the bony structure, including the type of joint and the shape of the bones. This is a major stability factor in some joints, such as the elbow and hip, but of far less importance in others, for example the knee and shoulder joints.
- The ligamentous arrangement, including the joint capsule, which is crucial in, for example, the knee joint.
- The arrangement of fascia, tendons and aponeuroses.
- Position – joints are more stable in the close-packed position, with maximal contact between the articular surfaces and with the ligaments taut, than in the loose-packed position.
- Atmospheric pressure, providing it exceeds the pressure within the joint, as in the hip joint.
- Muscular contraction – depending on the relative positions of the bones at a joint, muscles may have a force component capable of pulling the bone into the joint (see Figure 6.13); this is particularly important when the bony structure is not inherently stable, as in the shoulder joint.

Joint mobility or flexibility is widely held to be desirable for sportsmen and sportswomen. It is usually claimed to reduce injury. Although this is probably true, excessive mobility can sacrifice important joint stability and predispose to injury. It is also sometimes claimed that improved mobility enhances performance; although this is impeccably logical it is not well substantiated. Mobility is highly joint specific and is affected by body build, heredity, age, sex, fitness and exercise. Sports participants are usually more flexible than non-participants owing to the use of joints through greater ranges of movement, avoiding adaptive short-ening of muscles. Widely differing values are reported in the scientific literature for normal joint ranges of movement. The discrepancies may be attributable to unreliable in-strumentation, lack of standard experimental protocols and inter-individual differences.

MUSCLES – THE POWERHOUSE OF MOVEMENT

Muscles are structures that convert chemical energy into mechanical work and heat energy. In studying sport and exercise movements biomechanically, the muscles of interest are the skeletal muscles, used for moving and for posture. This type of muscle has striated muscle fibres of alternating light and dark bands. Muscles are extensible, that is they can stretch or extend, and elastic, such that they can resume their resting length after extending. They possess excitability and contractility. Excitability means that they respond to a chemical sti-mulus by generating an electrical signal, the action potential, along the plasma membrane. Contractility refers to the unique ability of muscle to shorten and hence produce move-ment. Skeletal muscles account for approximately 40–50 per cent of the mass of an adult of normal weight; they exist as about 75 pairs. The main skeletal muscles are shown in Figure 6.4. The proximal attachment of a muscle, that nearer the middle of the body, is known as the origin and the distal attachment as the insertion. The attachment points of skeletal muscles to bone and the movements they cause are not listed here but

Figure 6.4 Main superficial skeletal muscles. Left: (a) anterior view; Right: (b) posterior view.

can be found in many books dealing with exercise physiology and anatomy (for example, Marieb and Hoehn, 2012; see Further Reading) as well as in the Interactive eTextbook.

Muscle structure

Each muscle fibre is a highly specialised, complex, cylindrical cell. The cell is elongated and multinucleated, 0.01–0.1 mm in diameter and seldom more than a few centimetres long. The cytoplasm of the cell is known as the sarcoplasm. This contains large amounts of stored glycogen and a protein, myoglobin, which is capable of binding oxygen and is unique to muscle cells. Each fibre contains many smaller, parallel elements, called myofibrils, which run the length of the cell and are the contractile components of skeletal muscle cells. The sarcoplasm is surrounded by a delicate plasma membrane called the sarcolemma. The sarcolemma is attached at its rounded ends to the endomysium, the fibrous tissue surrounding each fibre. Units of 100–150 muscle fibres are bound in a coarse, collagenic fibrous tissue, the perimysium, to form a fascicle. The fascicles can be much longer than individual muscle fibres, for example around 250 mm long for the hamstring muscles. Several fascicles are bound into larger units enclosed in a covering of yet coarser, dense fibrous tissue, the deep fascia, or epimysium, to form muscle. The epimysium separates the muscle from its neighbours and facilitates frictionless movement.

The contractile cells are concentrated in the soft, fleshy central part of the muscle, called the belly. Towards the ends of the muscle the contractile cells finish but the perimysium and epimysium continue to the bony attachment as a cordlike tendon or flat aponeurosis, in which the fibres are plaited to distribute the muscle force equally over the attachment area. If the belly continues almost to the bone, then individual sheaths of connective tissue attach to the bone over a larger area.

The strength and thickness of the muscle sheath varies with location. Superficial muscles, particularly near the distal end of a limb, have a thick sheath with additional protective fascia. The sheaths form a tough structural framework for the semi-fluid muscle tissue. They return to their original length even if stretched by 40 per cent of their resting length. Groups of muscles are compartmentalised from others by intermuscular septa, usually attached to the bone and to the deep fascia that surrounds the muscles.

Muscle activation

Each muscle fibre is innervated by cranial or spinal nerves and is under voluntary control. The terminal branch of the nerve fibre ends at the neuromuscular junction or motor end-plate, which touches the muscle fibre and transmits the nerve impulse to the sarcoplasm. Each muscle is entered from the central nervous system by nerves that contain both motor and sensory fibres, the former of which are known as motor neurons. As each motor neuron enters the muscle, it branches into terminals, each of which forms a motor end-plate with a single muscle fibre. The term 'motor unit' is used to refer to a motor neuron and all the muscle fibres that it innervates, and these can be spread over a wide area of the muscle. The motor unit can be considered the fundamental functional unit of neuromuscular control. Each nerve impulse causes all the muscle fibres of the motor unit to contract fully and almost simultaneously. The number of fibres per motor unit is sometimes called the innervation ratio. This ratio can be less than 10 for muscles requiring very fine control and greater than 1000 for the weight-bearing muscles of the lower extremity. Muscle activation is regulated through motor unit recruitment and the motor unit stimulation rate (or rate-coding). The former is an orderly sequence based on the size of the motor neuron. The smaller motor neurons are recruited first; these are typically slow twitch, with a low maximum tension and a long contraction time. If more motor units can be recruited, then this mechanism dominates; smaller muscles have fewer motor units and depend more on increasing their stimulation rate.

Naming muscles

As noted in the introduction to this chapter, in the scientific literature muscles are nearly always known by their Latin names. The full name is musculus, which is often omitted or abbreviated to m. or M., followed by adjectives or genitives of nouns. The name may refer to role, location, size or shape of the muscle. An example of a muscle named after its location is the latissimus dorsi – the broadest (latissimus) muscle of the back. The flexor digitorum profundus is named after its role – the deep (profundus) flexor of the fingers. The trapezius muscle – the English name is identical to the Latin one for this, but this is true for only a few other muscles – is named after its trapezoidal shape. Some English names have become accepted, such as the anterior deltoid; obvious English translations of the Latin names, for example the deep flexor of the fingers (see above) are – somewhat sadly in my view – not commonly encountered in most scientific literature.

Muscles are often described by their role, such as the flexors of the knee and the abductors of the humerus. Most muscles have more than one role in movement; multi-joint muscles have roles at more than one joint.

Structural classification of muscles

The internal structure or arrangement of the muscle fascicles is related to both the force of contraction and the range of movement and, therefore, serves as a logical way of classifying muscles. There are two basic types, each of which is further subdivided.

Collinear muscles (Figure 6.5(a) to (e)) have muscle fascicles that are more or less parallel. A collinear muscle is capable of shortening by about one-third to one-half of

Figure 6.5 Structural classification of muscles. Collinear muscles: (a) longitudinal; (b) quadrate rhomboidal; (c) quadrate rectangular; (d) fan shaped; (e) fusiform. Pennate muscles: (f) unipennate; (g) bipennate; (h) multipennate.

its belly's length. Such muscles have a large range of movement, which is limited by the fraction of the muscle length that is tendinous. These muscles are very common in the limbs and are further divided as follows:

- Longitudinal muscles consist of long, strap-like fascicles parallel to the long axis, as shown schematically in Figure 6.5(a); examples are the rectus abdominis muscle of the abdominal wall and the sartorius, the longest muscle in the human body, which crosses the hip and knee joints across the front of the thigh.
- Quadrate muscles are four sided, usually flat, with parallel fascicles, as in Figure 6.5(b) and (c). They may have a rhomboid shape, as in the schematic representation of the rhomboideus major – a muscle of the scapula – in Figure 6.5(b), or rectangular, as, for example, the pronator quadratus, located on the anterior aspect of the forearm near the wrist and shown schematically in Figure 6.5(c).
- Fan-shaped muscles (Figure 6.5(d)) are relatively flat with almost parallel fascicles that converge towards the insertion point. A good example is the pectoralis major muscle on the upper anterior surface of the trunk.
- Fusiform muscles are usually rounded, tapering at either end (Figure 6.5(e)), and include the elbow flexors: brachialis, brachioradialis and biceps brachii. The location of the last of these is certainly familiar to most, if not all, sport and exercise science students. The brachialis lies directly underneath the biceps brachii, is a single joint muscle and is the main elbow flexor.

Pennate or penniform muscles (Figure 6.5(f) to (h)) have shorter fascicles than collinear muscles; the fascicles are angled away from an elongated tendon. This arrangement allows more fibres to be recruited, which provides a stronger, more powerful muscle at the expense of range of movement and speed of the limb moved. They account for 75 per cent of the body's muscles, mostly in the large muscle groups, including the powerful muscles of the lower extremity. This classification is further divided into the following groups:

- Unipennate muscles lie to one side of the tendon, extending diagonally as a series of short, parallel fascicles, as in Figure 6.5(f); the tibialis posterior muscle of the ankle is an example.
- Bipennate muscles (Figure 6.5(g)) have a long central tendon, with fascicles in diagonal pairs on either side. This group includes the rectus femoris muscle of the thigh and the flexor hallucis longus, which flexes the big toe (hallux).
- Multipennate muscles converge to several tendons, giving a herringbone effect (Figure 6.5(h)), for example the deltoid (deltoideus in Latin).

Types of muscle contraction

The term 'muscle contraction' refers to the development of tension within the muscle. The term is a little confusing, as contraction means 'becoming smaller' in much English usage. Some sport and exercise scientists would prefer the term 'action' to be used instead, but as this has yet to be widely adopted. I will use 'muscle contraction', of which there are three main types.

- In isometric, or static, contraction, the muscle develops tension with no change in overall muscle length, as when holding a dumbbell stationary in a biceps curl.
- In concentric contraction, the muscle shortens as tension is developed, as when a dumbbell is raised in a biceps curl.
- In eccentric contraction, the muscle develops tension while it lengthens, as in the lowering movement in a biceps curl.

Both concentric and eccentric contractions can, theoretically, be at constant tension (isotonic) or constant speed (isokinetic). However, most contractions normally involve neither constant tension nor constant speed.

Group action of muscles

When a fibre or muscle develops tension both ends tend to move; whether these movements actually occur depends on the resistance to movement and on the activity of other muscles. Furthermore, when a muscle develops tension, it tends to perform all of its possible actions at all joints it crosses. Because of these axioms, muscles act together rather than individually to bring about the movements of the human body, with each muscle playing a specific role – this is one important feature of coordinated movement. In such group actions, muscles are classified according to their role, as follows; please note that the muscle group terminology used here is that normally used in sports biomechanics, however many anatomists now prefer different names for these muscle group roles:

- The muscles that directly bring about a movement by contracting concentrically are known as the agonists, which means 'movers'. This group is sometimes divided into prime movers, which always contract to cause the movement, and assistant movers, which only contract against resistance or at high speed. However, electromyography (see below) does not usually support such a simple distinction. If we do accept such a distinction, then brachialis and biceps brachii would be prime movers for elbow flexion while brachioradialis would be generally considered an assistant mover. This distinction is closely related to the idea of spurt and shunt muscles touched on later in this section.
- Antagonists are muscles that cause the opposite movement from that of specified agonists. Their normal role in group action is to relax when the agonists contract, although there are many exceptions to this. At the elbow, the triceps brachii is antagonistic to brachialis and biceps brachii.
- Stabilisers contract statically to fix one bone against the pull of the agonists so that the bone at the other end can move effectively. Muscles that contract statically to prevent movements caused by gravity are sometimes called supporting muscles, for example the abdominal muscles in push-ups.
- Neutralisers prevent undesired actions of the agonists when the agonists have more than one function. They may do this by acting in pairs, as mutual neutralisers, when they enhance the required action and cancel the undesired ones. For example, the flexor carpi radialis flexes and abducts the wrist while the flexor carpi ulnaris flexes and adducts the wrist: acting together they produce only flexion. Such muscles are also sometimes called helping synergists. Neutralisers may also contract statically to prevent an undesired action of agonists that cross more than one joint (multi-joint muscles). The flexion of the fingers while the wrist remains in its neutral anatomical position involves static contraction of the wrist extensors to prevent the finger flexors from flexing the wrist. Such muscles are also sometimes called true synergists.

BOX 6.3 A SCHEMATIC MODEL OF SKELETAL MUSCLE

A simple schematic model of skeletal muscle is often used to represent its functionally different parts. The model used is normally similar to Figure 6.6, and has contractile, series elastic and parallel elastic elements. The contractile component is made up of the myofibril protein filaments of actin and myosin and their associated coupling mechanism.

THE ANATOMY OF HUMAN MOVEMENT

The series elastic element lies in series with the contractile component and transmits the tension produced by the contractile component to the attachment points of the muscle. The tendons account for by far the major part of this series elasticity, with elastic structures within the muscle cells contributing the remainder. The parallel elastic element comprises the epimysium, perimysium, endomysium and sarcolemma. The elastic elements store elastic energy when they are stretched and release this energy when the muscle recoils. The series elastic element is more important than the parallel elastic element in this respect. The elastic elements are important as they keep the muscle ready for contraction and ensure the smooth production and transmission of tension during contraction. They also ensure the return of the contractile component to its resting position after contraction. They may also help to prevent the passive overstretching of the contractile component when relaxed, reducing the risk of injury. In practice, the series and parallel elastic elements are viscoelastic rather than simply elastic, enabling them to absorb energy at a rate proportional to that at which force is applied and to dissipate energy at a rate that is time dependent; this would require the addition of a damping element to each elastic element in Figure 6.6. In toe-touching, the initial stretch is elastic followed by a further elongation of the muscle-tendon unit owing to its viscosity.

Figure 6.6 Simple schematic model of skeletal muscle.

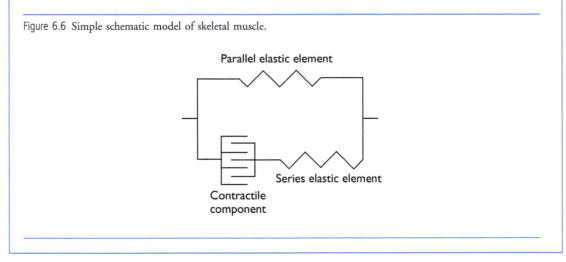

The mechanics of muscular contraction

This subsection will consider the gross mechanical response of a muscle to various neural stimuli. Much of this information is derived from *in vitro*, electrical stimulation of the frog gastrocnemius. However, we will assume that similar responses occur *in vivo* for the stimulation of human muscle by motor nerves. Although each muscle fibre can only respond in an all-or-none way, a muscle contains many fibres and can contract with various force and time characteristics.

The muscle twitch

The muscle twitch is the mechanical response of a muscle to a single, brief, low-intensity stimulus. The muscle contracts and then relaxes, as represented in Figure 6.7(a). After stimulation, there is a short period of a few milliseconds when excitation–contraction coupling occurs and no tension is developed. This can be considered as the time to take up the slack in the elastic elements and is known as the latency (or latent) period. The contraction time is the time from onset of tension development to peak tension (Figure 6.7(a)) and lasts 10–100 ms depending on the make-up of the muscle fibres. If the tension developed exceeds the resisting load, the muscle will shorten. During the following relaxation time the tension drops to zero. If the muscle had shortened, it now returns to its initial length. The muscle twitch is normally a laboratory rather than an *in vivo* event. In most human movement, contractions are long and smooth, and variations of the response are referred to as graded responses. These are regulated by two neural control mechanisms. The first – increasing the stimulation rate – involves increasing the rapidity of stimulation to produce wave summation. The second – increasing motor unit recruitment – involves recruitment of increasingly more motor units to produce multiple motor unit summation.

Wave summation and tetanus

The duration of an action potential is only a few milliseconds, which is very short compared with the following twitch. It is, therefore, possible for a series of action potentials, known as an action potential train, to be initiated before the muscle has completely relaxed. As the muscle is still partially contracted, the tension developed as a result of the second stimulus produces greater shortening than the first, as seen in Figures 6.7(b) and (c). The contractions are additive and the phenomenon is called wave summation. Increasing the stimulation rate will result in greater tension development as the relaxation time decreases until it eventually disappears. When this occurs, a smooth, sustained contraction called tetanus results (Figure 6.7(d)); this is the normal form of muscle contraction in the body. It should be noted that prolonged tetanus leads to an eventual inability to maintain the contraction and a decline in the tension to zero. This condition is termed muscle fatigue.

Multiple motor unit summation

The wide gradation of contractions within muscles is achieved mainly by the differing activities in their various motor units – in stimulation rate and in the number of units recruited. The repeated, asynchronous twitching of all the recruited motor units leads to brief summations or longer subtetanic or tetanic contractions of the whole muscle. For precise but weak movements only a few motor units will be recruited, while far more will be recruited for forceful contractions. The smallest motor units with the fewest muscle fibres, normally type I (see below), are recruited first. The larger motor units, normally type IIA then type IIB (see below), are activated only if needed. Both wave

Figure 6.7 Muscle responses: (a) muscle twitch; (b) wave summation; (c) incomplete and (d) complete tetanus.

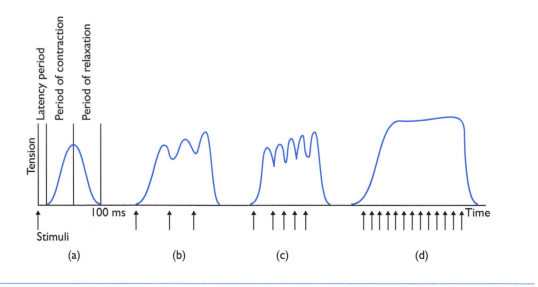

summation and multiple motor unit summation are factors in producing the smooth movements of skeletal muscle. Multiple motor unit summation is primarily responsible for the control of the force of contraction.

Treppe

The initial contractions in the muscle are relatively weak, only about half as strong as those which occur later. The tension development then has a staircase pattern called treppe, which is related to the suddenly increased availability of calcium ions. This effect, along with the increased enzymatic activity, the increase in conduction velocity across the sarcolemma and the increased elasticity of the elastic elements, which are all consequent on the rise in muscle temperature, leads to the pattern of increasingly strong contractions with successive stimuli. The effect could be postulated as a reason for warming up before an event, but this view is not universally accepted.

Development of tension in a muscle

The tension developed in a muscle depends upon:

- the number of fibres recruited and their firing (or stimulation) rate and synchrony
- the relative size of the muscle – the tension is proportional to the physiological cross-sectional area of the muscle; about 0.3 N force can be exerted per square milli-metre of cross-sectional area

Figure 6.8 Length–tension relationship for whole-muscle contraction. The dashed red line would be the continuation of active tension beyond the muscle's resting length in the absence of any passive tension.

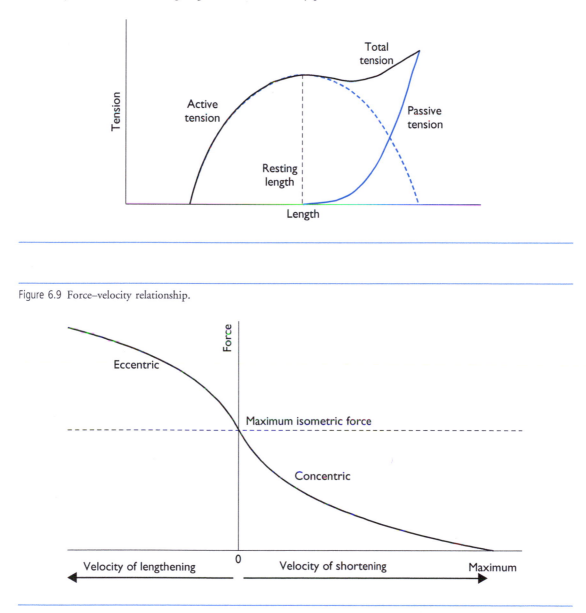

Figure 6.9 Force–velocity relationship.

- the temperature of the muscle and muscle fatigue
- the pre-stretch of the muscle – a muscle that develops tension after being stretched (the stretch–shortening cycle; see below) performs more work because of elastic energy storage and other mechanisms; the energy is stored mostly in the series elastic elements but also in the parallel elastic ones

Figure 6.10 Tension–time relationship.

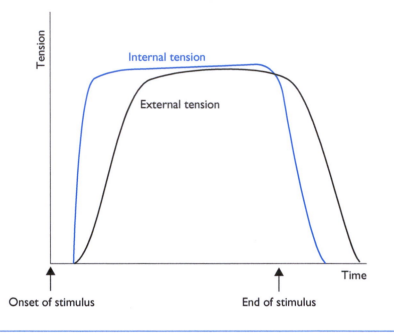

the mechanical properties of the muscle, as expressed by the length–tension, force–velocity and tension–time relationships (see below).

It should he noted that there are distinct differences in the rates of contraction, tension development and susceptibility to fatigue of individual muscle fibres. The main factor here is the muscle fibre type. Slow-twitch, oxidative type I fibres are suited to prolonged, low-intensity effort, as they are fatigue resistant because of their aerobic metabolism. However, they produce little tension as they are small and contract only slowly. Fast-twitch, glycolytic type IIB fibres have a larger diameter and contract quickly. They produce high tension but for only a short time, as they fatigue quickly because of their anaerobic, lactic metabolism. Fast-twitch, oxidative-glycolytic type IIA fibres are intermediate between the other two, being moderately resistant to fatigue because of their mainly aerobic metabolism. These fibres are able to develop high tension but are susceptible to fatigue at high rates of activity.

The length–tension relationship

For a single muscle fibre, the tension developed when it is stimulated to contract depends on its length. Maximum tension occurs at about the resting length of the fibre, because the actin and myosin filaments overlap along their entire length, maximising the number of cross-bridges attached. If the fibre is stretched, the sarcomeres lengthen and the number of cross-bridges attached to the thin actin filaments decreases. Conversely, the shortening of the sarcomeres to below resting length results in the overlapping of actin filaments from opposite ends of the sarcomere. In both cases the active tension is reduced. In a whole-muscle contraction the passive tension caused by the stretching of the elastic elements must be considered as well as the active tension developed by the contractile component, which is similar to the active tension of an isolated fibre (see Figure 6.8).

The total tension (Figure 6.8) is the sum of the active and passive tensions and depends upon the amount of connective tissue – the elastic elements – that the muscle contains. For single-joint muscles, such as brachialis, the amount of stretch is not usually sufficient for the passive tension to be important. In two-joint muscles, such as three of the four heads of the hamstrings – semitendinosus, semimembranosus and the long head of biceps femoris – the extremes of the length–tension relationship may be reached, with maximal total tension being developed in the stretched muscle, as in Figure 6.8.

The force–velocity relationship

As Figure 6.9 shows, the speed at which a muscle shortens when concentrically contracting is inversely related to the external force applied; it is greatest when the applied force is zero. When the force has increased to a value equal to the maximum force that the muscle can exert, the speed of shortening becomes zero and the muscle is contracting isometrically. The reduction of contraction speed with applied force is accompanied by an increase in the latency period and a shortening of the contraction time. A further increase of the force results in an increase in muscle length as the muscle contracts eccentrically; the speed of lengthening then increases with the force applied.

The tension–time relationship

The tension developed within a muscle is proportional to the contraction time. Tension increases with the contraction time up to the peak tension, as shown in Figure 6.10. Slower contraction enhances tension production as time is allowed for the internal tension produced by the contractile component, which can peak inside 10 ms, to be transmitted as external tension to the tendon through the series elastic elements; these have to be stretched, which may take about 300 ms. The tension within the tendon, and that transmitted to its attachments, reaches the maximum developed in the contractile component only if the duration of active contraction is sufficient. This only happens during prolonged tetanus.

Muscle stiffness

The mechanical stiffness of a muscle is the instantaneous rate of change of force with length – it is the slope of the muscle tension–length curve. Unstimulated muscles possess low stiffness (or high compliance). This rises with time during tension and is directly related to the degree of filament overlap and cross-bridge attachment. At high rates of change of force, such as occur in many sports, muscle is stiff, particularly in eccentric contractions, for which stiffnesses over 200 times those for concentric contractions have been reported. Stiffness is often considered to be under reflex control with regulation through both the length component of the muscle spindle receptors and the force–feedback component of the Golgi tendon organs. The exact role of the various reflex components in stiffness regulation in fast human movements in sport remains to be fully established, as do their effects in the stretch–shortening cycle (see below). It is clear, however, that the reflexes can almost double the stiffness of the muscles alone at some joints. Furthermore, muscle and reflex properties and the central nervous system interact in determining how stiffness affects the control of movement.

The stretch–shortening cycle

Many muscle contractions in dynamic movements in sport undergo a stretch–shortening cycle, in which the eccentric phase is considered to enhance performance in the concentric phase (Figure 6.11). The mechanisms thought to be involved are pre-load, elastic energy storage and release (mostly in tendons), and reflex potentiation. The stretch–shortening effect has not been accurately measured or fully explained. It is important not only in research but also in strength and power training for athletic activities. Some evidence shows that muscle fibres may shorten while the whole muscle–tendon unit lengthens. Furthermore, the velocity of recoil of the tendon during the shortening phase may be such that the velocity of the muscle fibres is less than that of the muscle–tendon unit. The result would be a shift to the right of the force–velocity curve (Figure 6.9) of the contractile component. These interactions between tendinous structures and muscle fibres may substantially affect elastic and reflex potentiation in the stretch–shortening cycle, whether or not they bring the muscle fibres closer to their optimal length and velocity. There have been alternative explanations for the phenomenon of the stretch–shortening cycle. Differences of opinion also exist on the amount of elastic energy that can be stored and its value in achieving maximal performance. Both the pre-load effect and greater elastic energy stored in the tendon are probably significant factors in the creation of larger muscle forces in, for example, a countermovement jump compared with a squat jump.

Muscle force components

In general, the overall force exerted by a muscle on a bone can be resolved into three force components, as shown in Figure 6.12. These are:

- A component of magnitude F_g, which tends to spin the bone about its longitudinal axis.
- A rotating component of magnitude F_t. In Figure 6.13 this is shown in one plane of movement only; in reality, this muscle force component may be capable of causing

Figure 6.11 Force potentiation in the stretch–shortening cycle in vertical jumps. Red curves show knee joint angle and black ones the vertical component of the ground reaction force: (a) concentric (+) knee extension in squat jump; (b) eccentric (−) contraction followed immediately by concentric (+) contraction in countermovement jump; (c) as (b) but with a 1 s pause between the eccentric and concentric phases. The angles and forces have been 'normalised' equally across the three jumps to fall within the ranges 0 to +1 and −1 to +1, respectively.

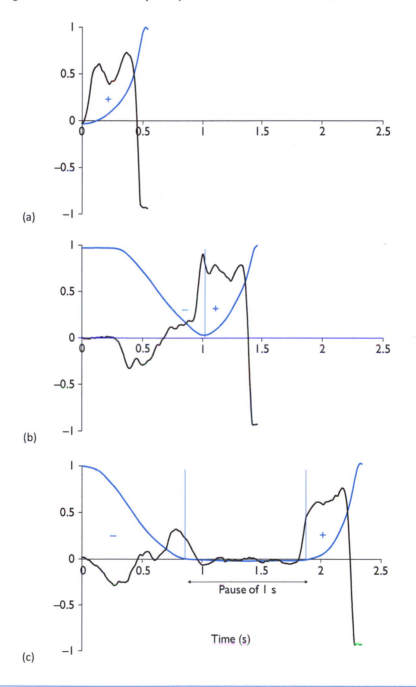

(a)

(b)

(c)

Figure 6.12 Three-dimensional muscle force components: (a) side view; (b) force components; (c) front view.

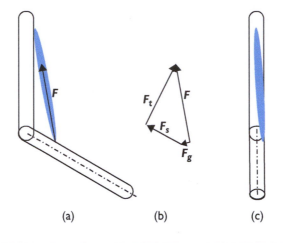

(a) (b) (c)

movement in both the sagittal and frontal planes, as, for example, flexor carpi ulnaris flexes and adducts the wrist.

- A component of magnitude F_s along the longitudinal axis of the bone, which normally stabilises the joint, as in Figures 6.13(c) and (d). This component may sometimes tend to dislocate the joint, as in Figure 6.13(f). Joint stabilisation is an important function of muscle force, particularly for shunt muscles (see below).

The relative importance of the last two components of muscle force is determined by the angle of pull (θ); this is illustrated for the brachialis acting at the elbow in Figure 6.13(a), assuming F_g to be zero. The optimum angle of pull is 90° when $F_t = F$ (Figure 6.13(e)) and all the muscle force contributes to rotating the bone. The angle of pull is defined as the angle between the muscle's line of pull along the tendon and the mechanical axis of the bone. It is usually small at the start of the movement, as in Figure 6.13(b), and increases as the bone moves away from its reference position, as in Figures 6.13(e) and (f).

For collinear muscles, the ratio of the distance of the muscle's origin from a joint to the distance of its insertion from that same joint (a/b in Figure 6.13(b)) is known as the partition ratio, p. It can be used to define two kinematically different types of muscle. Spurt muscles are muscles for which $p > 1$; the origin is further from the joint than is the insertion. The muscle force mainly acts to rotate the moving bone. Examples are the biceps brachii and brachialis for forearm flexion. Such muscles are often prime movers. Shunt muscles, by contrast, have $p < 1$ as the origin is nearer the joint than is the insertion. Even for rotations well away from the reference position, the angle of pull is always small. The force is, therefore, directed mostly along the bone so that these muscles act mainly to provide a stabilising rather than a rotating force. An example is brachioradialis in forearm flexion. Such muscles may also provide the

Figure 6.13 Two-dimensional muscle force components: (a) brachialis acting on forearm and humerus; (b) angle of pull; (c) stabilising and turning components of muscle force; (d) to (f) effect of angle of pull on force components. The magnitude and direction of the muscle force vector (*F*) have been kept constant through (a) to (f).

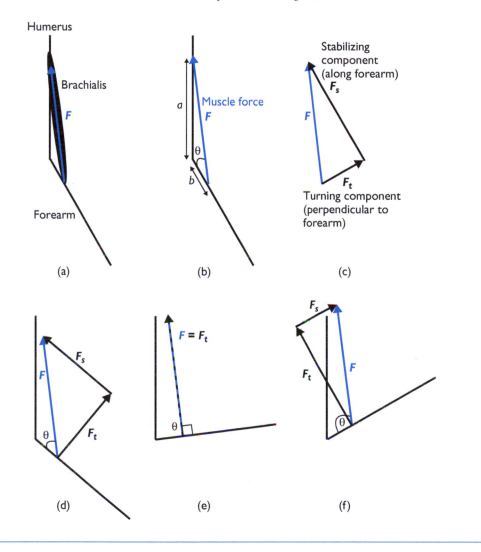

centripetal force, which is largely directed along the longitudinal axis of the bone towards the joint, for fast movements. Two-joint muscles are usually spurt muscles at one joint, as for the long head of biceps brachii acting at the elbow, and shunt muscles for the other joint, as for the long head of biceps brachii acting at the shoulder.

Within the human musculoskeletal system, anatomical pulleys serve to change the direction in which a force acts by applying it at a different angle and, sometimes, achieving an altered line of movement. The insertion tendon of peroneus longus is one such example. This muscle runs down the lateral aspect of the calf and passes around the lateral malleolus of the fibula to a notch in the cuboid bone of the foot. It then turns under the foot to insert into the medial cuneiform bone and the first metatarsal bone. The pulley action of the lateral malleolus and the cuboid accomplishes two changes of direction. The result is that contraction of this muscle plantar flexes the foot about the ankle joint (among other actions). Without the pulleys, the muscle would insert anterior to the ankle on the dorsal surface of the foot and would be a dorsiflexor. An anatomical pulley may also provide a greater angle of pull, thus increasing the turning component of the muscle force. The patella achieves this effect for quadriceps femoris, improving the effectiveness of this muscle as an extensor of the knee joint.

ELECTROMYOGRAPHY – WHAT MUSCLES DO

This and the next two sections are intended to provide you with an appreciation of the applications of electromyography to the study of muscle activity in sports movements. This includes the equipment and methods used and the processing of electromyographic data. We will also touch on the important relationship between muscle tension and the recorded signal, known as the electromyogram (abbreviation EMG, which is also, somewhat loosely, used as an abbreviation for electromyography). Electromyography is the technique for recording changes in the electrical potential of a muscle when it is caused to contract by a motor nerve impulse. The neural stimulation of the muscle fibre at the motor end-plate results in a reduction of the electrical potential of the cell and a spread of the action potential through the muscle fibre. The motor action potential (MAP), or muscle fibre action potential, is the name given to the waveform resulting from this depolarisation wave. This propagates in both directions along each muscle fibre from the motor end-plate before being followed by a repolarisation wave. The summation in space and time of motor action potentials from the fibres of a given motor unit is termed a motor unit action potential (MUAP; Figure 6.14). A sequence of MUAPs, resulting from repeated neural stimulation, is referred to as a motor unit action potential train (MUAPT). The physiological EMG signal is the sum, over space and time, of the MUAPTs from the various motor units (Figure 6.14).

Electromyography is the only method of objectively assessing when a muscle is active. It has been used to establish the roles that muscles fulfil both individually and in group actions. The electromyogram provides information on the timing, or sequencing, of the activity of various muscles in sports movements. By studying the sequencing of muscle activation, the sports biomechanist can focus on several factors which relate to skill, such as any overlap of agonist and antagonist activity and the onset of antagonist activity at the end of a movement. It also allows the sports biomechanist to study changes in muscular activity during skill acquisition and as a result of training. Electromyography can also be used to validate assumptions about muscle activity that are made when calculating the internal forces in the human musculoskeletal system. It should, however, be noted that the electromyogram cannot necessarily reveal what a muscle is doing, particularly in the fast multi-segment movements that predominate in sport.

Figure 6.14 Schematic representation of the generation and recording of the EMG signal.

Recording the myoelectric (EMG) signal

A full understanding of electromyography and its importance in sports biomechanics requires knowledge from the sciences of anatomy and neuromuscular physiology as well as consideration of many aspects of signal processing and recording, including instrumentation. A schematic representation of the generation of the (unseen) physiological EMG signal and its modification to the observed electromyogram is shown in Figure 6.14 – the electromyogram varies over time, as can be seen in this figure. So, we have another 'time series', which could be seen as another 'movement' pattern that could be useful to qualitative as well as quantitative movement analysts. Because of the complexity of the signal, it has rarely, if ever, been used in this way. Indeed, even quantitative biomechanical analysts often use it as no more than an 'on–off' indication of whether a muscle is contracting. As with kinematic data (Chapter 4), the electromyogram also consists of a range of frequencies, which can be represented by the EMG frequency spectrum (see below).

The physiological EMG signal is not the one recorded, as its characteristics are modified by the tissues through which it passes in reaching the electrodes used to detect it. These tissues act as a low-pass filter (see Appendix 4.1), rejecting some of the high frequency components of the signal. The electrode-to-electrolyte interface acts as a high-pass filter, discarding some of the lower frequencies in the signal. The two-electrode, or bipolar, configuration, which is normal for sports electromyography, changes the two-phase depolarisation–repolarisation wave to a three-phase one and removes some low frequency and some high frequency signals – it acts as a 'band-pass' filter. Modern, high quality EMG amplifiers should not unduly affect the frequency spectrum of the signal but the recording device may also act as a band-pass filter.

Many factors influence the recorded EMG signal. The intrinsic factors, over which the electromyographer has little control, can be classified as in Box 6.4.

BOX 6.4 INTRINSIC FACTORS THAT INFLUENCE THE ELECTROMYOGRAM

- Physiological factors, which include: the firing rates of the motor units; the type of fibre; the conduction velocity of the muscle fibres; and the characteristics of the volume of muscle from which the electrodes detect a signal (the detection volume) – such as its shape and electrical properties.
- Anatomical factors, which include the muscle fibre diameters and the positions of the fibres of a motor unit relative to the electrodes – the separation of individual motor unit action potentials becomes increasingly difficult as the distance to the electrode increases.

Extrinsic factors, by contrast, can be controlled. These include the location of the electrodes with respect to the motor end-plates, the orientation of the electrodes with respect to the muscle fibres and the electrical characteristics of the recording system (see below). The use of equipment with appropriate characteristics is vitally important and will form the subject of the rest of this section. The electrical signals that are to be recorded are small – of the order of 10 μV to 5 mV. To provide a signal to drive any recording device, we require signal amplification. The general requirement is to detect the electrical signals (electrodes), modify the signal (amplifier) and store the resulting waveform (recorder; compare with the force platform system of Chapter 5). All of this should be done linearly and without distortion. The following subsections summarise the important characteristics of EMG instrumentation.

EMG electrodes

The electrodes are the first link in the EMG recording chain. Their selection and placement are of considerable importance. Those used in sports biomechanics are predominantly surface electrodes, which can be passive, having no electrical power supply, or active, having a power supply. Indwelling electrodes are mainly used in clinical research. Few students have the luxury of choosing which type of electrode they will use and they will normally use passive surface electrodes, which are the focus of the rest of these three EMG subsections. It is worth noting that, compared with indwelling electrodes, surface electrodes are not only safer, easier to use and more acceptable to the person to whom they are attached, they also, for superficial muscles, provide quantitative repeatability that compares favourably with indwelling ones. Many of the principles and procedures covered will also apply to active surface electrodes; other equipment and data processing is common to all types of electrode (see Burden, 2008, listed in Further Reading).

The *European Recommendations for Surface Electromyography* (Hermens *et al.*, 1999; see Further Reading), called the SENIAM (Surface Electromyography for the Non-Invasive Assessment of Muscles) recommendations in the rest of this chapter, have attempted to standardise EMG assessment procedures. They recommend that only bipolar electrodes of pre-gelled silver–silver chloride material should be used, which conforms to standard practice in sports biomechanics. They also recommend a fixed distance of 20 mm between the centres of the two electrodes (as for the electrodes in Figure 6.17). The authors of the recommendations found no objective reason to recommend any particular shape of electrode, instead advising that users should always report the type, manufacturer and shape of the electrodes used.

EMG cables

Electrical cables are needed to connect the EMG electrodes to the amplifier or pre-amplifier. These can cause problems, known as cable or movement artefacts, which have frequencies in the range 0–10 Hz. The use of high-pass filtering, high quality electrically shielded cables and careful taping to reduce cable movement can minimise these problems. Cable artefacts can be reduced by using pre-amplifiers mounted on the skin near the detection electrodes and by good experimental procedures (see the next section). The use of active surface electrodes can virtually eliminate cable artefacts.

The effect of high-pass filtering at 10 Hz is shown in Figure 6.15, where Figures 6.15 (a) and (b) are the unfiltered and filtered signals respectively. The SENIAM recommendations for filtering the signal are to use a high-pass filter of 10 Hz if the signal is to be analysed in the frequency domain (see below and Chapter 4) and 10–20 Hz if the signal is only to be used for movement analysis. To reduce high frequency noise and aliasing, they also recommend a low-pass filter with a cut-off frequency of about 500 or 1000 Hz, at sampling frequencies, respectively, of 1000–2000 and 4000 Hz, depending on the application. Signal aliasing (see Chapter 4) will occur if the sampling frequency is less than twice the highest frequency in the power spectrum of the sampled signal.

EMG amplifiers

These are the heart of an EMG recording system. They should provide linear amplification over the whole frequency and voltage range of the EMG signal. Noise must be minimised and interference from the electrical mains supply (mains hum) must be removed as far as possible. The input signal will be around 5 mV with surface electrodes (or 10 mV with indwelling electrodes). The most important amplifier characteristics are described below.

Figure 6.15 Effect of high-pass (10 Hz) filter on cable artefacts. Top: (a) before filtering; Bottom: (b) after filtering.

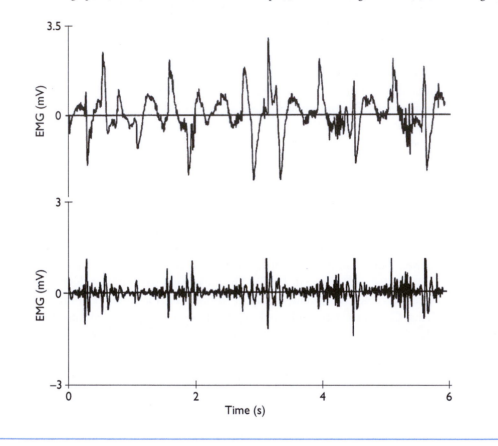

Figure 6.16 EMG signals without mains hum; v_a and v_b are biphasic motor unit action potentials recorded from two monopolar electrodes, $v_a - v_b$ is the triphasic differential signal from using the two electrodes in a bipolar configuration.

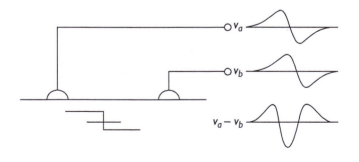

Gain

This is the ratio of output voltage to input voltage, and should be large and, ideally, variable in the range 100–10,000.

Input impedance

We can reduce the importance of obtaining a low electrical resistance of the skin by using an amplifier with a high input impedance – by which we mean a high resistance to the EMG signal. This impedance should be at least 100 times the skin resistance to avoid attenuation of the input signal. This can be seen from the relationship between the ratio (e_{emg} / e_i) of the detected signal (e_{emg}) to the amplifier input signal (e_i), and the amplifier input impedance (R_i) and the two skin plus cable resistances $(R_1$ and $R_2)$: $e_i / e_{emg} = R_i / (R_i + R_1 + R_2)$. The SENIAM recommendation for the minimum input impedance of an amplifier for use with passive surface electrodes is 100 MΩ (10^8 Ω). Input impedances for high performance amplifiers – used with active electrodes – can be as high as 10 GΩ (10^{10} Ω).

Frequency response

The ability of the amplifier to reproduce the range of frequencies in the signal is known as its frequency response. The required frequency response depends upon the frequencies contained in the EMG signal. This is comparable with the requirement for audio amplifiers to reproduce the range of frequencies in the audible spectrum. Typical values of EMG frequency bandwidth are 10–1000 Hz for surface electrodes and 20–2000 Hz for indwelling electrodes. Most modern EMG amplifiers easily meet such bandwidth requirements. About 95 per cent of the EMG signal is normally in the range up to 400 Hz, which explains why SENIAM recommend the use of a low-pass filter to remove higher frequencies. This signal range unfortunately also contains mains hum at 50 or 60 Hz. Also, SENIAM recommends that the input-referred voltage and current noise, respectively, should not exceed 1 µV and 10 pA.

Common mode rejection

Use of a single electrode would result in the generation of a two-phase depolarisation–repolarisation wave (Figure 6.16). It would also contain common mode mains hum. At approximately 100 mV, the hum is considerably larger than the EMG signal. This is overcome by recording the difference in potential between two adjacent electrodes, known as bipolar electrodes, using a differential amplifier. The hum is then largely eliminated as it is picked up commonly at each electrode because the body acts as an aerial – hence the name 'common mode'. The differential wave becomes triphasic (it has three phases, as in Figure 6.16). The smaller the electrode spacing, the more closely does the triphasic wave approximate to a time derivative of the single-electrode wave. In practice, perfect elimination of mains hum is not possible and the success of its removal is expressed by the common mode rejection ratio (CMRR). This should be 10,000 or greater. The overall system CMRR can be reduced to a figure lower than that of the amplifier by any substantial difference between the two skin plus cable resistances. The effective system common mode rejection ratio in this case can be downgraded to a value of $R_i / (R_1 - R_2)$; cables longer than 1 m often exacerbate this problem. For passive electrodes, the attachment of the pre-amplifier to the skin near the electrode site reduces noise pick-up and minimises any degradation of the CMRR arising from differences between the cable resistances.

Recorders

At present, A–D conversion and computer processing are by far the most commonly used recording methods. An A–D converter with 12- (1 in 4096) or 16-bit resolution is recommended by SENIAM. High sampling frequencies are needed to reproduce the signal successfully in digital form; telemetered systems do not always provide a sufficiently high sampling frequency.

EMG and muscle tension

Obtaining a predictive relationship between muscle tension and the electromyogram could solve a major problem for quantitative biomechanical analysis. This problem arises because the equations of motion at a joint cannot be solved because the number of unknown muscle forces exceeds the number of equations available. The problem is often known as muscle redundancy or muscle indeterminacy. If a solution could be found to this problem, it would allow the calculation of forces in soft tissue structures and between bones. It is not surprising, therefore, that the relationship between the EMG signal and the tension developed by a muscle has attracted the attention of many researchers.

The EMG provides a measure of the excitation of a muscle. Therefore, if the force in the muscle depends directly upon its excitation, a relationship should be expected between this muscle tension and suitably quantified EMG. A muscle's tension is regulated by varying the number and the firing rate of the active fibres; the amplitude of the EMG signal depends on the same two factors. It is, therefore, natural to speculate that a relationship does exist between EMG and muscle tension. We might further expect that this relationship would only apply to the active state of the contractile component, and that the contributions to muscle tension made by the series and parallel elastic elements would not be contained in the EMG (for a diagrammatic model of these elements of skeletal muscle, see Figure 6.6).

However, discrepancies exist between research studies even for isometric contractions, which should not lead us to expect a simple relationship between EMG and muscle tension for the fast, voluntary contractions that are characteristic of sports movements. For such movements, the relationship between EMG and muscle tension still remains elusive, although the search for it continues to be worthwhile.

Additionally, in complex multi-segmental movements, such as those we observe in sport, muscles influence other joints as well as the ones they cross. This means that, in sports movements, the electromyogram tells us when a muscle is active but not, generally, what that muscle is doing. This is a very important limitation to the use of EMG.

EXPERIMENTAL PROCEDURES IN ELECTROMYOGRAPHY

The results of an electromyographic investigation can only be as good as the preparation of the electrode attachment sites. Although skin resistance ceases to be a problem if active electrodes are used, many EMG studies in sports biomechanics currently use passive surface electrodes; good surface preparation is, therefore, still beneficial.

The location of the electrodes is the first consideration. For the muscles covered by their recommendations, the advice on electrode placements in the SENIAM report is well illustrated and simple (see Box 6.5 for a few examples). The separation of the electrodes was discussed above. For muscles not covered by these recommendations, simple advice is that:

- the two detector electrodes – or the detector pair – should be placed over the mid-point of the muscle belly
- the orientation of the electrode pair should be on a line parallel to the direction of the muscle fibres (for example Box 6.5)
- if the muscle fibres are neither linear nor in a parallel arrangement, the line between the two electrodes should point to the origin and insertion of the muscle for consistency.

The following is good experimental practice for skin preparation to improve the electrode-to-skin contact, thereby reducing noise and artefacts:

- The area of the skin on which the electrodes are to be placed is shaved if necessary.
- The attachment area is then cleaned and degreased using an alcohol wipe, the alcohol being allowed to evaporate before the electrodes are attached to the skin. None of the procedures used historically, requiring abrasion with sandpaper or a lancet to scratch the skin surface, are recommended by SENIAM; such procedures raise ethical, or health and safety, issues at many institutions and are not necessary if the amplifier input impedance conforms to that recommended in the previous section.
- The electrodes should preferably be pre-gelled; if they are not then, after the electrodes have been attached, electrode gel should be injected into them; any excess gel should be removed.
- It should not normally be necessary to check the skin resistance; however, if using older equipment, a simple DC ohmmeter reading of skin resistance should be taken. The resistance should be less than 10 kΩ and, preferably, less than 5 kΩ. If the resistance exceeds the former value, the electrodes should be removed and the preparation repeated.

- The reference electrode, also known as the earth or ground electrode, should be placed on electrically inactive tissue near the site of the recording electrodes or electrode pair. These sites are specific to each electrode (see the examples in Box 6.5) and are usually on a bony prominence.
- After the electrodes have been attached to the skin, the electrodes and cables usually need to be fixed to prevent cable-movement artefacts and pulling of the cables; SENIAM recommends the use of rubber (elastic) bands or double-sided tape or rings for this purpose. They also recommend a clinical test for each individual muscle, performed from the starting posture, to ensure satisfactory signals; a few examples of these tests are shown in Box 6.5.

After use, the electrodes should be sterilised or disposed of.

BOX 6.5 SOME ELECTRODE PLACEMENTS (ADAPTED FROM SENIAM)

Biceps brachii

Starting posture:	Seated on a chair; elbow at a right angle; palm facing up.
Electrode location:	On a line between the medial aspect of the acromion process and the cubital fossa, at one-third of the distance from the latter (Figure 6.17(a)) in the direction of the muscle fibres.
Reference electrode:	On or around the wrist.
Clinical test:	With one hand under the elbow, flex the elbow slightly below, or at, a right angle with the forearm supinated, and press against the forearm to extend the elbow.

Triceps brachii – long head

Starting posture:	Seated on a chair; shoulder about 90° abducted; elbow flexed at a right angle; palm facing down.
Electrode location:	Midway along a line between the posterior crest of the acromion process and the olecranon process, at two finger widths medial to that line (Figure 6.17(b)) in the direction of the muscle fibres.
Reference electrode:	On or around the wrist.
Clinical test:	Extend the elbow while applying pressure that would tend to flex it.

Rectus femoris

Starting posture:	Seated on a table; knees slightly flexed; upper body slightly bent backwards.
Electrode location:	Midway along the line from the anterior superior iliac spine to the superior aspect of the patella (Figure 6.17(c)) in the direction of the muscle fibres.

Reference electrode:	On or around the ankle or on the spinous process of the seventh cervical vertebra.
Clinical test:	Extend the knee – with no rotation of the thigh – against pressure.

Biceps femoris

Starting posture:	Lying prone with thighs on table; knees flexed by less than 90° from fully extended position; thigh and shank both slightly rotated externally.
Electrode location:	Midway along the line from the ischial tuberosity to the lateral epicondyle of the tibia (Figure 6.17(d)) in the direction of that line.
Reference electrode:	On or around the ankle or on the spinous process of the seventh cervical vertebra.
Clinical test:	Extend the knee against pressure applied to the leg proximal to the ankle.

Figure 6.17 Electrode locations based on SENIAM recommendations: (a) biceps brachii; (b) triceps brachii; (c) rectus femoris; (d) biceps femoris.

(a)

(b)

(c)

(d)

EMG DATA PROCESSING

Much kinesiological, physiological and neurophysiological electromyography simply uses and analyses the raw electromyogram. The amplitude of this signal, and all other EMG data, should always be related back to the signal generated at the electrodes, not given after amplification. Further EMG signal processing is often performed in sports biomechanics in an attempt to make comparisons between studies. It can also assist in correlating the EMG signal with mechanical actions of the muscles or other biological signals.

Although EMG signal processing can provide additional information to that contained in the raw signal, care is needed for several reasons. First, to distinguish between artefacts and signal, it is essential that good recordings free from artefacts are obtained. Second, the repeatability of the results needs consideration; non-exact repetition of EMGs is likely even from a stereotyped activity such as treadmill running. The siting of electrodes, skin preparation and other factors can all affect the results. Even the activity or inactivity of one motor unit near the pick-up site can noticeably change the signal. Third, such experimental factors make it difficult to compare EMG results with those of other studies. However, normalisation has been developed to facilitate such comparisons. This involves the expression of the amplitude of the EMG signal as a ratio to the amplitude of a contraction deemed to be maximal, usually a maximum voluntary contraction (MVC), from the same site. No consensus at present exists as to how to elicit an MVC and it is not always an appropriate maximum (for elaboration of this point, see Burden, 2008, listed in Further Reading).

Temporal processing and amplitude estimation (time domain analysis)

Temporal processing relates to the amplitude of the signal content, or the 'amount of activity'. It is often referred to as amplitude estimation. Such quantification is usually preceded by full-wave rectification as the raw EMG signal (Figure 6.18(a)) would have a mean value of about zero, because of its positive and negative deviations. Full-wave rectification (Figure 6.18(b)) simply involves making negative values positive; the rectified signal is expressed as the modulus of the raw EMG. Various terms have been, and are, used to express EMG amplitude, usually over a specified time interval, known as the epoch duration, such as the duration of the contraction or one running stride. The SENIAM recommendations specify epoch durations of 0.25–2 s for isometric contractions, 1–2 s for contractions less than 50 per cent of a maximal voluntary contraction (MVC) and 0.25–0.5 s for contractions greater than 50 per cent MVC. Such epoch durations considerably exceed the durations of muscle activity in many fast sports movements.

Figure 6.18 Time domain processing of EMG. Top: (a) raw signal; Middle: (b) full-wave rectified (FWR) EMG; Bottom: (c) smoothed, rectified EMG using a 6 Hz low-pass filter (linear envelope).

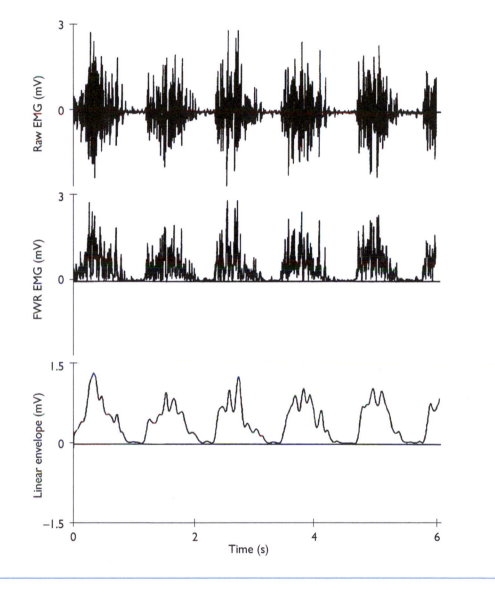

Average rectified EMG

The average rectified EMG is the average value of the full-wave rectified EMG, and is easily computed from a digital signal by adding the individual EMG values for each sample and dividing by the sample time. This is recommended by SENIAM for amplitude estimation of the EMG in non-dynamic contractions. The average rectified EMG is closely related to the integrated EMG (see below). As for other amplitude estimators of the electromyogram, the average rectified EMG is affected by the number of active motor units; the firing rates of motor units; the amount of signal cancellation by super-position; and the waveform of the motor unit action potential. The last of these depends upon electrode position, muscle fibre conduction velocity, the geometry of the detecting electrode surfaces and the detection volume.

Root mean square EMG (RMS EMG)

The RMS EMG is the square root of the average power (voltage squared) of the signal in a given time. It is easily computed from a digital signal by adding the squares of the individual EMG values for each sample, then taking the square root of the sum before dividing by the sample time. It is considered to provide a measure of the number of recruited motor units during voluntary contractions where there is little correlation among motor units. This is also recommended by SENIAM for amplitude estimation of the EMG in non-dynamic contractions.

Integrated EMG

This is simply the area under the rectified EMG signal. It is not recommended at all by SENIAM and is mentioned here only because of its wide use – and abuse – in earlier research.

Smoothed, rectified EMG

The standard way of obtaining the smooth, rectified EMG is by the use of a linear envelope detector (hence another name for this estimator, the 'linear envelope'), comprising a full-wave rectifier plus a low-pass filter. This is a simple method of quantifying signal intensity and gives an output (Figure 6.18(c)) that, it is claimed, follows the trend of the muscle tension curve with no high frequency components. It is the only intensity detector recommended by SENIAM for dynamic contractions – which predominate in sport – because of the statistical properties of such contractions.

The main issue with this estimator is the choice of the epoch duration, which, for this estimator, is related to the filter cut-off frequency (see also Chapter 4). A low cut-off frequency gives a reliable estimate of the signal intensity for 'stationary' activation of the muscle – this is a statistical term meaning, roughly, that the statistical properties of the activation signal do not change with time, not that the activation is constant. However, the amplitude estimates with a low cut-off frequency are inaccurate if the activation is non-stationary, when the statistical properties of the signal vary with time. A high cut-off frequency results in a noisy estimator for stationary activations and a linear envelope that follows closely the changes in the EMG. Typical values of the cut-off frequency are around 2 Hz for slow movements such as walking, and around 6 Hz for faster movements such as running and jumping. Also, SENIAM recommends that the cut-off frequency used should always be reported along with the type and order of filter. Most software packages for EMG analysis in sports biomechanics use a standard fourth-order Butterworth filter (as for filtering kinematic data; see Appendix 4.1).

A development of this approach is the use of an ensemble average calculated over several repetitions of the movement. This procedure theoretically – for physiologically identical movements – reduces the error in the amplitude estimation by a factor equal to the square root of the number of cycles. It is often used in clinical gait analysis but ignores the variability of movement patterns. It appears inappropriate for fast sports movements. The recommendations of SENIAM are that, if used, the number of cycles over which the ensemble average is calculated should be reported along with the standard error of the mean, to show up any movement variability.

Frequency domain analysis (spectral estimation)

Unless the data are explicitly time limited, as in a single action potential, the EMG signal can be transformed into the frequency domain (as for kinematic data; see Chapter 4). The EMG signal is then usually presented as a power spectrum (power equals amplitude squared) at a series of discrete frequencies, although it is often represented as a continuous curve, as in Figure 6.19. The epoch duration – over which the transformation of the time domain signal into the frequency domain occurs – which is recommended by SENIAM is 0.5–1.0 s. Again, these epoch durations considerably exceed the durations of muscle activity in many fast sports movements.

The central tendency and spread of the power spectrum are best expressed by the use of statistical parameters, which depend upon the distribution of the signal power over its constituent frequencies. Two statistical parameters are used to express the central tendency of the spectrum. These are comparable to the familiar mean and median in statistics. For a spectrum of discrete frequencies, the mean frequency is obtained by dividing the sum of the products of the power at each frequency and the frequency, by the sum of all of the powers. The median frequency is the frequency that divides the spectrum into two parts of equal power – the areas under the power spectrum to the two sides of the median frequency are equal. The median is less sensitive to noise than is the mean. The spread of the power spectrum can be expressed by the statistical bandwidth, which is calculated in the same way as a standard deviation.

The EMG power spectrum can be used, for example, to indicate the onset of muscle fatigue. This is accompanied by a noticeable shift in the power spectrum towards lower frequencies (Figure 6.20) and a reduction in the median and mean frequencies. This frequency shift is caused by an increase in the duration of the motor unit action potential. This results either from a lowering of the conduction velocity of all the action potentials or through faster, higher frequency motor units switching off while slower, lower frequency motor units remain active.

Figure 6.19 Idealised EMG power spectrum; f_m is the median and f_{av} the mean frequency.

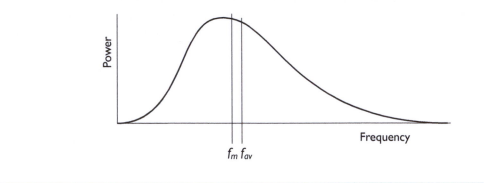

Figure 6.20 EMG power spectra at (a) the start and (b) the end of a sustained, constant force contraction.

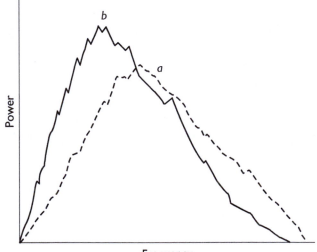

ISOKINETIC DYNAMOMETRY

The measurement of the net muscle torque at a joint using isokinetic dynamometry is very useful in providing an insight into muscle function and in obtaining muscle performance data for various modelling purposes ('isokinetic' is derived from Greek words meaning 'constant velocity'). Isokinetic dynamometry is used to measure the net muscle torque (called 'muscle torque' in the rest of this section) during isolated joint movements, as in Figure 6.21. A variable resistive torque is applied to the limb segment under consideration; the limb moves at constant angular velocity once the preset velocity has been achieved, providing the person being measured is able to maintain that velocity in the specified range of movement. This allows the measurement of muscle torque as a function of joint angle and angular velocity, which, at certain joints, may then be related to the length and contraction velocity of a predominant prime mover, for example the quadriceps femoris in knee extension. By adjusting the resistive torque, both muscle strength and endurance can be evaluated. Isokinetic dynamometers are also used as training aids, although they do not replicate the types and speeds of movement in sport.

Figure 6.21 Use of an isokinetic dynamometer for Top: (a) knee extension; Bottom: (b) elbow flexion.

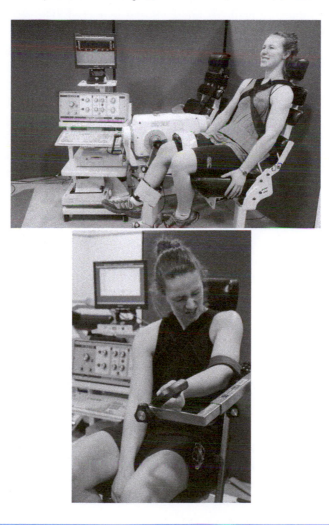

Passive isokinetic dynamometers operate using either electromechanical or hydraulic components. In these devices, resistance is developed only as a reaction to the applied muscle torque, and they can, therefore, only be used for concentric movements. Electromechanical dynamometers with active mechanisms allow for concentric and eccentric movements with constant angular velocity; some systems can be used for concentric and eccentric movements involving constant velocity, linearly changing acceleration or deceleration, or a combination of these.

Several problems affect the accuracy and validity of measurements of muscle torque using isokinetic dynamometers. Failure to compensate for gravitational force can result in significant errors in the measurement of muscle torque and in data derived from those measurements. These errors can be avoided by the use of gravity compensation methods, which are an integral part of the experimental protocol in most computerised dynamometers. The development and maintenance of a preset angular velocity is another potential problem. In the initial period of the movement, the dynamometer is accelerated without resistance until the preset velocity is reached. The resistive mechanism is then activated and slows the limb down to the preset velocity. The duration of the acceleration period, and the magnitude of the resistive torque required to decelerate the limb, depend on the preset angular velocity and the athlete being evaluated. The dynamometer torque during this period is clearly not the same as the muscle torque accelerating the system. If the muscle torque during this period is required, it should be calculated from the moment of inertia and angular acceleration data. The latter should be obtained either from differentiation of the angle–time data or from accelerometers if these are available.

Errors can also arise in muscle torque measurements unless the axis of rotation of the dynamometer is aligned with the axis of rotation of the joint, estimated using anatomical landmarks (see, for example, Box 6.2). For normal individuals and small misalignments, the error is very small and can be neglected. Periodic calibration of the dynamometer system is necessary for both torque and angular position, the latter using an accurate goniometer. Torque calibration should be carried out statically, to avoid inertia effects, under gravitational loading.

Accurate assessment of isokinetic muscle function requires the measurement of torque output while the angular velocity is constant; computation of angular velocity is, therefore, essential. Most isokinetic dynamometers output torque and angle data in digital form. Angular velocity and acceleration can be obtained by differentiation of the angle–time data after using appropriate noise reduction techniques (see Chapter 4). Instantaneous joint power ($P = T.\omega$) can be calculated from the torque (T) and angular velocity (ω) when the preset angular velocity has been reached.

Data processing in isokinetic dynamometry

The following parameters can normally be obtained from an isokinetic dynamometer to assess muscle function (for further information, see Baltzopoulos, 2008, listed in Further Reading).

The maximum torque

The isokinetic maximum torque is used as an indicator of the muscle torque that can be applied in dynamic conditions. It is usually evaluated from two to six maximal repetitions and is taken as the maximum single torque measured during these repetitions. The maximum torque depends on the angular position of the joint. Maximum power can also be calculated.

The reciprocal muscle group ratio

The reciprocal muscle group ratio is an indicator of muscle strength balance around a joint, which is affected by age, biological sex and physical fitness. It is the ratio of the maximum torques recorded in antagonist movements, usually flexion and extension – for example the quadriceps femoris to hamstrings muscle group ratio.

The maximum torque position

The maximum torque position is the joint angle at maximum torque and provides information about the mechanical properties of the activated muscle group. It is affected by the angular velocity. As the angular velocity increases, the maximum torque position tends to occur later in the range of movement and not in the mechanically optimal joint position. It is, therefore, crucial to specify the maximum torque position as well as the maximum torque.

Muscular endurance under isokinetic conditions

Muscular endurance under isokinetic conditions is usually assessed through a 'fatigue index'. It provides an indication of the muscle group's ability to perform the movement at the preset angular velocity over time. Although there is no standardised testing protocol or period of testing, it has been suggested that 30–50 repetitions or a total duration of 30–60 s should be used. The fatigue index can then be expressed as the ratio of the maximum torques recorded in the initial and final periods of the test.

SUMMARY

In this chapter, we focused on the anatomical principles that relate to movement in sport. The functions of the skeleton, the types of bone, the process of bone fracture and typical surface features of bone were covered. We then looked at the tissue structures involved in the joints of the body, joint stability and mobility, and the identification of the features and classes of synovial joints. The features and structure of skeletal muscles were considered, along with the ways in which muscles are structurally and functionally classified, the types and mechanics of muscular contraction, how tension is produced in muscle and how the total force exerted by a muscle can be resolved into components depending on the angle of pull. The use of electromyography in the study of muscle activity in sports biomechanics was considered, including the equipment and methods used, and the processing of EMG data. Consideration was given to why the EMG is important in sports biomechanics and why the recorded EMG differs from the physiological EMG. We saw that electromyography shows us when a muscle is active but not, in complex multi-joint sports movements, what the muscle does. We covered the relevant recommendations of SENIAM and the equipment used in recording the EMG, along with the main characteristics of an EMG amplifier. The processing of the raw EMG signal was considered in terms of its time domain descriptors, and the EMG power spectrum and the measures used to define it. We concluded by examining how isokinetic dynamometry can be used to record the net muscle torque at a joint.

STUDY TASKS

Many of the following tasks can be attempted simply after reading the chapter. For some of the tasks, a skeleton, or a good picture of one, is helpful, while tasks involving movements will require you to observe yourself or a partner. These observations will be easier if your experimental partner is dressed only in swimwear. If you are observing yourself, a mirror will be required.

Q

1 Answer all of the multiple-choice questions for Chapter 6 in the Interactive eTextbook.
   Hint: Keep repeating this until you have answered all of the questions correctly.

2 With an experimental partner, perform the following activities for each of these synovial joints – the shoulder, the elbow, the radioulnar joints of the forearm, the wrist, the thumb carpometacarpal joint, the metacarpophalangeal and interphalangeal joints of the thumb and fingers, the hip, the knee, the ankle, the subtalar joint (rear foot), and the metatarsophalangeal and interphalangeal joints of the toes.

   a) Identify the joint's class and the number of axes of rotation (non-axial, uniaxial, biaxial or triaxial).

   b) Name and demonstrate all the movements at that joint.

   c) Estimate – from observation only – the range (in degrees) of each movement, to the nearest 10°.

   d) Seek to identify the location of the axis of rotation for each movement and find a superficial anatomical landmark or landmarks (usually visible or palpable bony landmarks) that could be used to define this location – for example, you may find the flexion–extension axis of the shoulder to lie 5 cm inferior to the acromion process of the scapula.
   Hint: You should re-read the sections on 'Movements in the cardinal planes' in Chapter 1, and 'The skeleton and its bones' and 'The joints of the body' in this

chapter before and while undertaking this task. You will also find information on the location of joint axes of rotation from anatomical landmarks in Box 6.2.

3   Name the types of muscular contraction; demonstrate and sketch each in a weight-training activity, such as a biceps curl. Palpate the relevant musculature to ascertain which muscles are contracting.

Hint: You may wish to re-read the subsections on 'Types of muscle contraction' and 'Group action of muscles', and consult relevant material on muscle origins and insertions and prime mover roles of muscles in the Interactive eTextbook, or relevant sections in Marieb and Hoehn (2012; see Further Reading) before and while undertaking this task.

4   With reference to Figure 6.4 and using an experimental partner, locate and palpate all the superficial muscles in Figure 6.4. By movements against a light resistance only, seek to identify each muscle's prime mover roles.

Hint: You may wish to consult the material on muscle origins and insertions and prime mover roles of muscles in the Interactive eTextbook, or relevant sections in Marieb and Hoehn (2012; see Further Reading) before and while undertaking this task.

5   How does the information contained in each of the time domain processed EMG signals differ from that in the raw EMG? What additional information might this provide for the sports biomechanist and what information might be lost?

Hint: You may wish to consult the section on 'EMG data processing' before undertaking this task.

6   Outline the uses of the EMG power spectrum and the applications and limitations of the various measures used to describe it.

Hint: You may wish to consult the section on 'EMG data processing' before undertaking this task.

7   Explain the main characteristics required of an EMG amplifier. Log on to any EMG manufacturer's website (accessed through a search engine or through one of the web addresses in the Interactive eTextbook). Obtain the technical specification of that manufacturer's EMG amplifier, and ascertain whether this conforms to the recommendations of this chapter.

Hint: You may wish to consult the subsection on 'EMG amplifiers' before undertaking this task.

8   Imagine that you are to conduct an experiment in which surface electrodes will be used to record muscle activity from biceps brachii, triceps brachii, rectus femoris and biceps femoris. Using a fellow student or friend to identify the muscles, and the recommendations of Box 6.5 for electrode placement, mark the sites at which you would place the detecting and ground electrodes for each of these muscles.

Hint: You may wish to consult the section on 'Experimental procedures in electromyography', as well as Box 6.5, before undertaking this task.

9   Imagine that you are to conduct an experiment in which measurements are to be taken from an isokinetic dynamometer on the quadriceps femoris and hamstrings muscle groups. What measurements would you make and why?

Hint: You may wish to re-read the section on 'Isokinetic dynamometry' and to consult Baltzopoulos (2008; see Further Reading) before undertaking this task.

10 **Case study**.

a) Answer the five multiple-choice questions for this study task in the Interactive eTextbook.

b) If you have access to EMG equipment, and with appropriate supervision if necessary, perform the preparation, electrode siting and so on from Study Task 8. (This will form the methods section of your case study report.)

c) Then carry out experiments to record EMGs as follows:

   i) From biceps brachii and the long head of triceps brachii during the raising and lowering phases of a biceps curl with a dumbbell and from an isometric contraction with the dumbbell held at an elbow angle of about 90°. Check that you are obtaining good results and repeat the preparation if not. Graph the results (this will form part of the results section of your case study report). Comment on the results you obtain (this will form part of the discussion section of your case study report).

   ii) From the same two muscles as in (i), throwing a dart – or similar object – at normal speed, much more slowly, and much more quickly. Graph the results (this will form part of the results section of your case study report). Comment on the results you obtain (this will form part of the discussion section of your case study report).

   iii) From the rectus femoris and biceps femoris during rising from and lowering onto a chair. Again, check that you are obtaining good results, and repeat the preparation if not. Graph the results (this will form part of the results section of your case study report). Explain the apparently paradoxical nature of the results (this is known as Lombard's paradox; this will form part of the discussion section of your case study report).

(If you do not have access to EMG equipment, you can obtain EMG data from these experiments in the Excel file 'EMG Data' in the Interactive eTextbook. You will need to plot graphs of these data. In this case, you will need to base the methods section of your case study report on information in the section 'Experimental procedures in electromyography' in this chapter.)

d) Write a report of your case study in no more than 1000 words with no more than eight graphs. This will comprise methods, results and discussion sections, with contents as above.

Hint: You are strongly advised to consult, and follow under supervision, the section on 'Experimental procedures in electromyography', as well as Box 6.5, before and while undertaking this task.

SORTING AND LABELLING ACTIVITIES (INTERACTIVE ETEXTBOOK ONLY)

Sorting activity.
Labelling activity.

FURTHER READING

Baltzopoulos, V. (2008) Isokinetic dynamometry, in C.J. Payton and R.M. Bartlett (eds) *Biomechanical Evaluation of Movement in Sport and Exercise*, London: Routledge, pp. 103–128. Chapter 6 provides comprehensive coverage of all aspects of isokinetic dynamometry.

Bartlett, R.M. and Bussey, M. (2012) *Sports Biomechanics: Reducing Injury Risk and Improving Sports Performance*, London: Routledge. Chapters 1–3 deal with factors leading to bone fracture, and other injuries, in sport.

Basmajian, J.V. and De Luca, C.J. (1985) *Muscles Alive: Their Functions Revealed by Electromyography*, Baltimore, MD: Williams and Wilkins. This is a classic text in its fifth edition, although the sixth edition is now far too long overdue. You should be able to find a copy in your university library. Chapters 12–17 provide a vivid description of the actions of muscles as revealed by electromyography, and are highly recommended. Other chapters, for example, cover motor control, fatigue and posture, but are now rather out of date.

Burden, A.M. (2008) Surface electromyography, in C.J. Payton and R.M. Bartlett (eds) *Biomechanical Evaluation of Movement in Sport and Exercise*, London: Routledge, pp. 77–102. Chapter 5 provides comprehensive coverage of many aspects of electromyography related to sports movements.

Hermens, H.J., Freriks, B., Merletti, R., Stegeman, D., Blok, J., Rau, G., Disselhorst-Klug., C. and Hägg, G. (1999) *SENIAM: European Recommendations for Surface Electromyography,* Enschede: Roessingh Research and Development. One of the most recent attempts to standardise procedures for electromyography. A very valuable reference source, although it is spoilt somewhat by typographical, punctuation and grammatical errors and is rather turgid. There are also some bizarre omissions of superficial muscle placement sites, such as those for all the muscles that originate in the forearm; however, the placement sites recommended are very useful for both students and researchers.

Marieb, F.N. and Hoehn, K. (2012) *Human Anatomy and Physiology*, San Francisco, CA: Benjamin/Cummings. See Chapters 6–10. Many anatomy and physiology texts contain supplementary information about, for example, the attachment points and actions of specific muscles. This one, the ninth edition of the text, is highly recommended and readable, with glorious colour illustrations.

Glossary of important terms

Analogue Any signal continuous in both time and amplitude. See also **digital**.

Angle–angle diagram A graph in which the angle of one joint or body segment is plotted as a function of the angle of another joint or body segment. Conceptually, these can also be three-dimensional – involving three joints.

Axes The imaginary lines of a **reference system** along which position is measured.

Axis of rotation An imaginary line about which a body or body segment rotates.

Ballistic Rapid movements initiated by muscular contraction but continued by momentum.

Bernoulli's principle A low-pressure zone is created in a region of high fluid flow velocity, and a high pressure zone is created in a region of low fluid flow velocity. This can give rise to **lift**.

Boundary layer The thin layer of fluid that is adjacent to the surface of a body moving through a fluid. The fluid flow in the boundary layer may be **laminar** or **turbulent**.

Buoyancy force The upward force exerted on an immersed, or partially immersed, body by the fluid it displaces.

Calibration This refers to the process of determining the relationship between the output (or response) of a measuring instrument and the value of the input quantity or attribute used as a measurement standard. In motion analysis, calibration usually refers to the process of relating the recorded image coordinates to those of the real-world space in which the movement occurred.

Central tendency Measures of the location of the middle or the centre of a distribution of values.

Centre of mass (whole body) The imaginary point about which all of the mass particles of the body are evenly distributed. In the context of movement analysis, effectively coincident with the centre of gravity.

Centre of percussion That point in a body moving about a fixed axis of rotation at which it may strike an obstacle without transmitting an acceleration (or shock) to that axis.

Centre of pressure The effective point of application of a force distributed over a surface.

Cinematography Motion picture photography. See also **videography**.

Collinear forces Forces whose lines of action are the same.

Continuous relative phase (CRP) A graph of the **relative phase angle** as a function of time.

Countermovement A movement made in the direction opposite to that of the desired direction of motion – as in a countermovement jump.

Close-packed position The joint position with maximal contact between the articular surfaces and in which the ligaments are taut. See also **loose-packed position**.

Cross-correlation A correlation of variables from two different time series. See also **cross-correlation function**.

Cross-correlation function The graph of the cross-correlation coefficient between two different **time series** as a function of the (phase or time) lag between the two time series, as we vary the lag, often within prescribed limits.

Cross-sectional (study) The observation of a defined population at an instant in time or across a specified – usually short – time interval. See also **longitudinal study**.

Curvature A complex concept to 'tie down' mathematically. Here, we use it in the context that curvature is the amount by which a line deviates from being straight; the more the deviation, the greater the curvature. Curvature, in this context, turns out to be directly related to the acceleration of a point or angle, if the line graph is a graph of the displacement of that point or the angle over time.

Damping Any effect that tends to reduce the amplitude of the oscillations of an oscillatory system.

Degrees of freedom Used in movement analysis for the set of independent displacements that specify completely the displaced or deformed position of the body or system. Used more broadly in motor learning and control.

Depolarisation A reduction in the **electrical potential** of a membrane.

Deterministic model A model (sometimes referred to as a hierarchical model) linking biomechanical variables with the goal of the movement; such models are used in both qualitative and quantitative biomechanical analysis. Variables at one level of the model completely determine (hence the name) the variable to which they are linked at the level above.

Differentiation Expresses the rate at which a variable changes with respect to the change in another variable (in biomechanics, normally time) with which it has a functional relationship.

Digital Uses discrete values (often electrical voltages), rather than a continuous spectrum of values, as in an analogue system, particularly those represented as binary numbers. A digital transmission (as for digital radio or television) is considered less 'noisy' because slight variations do not matter – they are ignored when the signal is received. See also **analogue**. In motion analysis, a digital image is made up of a two-dimensional array of discrete 'picture cells' or 'pixels'.

Digitising, digitisation This term is normally used in sports biomechanics to refer to the process of specifying or measuring the horizontal and vertical (x and y) image coordinates of points on a sports performer's body when displayed on a video frame; more strictly called coordinate digitising.

Drag The mechanical force generated by a solid object travelling through a fluid that acts in the direction opposite to the movement of the object; any object moving through a fluid experiences drag. See also **lift**.

Dynamometry The measurement of force or torque output; used as an estimate of muscular strength.

Ecological motor control Holds that all movements and actions are influenced or constrained by the environment. Environmental information is necessary to shape or modify the characteristics of movement to achieve specific actions or tasks.

Ecological validity The notion that sports movements studied in their natural environment are more valid representations of what happens during performance of the sport than movements replicated in a controlled laboratory environment. See also **validity**.

Efficacy The ability to produce a desired amount of a desired effect.

Elasticity The property of a material that enables it to return to its original size and shape. In contrast, plasticity refers to the condition of connective tissue (ligaments or tendons) which has been stretched past its elastic limit and will no longer return to its original shape. See also **viscoelastic**.

Electrical potential The voltage across a membrane at steady-state conditions.

Energy The capacity of a system to do work. See also **kinetic energy** and **potential energy**.

Equilibrium The state of a system whose acceleration is unchanged; a state of balance between various physical forces. Equilibrium can be: neutral, in which the body will remain in a position if displaced from another position; stable, in which the body will return to its original position if it is displaced; or unstable, in which the displacement of the body continues to increase once it has been displaced.

Force plate, force platform A device that measures the contact force between an object and its surroundings, usually the ground reaction force.

Frame rates and field rates for video cameras Most video cameras, or camcorders, to which you are likely to have routine access, use two interlaced fields to make up a video frame. The fields are half the inter-frame interval apart in time and use half of the horizontal lines of pixels which, when interlaced, make up the whole frame. The standard frame rate is 25 per second (25 Hz) for PAL cameras (used in Europe and Australasia, for example) and approximately, but not exactly, 30 per second (30 Hz) in NTSC cameras (mostly used in North America). Theoretically the two fields can be displayed separately but not all camcorders can do this, neither can some biomechanical analysis software packages for particular video formats. Progressive video cameras and camcorders are now becoming more widely available. These sample at the same frame rates as above but are not interlaced; each frame uses all of the horizontal lines of pixels sampled simultaneously. Interlaced cameras often have an 'i' in their specification, along with the number of horizontal lines of pixels, for example, 1080i, and progressive cameras have a 'p', for example, 1080p. The slow frame rates of these video cameras and camcorders are a serious drawback to their use in sports biomechanics, particularly for fast movements and for quantitative analysis. Video cameras with higher frame rates (up to thousands of frames per second) are available, but are far more expensive than camcorders.

Free-body diagram A diagram in which the object of interest is isolated from its surroundings and all of the force vectors acting on the body are shown.

Frequency domain A representation of a signal in which the power (or amplitude) of the signal is plotted as a function of the frequencies within the signal. See also **power spectrum** and **time domain**.

Genlock A common technique in which the video output of one source, or a specific reference signal, is used to synchronise other picture sources so that images are captured simultaneously. Rarely found, at the time of writing of this book, on digital camcorders.

Geometry Branch of knowledge dealing with spatial relationships.

Gradient The inclination of a line or surface along a given direction. In movement analysis, effectively the same as the **slope**.

High definition digital video cameras My favourite specification of high definition (HD) video cameras is that they have a higher resolution (definition) than standard definition (SD) cameras! There is no universally agreed specification for HD cameras. The definition of a video camera (also known as the resolution of the image) is the number of pixels in a horizontal scan line (the horizontal resolution) $\times$ the number of horizontal lines of pixels (the vertical resolution) which make up one frame. In a standard definition camera, both of those numbers are less than 1000 (say, for example, 720×480); in a high definition camera, one or both are greater than 1000 (say, for example, 1280×720). High definition cameras should give a clearer image than standard definition ones, which is useful in movement analysis. The higher resolution is beneficial, particularly in quantitative biomechanical analysis, in which a higher resolution should lead to more accurate data.

Impedance (electrical) The ratio of voltage to electric current; a measure of resistance to time-varying electric current in an electric circuit. Sometimes (but not always) identical to **resistance**.

Inertia The reluctance of a body to move. For linear motion, mass is the inertia; for angular motion (rotation), the **moment of inertia** is the important factor.

Innervation ratio In a muscle, the average number of muscle fibres innervated by a single motor neuron.

Integral The result of the process of **integration**; the area under a variable–time curve.

Integration The mathematical process of calculating an **integral**.

Inverse dynamics An analytical approach calculating forces and moments based on the accelerations of the object, usually computed from measured displacements and angular orientations from **videography** or automatic marker-tracking systems.

Isokinetic (exercise) An exercise or other activity in which concentric muscle contraction moves a limb against a device that is speed controlled. Theoretically, if not practically, the speed is constant (the meaning of the word 'isokinetic').

Isometric Muscle action in which tension develops but there is no visible or external change in joint position; no external work is produced. An isometric exercise loads the muscle in one joint position.

Isotonic Often used for muscle action in which tension is developed either by the lengthening (eccentric) or shortening (concentric) of muscle fibres. Theoretically, the tension is constant (the meaning of the word 'isotonic'). An isotonic exercise is one in which an eccentric or concentric muscle contraction is generated to move a weight through a range of motion.

Kinaesthetic From kinaesthesis, the ability to sense proprioceptively (from sensory receptors within the body) the movements of the limbs and body.

Kinematics The branch of mechanics that examines the spatial and temporal components of movement without reference to the forces causing the movement.

Kinetic energy The ability of a body to do work by virtue of its motion. See also **potential energy**.

Laminar flow At slow speeds, a fluid flows smoothly over the surface of an object. Laminar flow can be considered as a series of thin plates (or laminae, hence the name) sliding smoothly past each other. 'Information' is passed between the elements of the fluid at a microscopic scale. See also **turbulent flow**.

Lift The component of fluid force that acts perpendicular to the direction of movement of an object through the fluid. Arises when the object deflects the fluid flow asymmetrically. See also **drag**.

Longitudinal (study) A correlational research study that involves observations of the same people over relatively long time periods. Unlike **cross-sectional studies**, longitudinal studies track the same people and, therefore, the differences observed in those people are less likely to be the result of cultural differences across generations.

Loose-packed position The joint position with less than maximal contact between the articular surfaces, in which contact areas frequently change. See also **close-packed position**.

Low-pass filter A filter that passes low frequencies while attenuating (or, at least in principle, removing) frequencies above the cut-off frequency. In movement analysis, used mainly to remove high frequency 'noise' from a low frequency movement signal.

Magnus effect The curve in the path of a spinning ball caused by a pressure differential around the ball.

Maximum voluntary contraction (MVC) The maximal force that is exerted by a muscle, normally during a static contraction against an immovable resistance.

Moment of inertia The reluctance of a body to rotate; it depends not only on the mass of the body but on the distribution of that mass about the axis of rotation.

Motor end-plate A flattened expansion in the sarcolemma of a muscle that contains receptors to receive expansions from the axonal terminals; also called the **neuromuscular junction**.

Motor unit A motor neuron and all the muscle cells it stimulates; the fundamental functional unit of neuromuscular control.

Movement variability The variability that exists within a movement system, which is observable during movement; it is due to non-linear dynamical processes within the movement system.

Neuromuscular junction Region where the motor neuron comes into close contact with (innervates) skeletal muscle; also called the **motor end-plate**.

On-line motion analysis systems Systems that automatically track markers placed on a person's body during movement. They are generally far more expensive and complex than systems used for videography. 'On-line' is used in this context to mean under full computer control.

Pathological (movement) An exceptionally awkward or inconvenient atypical example of movement, usually linked to an underlying anatomical or physiological cause, such as injury or disease.

Pelvic girdle The two hip bones plus the sacrum, which can be rotated forwards, backwards and laterally to optimise positioning of the hip joint (see also Chapter 1).

Phase angle The angle formed between the x-axis of the **phase plane** and the vector of the phase plane trajectory. This angle quantifies where the trajectory is located in the phase plane as time progresses and is used to calculate the **relative phase (angle)**.

Phase plane, phase portrait Usually constructed, in movement analysis, by plotting the angular velocity of a joint or body segment against its angular position. It provides a qualitative picture of the organisation of the system. Conceptually, these can involve any two (or more) properties of a joint or body segment.

Piezoelectric The ability of crystals to generate a voltage in response to an applied mechanical stress.

Planes (of movement) A two-dimensional plane running through an object. Movement occurs in the plane or parallel to it. Movement in a single plane is often called planar.

Potential energy The ability of a body to do work by virtue of its position. See also **kinetic energy.**

Power spectrum A way of expressing the strength, or power, of the different frequencies that form a signal. See also **frequency domain.**

Projectile An object – or person – that has been projected into the air. See also **projection angle, projection height, projection velocity** and **trajectory.**

Projection angle (release angle, take-off angle) The angle at which a projectile is released. See also **projection height** and **projection velocity.**

Projection height (release height, take-off height) The difference between the height at which a projectile is released and the height at which it lands. See also **projection angle** and **projection velocity.**

Projection velocity (release velocity, take-off velocity) The velocity at which a projectile is released, which may be broken into horizontal and vertical components. The magnitude of the projection velocity, with no indication of its direction, is the projection (release or take-off) speed. See also **projection angle** and **projection height.**

Q angle The Q angle is formed from a line drawn from the anterior superior iliac spine (ASIS; the main origin of the rectus femoris muscle) to the centre of the kneecap, and from a second line drawn from the centre of the kneecap to the tibial tubercle (the insertion of the patellar tendon). The Q angle is the acute angle between those two lines. It is roughly 14° in men and 17° in women.

Range The horizontal distance a **projectile** travels.

Redundant In the context of motor control, this is the duplication of critical movements in a system to increase the versatility of the system – there is more than one way to locate a system or segment in a given position.

Reference system A system of coordinates used to locate a point in space.

Reflex Involuntary response to a stimulus.

Relative phase angle The difference between the **phase angles** of two joints or body segments; the convention is to subtract the more distal from the more proximal. See also **continuous relative phase**.

Reliability The consistency of a set of measurements or measuring instrument. When comparing the consistency of human operators, reliability usually refers to intra-individual consistency; inter-individual consistency is often called objectivity.

Resistance (electrical) A measure of the extent to which an object, such as the skin, opposes the passage of an electric current. Sometimes (but not always) identical to **impedance**.

Rigid body An idealisation of a body of finite size in which deformation is neglected. In other words, the distance between any two given points of a rigid body remains constant with time regardless of any external forces exerted on it.

Sequential coordination Movement coordination that involves the sequential action of a chain of body segments, often leading to high-speed motion of external objects through the production of a summed velocity at the end of the chain of segments.

Shear A force applied parallel to an object creates deformation internally in a direction at right angles to that of the applied force.

Shear stress The load per unit cross-sectional area applied parallel to the plane of cross-section of the loaded object. In contrast, the normal stress is the load per unit cross-sectional area applied perpendicular to the plane of cross-section of an object.

(Signal) amplitude A non-negative scalar measure of a signal's magnitude of oscillation; that is, the magnitude of the maximum disturbance during one wave cycle. See also **signal frequency**.

Signal frequency The number of times a repeated event occurs per unit of time. See also **signal amplitude**.

Slope The ratio of the 'rise' (change in the vertical component) to the 'run' (change in the time component) on a variable–time curve. In movement analysis, effectively the same as the **gradient**.

Spatial Refers to a set of **planes of movement** and **axes** defined in three-dimensional space. Movement in two or more planes is often called spatial.

Steady-state response The response of a system in **equilibrium**. The steady-state response does not necessarily mean that the response is a fixed value; it may be oscillatory. See also **transient response**.

Stretch–shortening cycle A common sequence of joint actions in which an eccentric (lengthening) muscle contraction, or pre-stretch, precedes a concentric (shortening) muscle contraction.

Stress Force per unit of area.

Tangent (of an angle) The ratio of the length of the side opposite to an angle to the side adjacent to the angle in a right (or right-angled) triangle.

Tangent (line) A line that touches but does not intersect a curved line or surface and that is perpendicular to the radius of curvature of the arc of the curve where the tangent touches the line or surface.

Tangential velocity For a body moving along a curved path, the tangential velocity is the change, per unit of time, in linear position along the instantaneous line tangent to the curve.

Telemetry (as in 'telemetered') Automatic transmission and measurement of data from remote sources by radio or other remote means.

Tetanus State of a muscle (or a muscle fibre) producing sustained maximal tension resulting from repetitive neural stimulation.

Three-dimensional Occurring in two or three planes; requires a minimum of three co-ordinates to describe, for example x-, y- and z-coordinates. See also **two-dimensional**.

Time domain A representation of a signal in which the signal is presented as a function of time (a time series); the more familiar way of displaying biomechanical variables. See also **frequency domain**.

Time series A list of numbers assumed to measure some process sequentially in time. Usually visualised as a graph made from the list of numbers plotted against time.

Trajectory The flight path of a **projectile** determined by the horizontal and vertical acceleration of the projectile and its projection speed, angle and height.

Transient response The response of a system before achieving equilibrium. See also **steady-state response**.

Turbulent flow Fluid flow characterised by a series of vortices or eddies. 'Information' is passed between the elements of the fluid at a macroscopic scale. This is by far the predominant fluid flow in nature. See also **laminar flow**.

Two-dimensional Occurring within a single plane (usually the sagittal plane for analysis in sports biomechanics); requires a minimum of two coordinates to describe, for example x- and y-coordinates. See also **three-dimensional**.

Validity Results that accurately reflect the concept being measured. An experiment is said to possess external validity if it results hold across different experimental settings, procedures and participants. An experiment is said to possess internal validity if it properly demonstrates a causal relation between two variables. See also **ecological validity**.

Videography The process of capturing images onto a videotape (or, more likely, a video cassette) or directly to a computer; also used to include the later analysis of these images, usually using quantitative video analysis software. See also **cinematography**.

Viscoelastic A material that exhibits non-linear properties on a stress–strain curve. See also **elasticity**.

Viscosity The measure of a fluid's resistance to flow.

Wake The disruption of fluid flow downstream of a body caused by the passage of the body through the fluid.

SI units used in this book

Quantity	Symbol	Unit name	Unit Symbol	Unit Derivation	Comments
Acceleration	a		m/s^2	(metre/second)/ second	
Angle, angular displacement	θ	radian	rad		Radians are non-dimensional; degree (°) is tolerated
Angular acceleration	α		rad/s^2	(radian/second)/ second	$°/s^2$ is tolerated
Angular momentum	L		$kg{\cdot}m^2/s$	kilogram·metre²/ second	
Angular velocity	ω		rad/s	radian/second	°/s is tolerated
Density	ρ		kg/m^3	kilogram/metre³	
Displacement, distance or position	r	metre	m		usually as x, y, z coordinates; mm preferred to cm as a subunit
Electrical current	I	ampere	A		picoamp (pA; 10^{-9}A)
Electrical potential	V	volt	V		millivolt (mV; 10^{-3}V); microvolt (µV; 10^{-6}V)
Electrical impedance or resistance	R	ohm	Ω	volt/amp	kilohm (kΩ; $10^{3}\Omega$); megohm (MΩ; $10^{6}\Omega$); gigaohm (GΩ; $10^{9}\Omega$)

(Continued)

Quantity	Symbol	Unit name	Unit Symbol	Unit Derivation	Comments
Energy	E	joule	J	N·m	
Force	F	newton	N		
Frequency	f	hertz	Hz		events/second; kilohertz (kHz; 10^3Hz)
Impulse of force	I		N·s	newton·second	
Impulse of moment of force	I		N·m·s	newton·metre·second	
Length	l	metre	m		
Mass	m	kilogram	kg		
Moment of force or torque	M		N·m	newton·metre	
Moment of inertia	I		kg·m^2	kilogram·metre^2	
Momentum (linear)	p		kg·m/s	kilogram·(metre/ second)	
Power	P	watt	W	J/s	
Pressure, stress	σ	pascal	Pa	N/m^2	
Time	t	second	s		hour (h) and minute (min) also used; millisecond (ms) main subunit
Velocity	v		m/s	metre/second	
Volume	V		m^3	metre^3	
Work	W	joule	J	N·m	

Index

Locators in **bold** refer to figures, plates and tables